Traumatic Head Injury in Children

Traumatic Head Injury in Children

EDITED BY

Sarah H. Broman
Mary Ellen Michel

New York   Oxford
OXFORD UNIVERSITY PRESS
1995

Oxford University Press

Oxford   New York
Athens   Auckland   Bangkok   Bombay
Calcutta   Cape Town   Dar es Salaam   Delhi
Florence   Hong Kong   Istanbul   Karachi
Kuala Lumpur   Madras   Madrid   Melbourne
Mexico City   Nairobi   Paris   Singapore
Taipei   Tokyo   Toronto

and associated companies in
Berlin   Ibadan

Copyright © 1995 by Oxford University Press, Inc.

Published by Oxford University Press, Inc.
198 Madison Avenue, New York, New York 10016

Oxford is a registered trademark of Oxford University Press

Library of Congress Cataloging-in-Publication Data
Traumatic head injury in children / edited by Sarah H. Broman,
Mary Ellen Michel.
p. cm.   Includes bibliographical references and index.
ISBN 0-19-509428-X
1. Brain-damaged children.   2. Brain—Wounds and injuries—
Complications.   I. Broman, Sarah H.   II. Michel, Mary Ellen.
[DNLM: 1. Brain Injuries—in infancy & childhood.   WL 354 T7773 1995]
RJ496.B7T73   1995
617.4'81044'083—dc20
DNLM/DLC for Library of Congress   94-45129

1 3 5 7 9 8 6 4 2

Printed in the United States of America
on acid-free paper

Foreword

This volume on traumatic head injury in children appears at a crucial time when there is not only a growing public health problem represented by pediatric head trauma, but the "Decade of the Brain" has opened up possibilities for sophisticated approaches to human brain-behavior relationships. When we speak of head injury, it is the trauma to the brain and the sequelae thereof, the ability of the brain to heal and/or compensate, that concern us. Of the methodological advances most immediately applicable to the characterization of deficits and outcomes, the statistical and neuropsychological expertise of contributors to this volume stand out most clearly: for example, Fletcher and his colleagues' "call to arms" for outcome analyses in terms of individual child-specific recovery curves; Levin and his colleagues' increasingly sensitive and norm-referenced frontal lobe measures; and Dennis and her colleagues' approach to fractionation of attentional processes. With the aid of computer technology, clinical data can now be collected and analyzed with greater capacity to filter out task-related confounding factors and group-related confounding factors that obscure individual changes. The ability to handle more complex statistical models will allow researchers to incorporate environmental and psychosocial variables into the profiles of children's deficits and outcomes, as advocated by Taylor and his coworkers.

Oddly, the more "physical" advances in brain science technology may make matters somewhat *less* clear in the short run; already researchers are grappling with revelations from structural magnetic resonance images that increase the visible numbers and locations far beyond what the "old" computerized tomography or even the first-generation MRI showed. Neat subdivisions of the head-injured population into "frontal" and "extrafrontal" are subverted by the sensitivity of the structural MRI, necessitating the use of volumetrics (e.g., percent of lesional volume that is frontal) and the insertion of qualifying adjectives like "predominantly" before designations of anatomic grouping. Lest one jump ahead to thinking of functional MR (fMR) as the salvation of the brain researcher, caution must be sounded: physiological techniques are difficult to interpret without excellent cognitive neuroscience and statistical methodology; moreover, normative data bases are now scarce.

Besides methodological issues, an overview of this volume reveals significant clinical concern regarding (1) the adequacy of our indices of initial *severity* of traumatic head injury and (2) outcome after the majority of pediatric traumatic head injuries that are currently called "mild." Obviously, the issues are linked; if the criteria for initial severity change, then the number and/or percentage of "mild" cases will also change. Several contributors to this volume raise the issue of the adequacy of coma scales as severity indices. The sensitivity of MRI (structural) and possibly, once we know where best to measure it, of fMR (physiological) can add to initial severity rankings findings implicating brain impairment. For example, finding structural changes on MRI might shift what is now a "mild" case (on the basis of Glasgow Coma Scale) into the "moderate" category.

Assuming that in the future a substantial number of cases will still be designated as "mild" among children with traumatic head injury, the definitive study of residual deficits is yet to be undertaken. It may be argued that the appropriate controls for the "mild" cases are same-gender siblings rather than unrelated controls since a sibling is socioeconomically, psychosocially, and, in terms of IQ, cognitively the best premorbid match for subtle effects of brain injury. Beyond this step we must address the real clinical problem of traumatic brain injury occurring nonrandomly, that is, more often in those who premorbidly carried the developmental burdens currently labeled as "learning-disabled" and "attention-deficit hyperactivity–disordered." To date, the most elegant research (like that of Levin's group) has scrupulously eliminated such premorbidly complicated subjects from research on the effects of traumatic brain injury. Yet it may be argued that it is upon the premorbidly impaired that mild head injury is most likely to inflict the critical lesion(s) that lead to decompensation; hanging on by a thread, as it were, the premorbidly learning-disabled who sustain head injury may drop down into a more serious disability category. Researchers may need to examine the impact of mild traumatic brain injury upon the premorbidly developmentally disordered as compared with the premorbidly "clean" cases before declaring with confidence that "mild" cases have good outcomes. Certainly, socioeconomic adversity will be a confounding factor; indeed, socioeconomic adversity itself will correlate highly with manifest (as opposed to *compensated*) developmental disorder since higher socioeconomic status confers a greater likelihood of compensating for pre-existing behavioral deficits. Only with large numbers of subjects allowing representation of a range in both socioeconomic status and premorbid status can this hypothesis about sequelae of mild head trauma be tested.

Finally, the developmental perspective must inform the reading of this volume. "Children" is a plural noun encompassing a biological spectrum in which heterogeneity exceeds what the plural provides—not just "more than one child" but a panoply of chronologically aged and developmentally staged individual children. It is on this very heterogeneous group that traumatic injuries have their also-heterogeneous impacts.

This volume properly places the field at the crossroads of accumulated knowledge and questions yet to be asked. It is an outstanding contribution to the literature on head injury in children providing information not readily available in any other source. It makes an equally valuable contribution in pointing out directions for future research on the brain's continuous responsiveness to external and internal challenges.

MARTHA BRIDGE DENCKLA

Preface

It is a well-established principle that advances in scientific knowledge—resulting from the most basic studies of subcellular processes to studies of physiological and neurobehavioral systems—can contribute to more effective treatment of human diseases and disorders, sometimes almost immediately. The flow of knowledge also goes the other way. So-called experiments of nature, such as the developmental disorder of Williams syndrome (Broman & Grafman, 1994) and serious trauma to the head, a subject of this book, can affect cognition adversely and selectively and provide useful human models for the study of brain function.

This volume focuses on the consequences of traumatic closed head injury in children, the methods used to study these outcomes, and implications for future study and interventions. A major goal of the authors is to explore ways of identifying sources of unexplained variability in outcome, an objective that could improve treatment and rehabilitation of head-injured children and expand our knowledge of relations between the functional and anatomic organization of the developing brain and behavior.

Head trauma is a major public health problem in children. It is the leading cause of death and a major contributor to a spectrum of morbidity involving cognition and other adaptive behaviors associated with brain injury. The problems experienced by children with severe head injury are persistent and often evolve over time, requiring long-term follow-up for accurate description and appropriate intervention. But the vast majority of head trauma in young children is mild head injury. Relatively few studies have been conducted in this group, however, and the findings are conflicting.

The purpose of this book, and the 1993 conference at the National Institute of Neurological Disorders and Stroke from which it evolved, is to evaluate the current state of knowledge about consequences of traumatic head injury in childhood and to identify sources of variability in outcome found in studies of both severe and mild injury. Such unaccounted-for variability indicates that poorly understood or presently unknown factors are affecting outcome during the course of recovery from childhood traumatic head injury. It is also an indicator of the need for better-defined, more uniform research methodologies, including more precise definitions of degrees of severity of injury, sample selection techniques that minimize ascertainment biases, the development of reliable and valid outcome measures, and more extensive postinjury longitudinal follow-up. Many of these methodological problems and gaps in knowledge have surfaced in the work of a relatively small but active group of investigators. Now is a favorable time to review research findings in this important area and to encourage the expansion of research efforts by developmentalists in the biomedical, behavioral, and public health fields.

This volume is organized into four parts: the first covers basic conceptual, epidemiological, and pathophysiological issues related to the study and treatment of childhood head injury; the second, empirical data from outcome studies of traditional but relatively limited duration; the third, life-span effects, rehabilitative interventions, and treatment; and fourth, commentaries from a biomedical and a behavioral perspective. Certain themes figure prominently in most of the chapters. They are the problems of classification or assessment of both the characteristics of the injury (severity, localization) and the quality of the outcome (behavioral functions evaluated, level of difficulty of tasks administered, length of follow-up); determining the effects of preinjury characteristics of the child and his or her environment; postinjury environmental effects; and, indirectly, the relatively few resources devoted to research and intervention for the head-injured child compared with the head-injured adult. Promising developments that address some of these problems are improved technologies for imaging the structure and function of the brain and the increasing rigor of the experimental designs used to evaluate outcomes and interventions, including those proposed for future clinical trials.

Finally, a word about terminology. Although "traumatic brain injury (TBI)" is used frequently by most of the authors, we have titled the book *Traumatic Head Injury in Children*. This is because it cannot always be assumed, especially in "mild" cases, that the brain is injured following trauma to the head.

Bethesda, Md.   S.H.B.
January 1995   M.E.M.

Reference

Broman, S. H., & Grafman, J. (Eds.) (1994). *Atypical cognitive deficits in developmental disorders*. Hillsdale, NJ: Erlbaum.

Contents

Contributors

Robert F. Asarnow, Department of Psychiatry, University of California at Los Angeles, Los Angeles, California

Arthur Benton, Department of Neurology, University of Iowa Hospitals, Iowa City, Iowa

Polly E. Bijur, Departments of Pediatrics and Epidemiology and Social Medicine, Albert Einstein College of Medicine, Bronx, New York

Sarah H. Broman, Developmental Neurology Branch, Division of Convulsive, Developmental, and Neuromuscular Disorders, National Institute of Neurological Disorders and Stroke, Bethesda, Maryland

Derek A. Bruce, Department of Neurosurgery, Children's Medical Center, Dallas, Texas

Sandra Bond Chapman, Callier Center for Communication Disorders, University of Texas at Dallas, Dallas, Texas

Campbell Clark, Department of Psychiatry, University of British Columbia, Vancouver, British Columbia, Canada

Martha Bridge Denckla, Department of Developmental Cognitive Neurology, The Kennedy-Krieger Institute, Baltimore, Maryland

Maureen Dennis, Department of Psychology, The Hospital for Sick Children, Toronto, Ontario, Canada

Dennis Drotar, Department of Psychiatry, Case Western Reserve University and MetroHealth Medical Center, Cleveland, Ohio

Howard M. Eisenberg, Division of Neurological Surgery, University of Maryland Medical System, Baltimore, Maryland

Linda Ewing-Cobbs, Department of Pediatrics, University of Texas Medical School, Houston, Texas

Jack M. Fletcher, Department of Pediatrics, University of Texas Medical School, Houston, Texas

David J. Francis, Department of Psychology, University of Texas, Houston, Texas

Jordan Grafman, Cognitive Neuroscience Section, Medical Neurology Branch, National Institute of Neurological Disorders and Stroke, Bethesda, Maryland

Mary Haslum, Faculty of Health and Community Studies, University of the West of England, Bristol, England

Robin P. Humphreys, Department of Neurosurgery, The Hospital for Sick Children, Toronto, Ontario, Canada

Susan Klein, Department of Psychology, Case Western Reserve University, Cleveland, Ohio

Harry Klonoff, Department of Psychiatry, University of British Columbia, Vancouver, British Columbia, Canada

Pamela S. Klonoff, Barrow Neurological Institute, St. Joseph's Hospital and Medical Center, Phoenix, Arizona

Lisa Koski, Department of Psychology, The Hospital for Sick Children, Toronto, Ontario, Canada

Jess F. Kraus, School of Public Health, University of California at Los Angeles, Los Angeles, California

Harvey S. Levin, Division of Neurological Surgery, University of Maryland Medical System, Baltimore, Maryland

Richard Lewis, Neuroscience Program, Pomona College, Pomona, California

Roger Light, Department of Psychiatry, University of California at Los Angeles, Los Angeles, California

Carol McCleary, Department of Neurology, University of Southern California, Los Angeles, California

Linda J. Michaud, Departments of Rehabilitation Medicine and Pediatrics, University of Pennsylvania School of Medicine, Philadelphia, Pennsylvania

Mary Ellen Michel, Division of Stroke and Trauma, National Institute of Neurological Disorders and Stroke, Bethesda, Maryland

Andres Salazar, Department of Clinical Investigation, Walter Reed Army Medical Center, Washington, D.C.

Paul Satz, Neuropsychiatric Institute, University of California Medical Center, Los Angeles, California

David Shaffer, Division of Child Psychiatry, New York State Psychiatric Institute, New York, New York

Bennett A. Shaywitz, Departments of Pediatrics and Neurology, Yale University School of Medicine, New Haven, Connecticut

Terry Stancin, Department of Pediatrics, Case Western Reserve University and MetroHealth Medical Center, Cleveland, Ohio

H. Gerry Taylor, Department of Pediatrics, Case Western Reserve University and Rainbow Babies and Children's Hospital, Cleveland, Ohio

Shari Wade, Department of Pediatrics, Case Western Reserve University and Rainbow Babies and Children's Hospital, Cleveland, Ohio

John David Ward, Division of Neurological Surgery, Medical College of Virginia, Richmond, Virginia

Margaret Wilkinson, Department of Psychology, The Hospital for Sick Children, Toronto, Ontario, Canada

Keith Yeates, Department of Pediatrics, The Ohio State University and Columbus Children's Hospital, Columbus, Ohio

Kenneth Zaucha, Neuropsychiatric Institute, University of California Medical Center, Los Angeles, California

I

THE ISSUES

1

Variability in Outcomes after Traumatic Brain Injury in Children: A Developmental Perspective

JACK M. FLETCHER, LINDA EWING-COBBS,
DAVID J. FRANCIS, and HARVEY S. LEVIN

Traumatic brain injury (TBI) in children is a major public health problem in the United States. Epidemiological studies indicate that the overall incidence of TBI in children is approximately 200 per 100,000 per year (Annegers, 1983; Kraus, this volume). Although most of these cases involve minor injuries, approximately 10 of these 200 children will die. One of every 30 newborn children will sustain a significant brain injury before 16 years of age (Annegers, 1983). Head injury is the leading cause of death in people under 35 years of age. In children under 15 years of age, half of all mortality is due to trauma, and injuries to the head account for half the trauma deaths. In contrast to patterns of research support, the incidence of death from TBI is five times higher than mortality from leukemia, the second leading cause of death in children.

The morbidity associated with TBI is also significant. Of the survivors, approximately 30 children per 100,000 sustain severe brain injuries. These children show a spectrum of disability ranging from persistent vegetative state through significant mental and physical disability to disrupted ability to learn efficiently and adjust to home and school. In one study of TBI survivors, 80% of severely injured children either failed a grade or were in a modified educational environment 2 years postinjury (Ewing-Cobbs et al., 1991). The National Pediatric Trauma Registry showed that 30% of children with mild to severe TBI had behavioral difficulties following discharge from a major trauma unit. Behavioral difficulties were reported in 73% of children with multiple functional impairments affecting activities of daily living (DiScala et al., 1991).

Despite the significance of TBI in children, there have been relatively few investigations of outcome. Since many outcome studies address only survival, studies of

3

morbidity are reported even less frequently. Pediatric TBI cases are rarely included in clinical intervention trials, and there are very few treatment studies specifically involving children with TBI (see Chapter 14). Outcome studies tend to be short in duration, rarely persisting beyond 1 year postinjury, and many studies provide only descriptive assessments of outcome. Only recently was TBI designated as an eligibility category for special education services in the public schools.

Available studies clearly establish a range of outcomes after pediatric TBI, and there is considerable variability in the outcomes between centers (Fletcher & Levin, 1988; Levin et al., 1982). The basis for this variability is unclear. The purpose of this chapter is to discuss issues underlying the assessment of outcomes in children with TBI. Particular attention is directed to variability in outcomes, which stems from at least three sources. The first source is how outcome is measured. The second source involves predictors of outcomes, including the mechanism of TBI, its varying effects at the level of the brain, and reciprocal effects between the injury and the child's environment. The third factor, which is unique to any study of children, is the variability inherent in development. This variability, reflecting the processes of change that represent development, distinguishes studies of children from studies of adults. In adults, a principal question for investigations of outcome is the extent to which the adult returns to premorbid levels of functioning. In children, the premorbid level of functioning is not equivalent to the child's final level of attainment of a skill, since in them injury interrupts ongoing development. The assessment of outcome will vary with the age at injury and the age at outcome assessment (Levin et al., 1984). Any measurement of children must take into account change over time, which represents a primary source of variability.

Many of the sources of variability in outcomes are listed in Table 1-1. Each is discussed below. It will be evident that a major source of variability is the way in which outcomes are measured and the model of change underlying the assessment. In addition, sampling, injury, and environmental factors are major sources of variability.

Measurement of Outcome

There are multiple purposes for assessing outcomes after pediatric TBI (Langfitt, 1978). The first is to predict the outcome, or prognosis, for an individual child.

TABLE 1-1.   Sources of Variability in Outcomes after Traumatic Brain Injury in Children

Measurement of outcomes—assessment devices
Injury characteristics: mechanism, severity, and pathophysiology
Environmental variables: premorbid characteristics (child and family), postinjury environment, and interventions
Model of change

The second is to develop standards for the evaluation of the effects of treatment and prevention efforts. A third purpose is to estimate the significance of TBI as a public health problem. Finally, a fourth purpose is to better understand how development proceeds in a child with brain injury. Analysis of outcomes provides information concerning how behavior is mediated by the normal and injured brain.

Assessment Devices

In addition to the assessment of survival, there are three principal methods for assessing outcomes after pediatric TBI. These methods include (1) *qualitative* assessments of outcome by clinical judgments; (2) psychometric tests, which are usually *quantitative* and continuous; and (3) rating scales and interviews, which typically take *qualitative* information and place the data on a *quantitative,* continuous scale.

1. *Clinical judgments.* It is very common for studies of pediatric TBI to use measures of outcome based on clinical judgments. These measures of outcome are examples of noncontinuous or *qualitative* changes in the child's recovery. The best example of a clinical judgment is *survival,* which can be represented as a dichotomous scale ("Survived," "Did Not Survive"). Other examples of outcome assessments that are basically qualitative are the Glasgow Outcome Scale (Jennett & Bond, 1975) and the Disability Rating Scale (Rappoport et al., 1982). There are also other measures based on clinical judgments. Since the Glasgow Outcome Scale is widely recognized, it will serve as our focus for instruments based on clinical judgments.

The Glasgow Outcome Scale was designed to measure qualitative change on an ordinal scale with minimal overlap across categories. The scale basically distinguishes death, persistent vegetative state, complete dependence, partial dependence, and independence. Designed for adults, the Glasgow Outcome Scale can be modified for children (see Table 1-2).

Most survivors of pediatric TBI have "Good Recovery" outcomes (see Table 1-2). However, there is substantial variability within this outcome category. Miner and coworkers (1986) found that 18 of 20 children with moderate to severe TBI had "Good Recovery" outcomes on the modified Glasgow Outcome Scale 3 months postinjury; the other 2 had "Severe Disability" outcomes (see Table 1-2). Of the 18 children with "Good Recovery" outcomes, one had a normal neuropsychological evaluation at 1 year postinjury, with the other 17 showing a variety of mild to moderate deficiencies. By 2 years postinjury, at least 80% of this sample of "Good" outcomes at 3 months had failed a grade or were involved in a modified educational program. Hence, the Glasgow Outcome Scale provides outcome information that is quite different from information provided by a neuropsychological examination. Moreover, the scale points on this measure mask significant variability in outcomes that may be apparent with other measures.

This variation in outcomes obtained using different assessment approaches is important. If survival rates or a modified Glasgow Outcome Scale are used to assess outcomes, children are more likely than adults to survive TBI and have less

TABLE 1-2.   Glasgow Outcome Scale for Children

Good Recovery: Resumption of preinjury activities and academic placement with minimal neurological deficit.

Moderate Disability: Able to function independently but at a reduced level relative to preinjury status—special education or rehabilitation services required.

Severe Disability: Unable to function independently and requiring substantial assistance with self-care skills.

Persistent Vegetative State

Death

Source: From Miner et al., 1986.

associated morbidity (Bruce, this volume). If psychometric tests or interviews/ rating scales are used to assess morbidity, the converse is true. In fact, outcomes for children injured between birth and 6 years of age look worse relative to adult outcomes when psychometric tests are used (Ewing-Cobbs et al., 1989). These assessment issues have important implications for models of recovery of function after brain injury, particularly if the study is interpreted to support models showing preferential recovery in more immature brains.

More generally, one form of assessment (e.g., clinical judgments versus psychometric tests) is not better than another. The purpose for which outcomes are assessed dictates selection of a particular index of outcome. However, the interpretation of outcomes will vary depending on the conceptualization of change. When change (recovery) is assessed with an instrument based on a qualitative model, the interpretation may differ from the interpretation provided by an instrument based on a quantitative conceptualization of change.

2. *Psychometric tests.* Neuropsychological tests are commonly used to assess outcomes after pediatric TBI. These tests measure different aspects of cognitive and sensorimotor ability; they generate metrics that are quantitative and continuous and that can be divided into categories through arbitrary subdivisions.

Figure 1-1 shows a score distribution from the Wechsler Intelligence Scale for Children—Revised (WISC-R) (Wechsler, 1974). The bell-shaped distribution of scores can be divided into "average" or "good" outcomes as well as varying levels of disability, paralleling division of outcomes into categories in many pediatric clinical trials. For example, WISC-R scores between 89 and 111 are usually considered average or "normal." Other designations could be marked according to dispersion from the average score of 100. The problems with this approach are (1) the arbitrariness of the subdivisions—a score of 85 is "abnormal" while a score of 90 is "normal"; (2) the amount of normal dispersion ("error") around any given score (on the WISC-R, $\pm$ 7 points) (Sattler, 1992); and (3) the loss of information involved when variability is artificially constrained. It is important to understand whether differences between scores of 85 and 90 are significant. More important, why does a child obtain a score of 85 some 3 months postinjury and 90 1 year postinjury? Is this change simply due to practice, is it a characteristic of recovery, or does it represent development due to maturation? Characterizing this change on a qualitative metric (abnormal to normal) scale may be very misleading, since the score distribution is continuous and the amount of change may or may not be meaningful.

3. *Rating scales and interviews.* The third approach to the assessment of outcome is to interview a caregiver concerning the child or have the caregiver rate the child's abilities or behavior on some type of scale. An example of an interview-based procedure is the Vineland Adaptive Behavior Scales (Vineland) (Sparrow et al., 1984). The Personality Inventory for Children—Revised (PIC-R) (Lachar, 1982; Wirt et al., 1990) is a good example of a rating scale.

The Vineland is a revision and restandardization of the Vineland Social Maturity scale. Adaptive behavior is measured in four domains: Communication, Socialization, Daily Living, and Motor. The Vineland, a nationally normed measure appropriate from birth to adulthood, is administered through a nondirective parental interview. Numerous validity studies are available, including previous studies of other populations of brain-injured children, showing that the Vineland may be more sensitive to the child's overall adaptation than traditional parent-based behavioral adjustment rating scales (Fletcher et al., 1990).

The PIC-R, a self-administered questionnaire, is completed by the parent; it is composed of items that were developed to tap the major dimensions of psychopathology in children. Extensive validity data have been published for the PIC-R (Lachar, 1993). The revised form of the PIC is a multidimensional measure of behavior and adjustment derived from adult informant responses to 280 brief inventory items (Lachar, 1982). These responses provide 20 scales, including 4 factor scales, 3 measures of informant response style, a general screening scale, and 12 scales measuring child behavior, affect, and family status. Of the latter

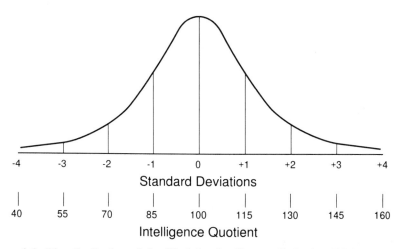

Figure 1-1. The distribution of the Wechsler Intelligence Scale for Children—Revised (Wechsler, 1974). Various categories representing intellectual levels could be interpreted as categorical outcomes as represented by the designations in the figure.

12 scales, 3 measure cognitive status (Achievement, Intellectual Screening, and Development). The other 9 scales measure behavioral adjustment. The 4 factor scales combine information from the 12 clinical scales and yield the following factors: undisciplined/poor self-control, social incompetence, internalization/somatic symptoms, and cognitive development.

The Vineland and the PIC-R provide different types of information. Available studies show that measures such as the Vineland are more sensitive to variations in outcome after TBI than the scales of the PIC-R that measure behavioral adjustment or another well-known behavior rating scale, the Child Behavior Checklist (Achenbach, 1991). Fletcher and coworkers (1990) compared 1-year outcomes on the Vineland and Child Behavior Checklist in children with mild, moderate, and severe TBI. Results revealed no differences in outcome at 1 year postinjury on the Child Behavior Checklist, with all groups obtaining ratings in the normal range. In contrast, children with severe TBI had significantly lower scores on the Vineland at 1 year postinjury relative to children with mild and moderate TBI (see Figure 1-2).

In a subsequent study comparing the Vineland and PIC-R, Fletcher and colleagues (submitted) found that the behavioral adjustment scales of the PIC-R were

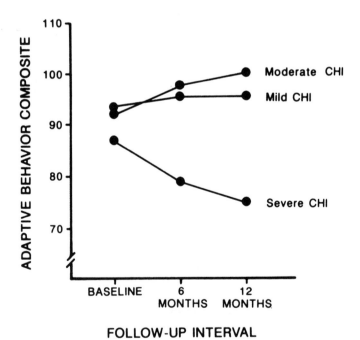

FOLLOW-UP INTERVAL

Figure 1-2. Vineland Adaptive Behavior Scales composite score by severity of closed head injury (CHI). The baseline evaluation is actually a premorbid assessment. The two follow-up evaluations at 6 and 12 months show no significant changes in children with mild and moderate CHI, but the severely injured group shows much lower scores over the follow-up interval.

not sensitive to variations in outcome. However, the Vineland and the scales of the PIC-R that ask questions about the child's cognitive functioning were lower in children with severe TBI than they were in children with mild/moderate TBI. These studies suggest that rating scales derived from a mental health framework are less sensitive to variations in outcome than rating scales or interviews that address the TBI child's cognitive or adaptive functioning.

Like psychometric tests, interviews and rating scales can be construed to assess qualitative or quantitative change. They often convert information that is qualitative to a continuous scale. Such a conversion may be required, because what is appropriate for the child in terms of behavior or independent functioning varies with age. This approach would be analogous to taking the categories of the Glasgow Outcome Scale, collecting normative data at different ages, and generating age-based standards. In this case, such an approach would be illogical because the categories from the Glasgow Outcome Scale are not conceptualized from a model of the child's development and are simply descriptive of end points that do not vary with development. It would be possible to take outcome measures such as the Vineland or PIC-R and convert them to qualitative rubrics. The issues involved in converting outcome measures from quantitative to qualitative scales are described above, in the section on psychometric tests. In addition, a major question is whether information is lost that could make the end-point assessment more sensitive to variations in outcome (Fletcher et al., 1991).

Conclusions: Assessment Devices

The examples discussed above show that variability in outcomes reflects in part the type of device that is used to measure outcome. Clinical judgments, psychometric tests, and interview/rating scales involve overlapping but different domains of assessment. A major question is how the device is scaled. In this respect, any decisions about scaling represent in part the underlying conceptualization of the change that follows injury. Survival is an obvious example of an area of outcome assessment where qualitative, noncontinuous change is assessed. When psychometric tests, interviews, and rating scales are used, the scaling is often quantitative. Problems may emerge when assessment devices that yield continuously distributed scales are used to create qualitative end points. Not only is the underlying model often inappropriate, but considerable information may be lost by ignoring reliable differences between individuals whose scores classify them within the same categorical end point.

Predictors of Outcome

Injury Characteristics

Methods used to characterize the nature and severity of TBI are major sources of variability in outcomes. This variability has at least three sources: (1) mechanism of injury; (2) measurement of severity; and (3) pathophysiological effects of injury on the brain.

1. *Mechanism of injury.* Children at different ages are subject to different causes of trauma. Infants and toddlers, for example, often sustain TBI from physical abuse or falls. Children in the 4- to 12-year-old range are commonly victims of falls, sporting accidents, and motor vehicle accidents. Any child can receive a TBI from the last of these, but the frequency increases with age. Adolescents are often involved in high-speed automobile accidents, which are also frequent causes of TBI in adults. Variability in outcome occurs across ages partly because these events vary in the amount of force affecting the head. Minor injuries are more likely to occur in accidents that do not involve motor vehicles. Penetrating injuries, particularly gunshot wounds, produce devastating injuries. These differences interact with the degree of brain development in the child (Jellinger, 1983). Any study of pediatric TBI should provide information on the mechanism of injury.

2. *Severity.* It is common to characterize the severity of TBI according to different indices of depth of coma. A major source of variability is how and when this assessment is made. The most widely used assessment device is the well-known Glasgow Coma Scale (Teasdale & Jennett, 1974; see Table 1-3). This scale, which has been extensively validated with adults, is clearly useful for children. However, there are problems with the use of the Glasgow Coma Scale with young children, particularly infants and toddlers who are preverbal. A Glasgow Coma Scale score in the moderate range for a preverbal child may portend a more severe injury than a similar score in a verbal child. Modifications of the Glasgow Coma Scale have been developed for young children but have not seen extensive use (see Bruce, this volume).

Another issue is at what time postinjury to assess the depth of coma (Levin et al., 1982). The Glasgow Coma Scale score in the emergency room can be higher than the score 24 hours later, particularly in children that deteriorate because of brain swelling or other problems. It is useful to report both scores, because children may be placed in different groups depending on when the Glasgow Coma Scale is obtained. This may account for some of the variations in outcome reported for patients with "mild" injuries, who may demonstrate deterioration after resuscitation.

Duration of impaired consciousness is also used to index severity. This variable most commonly reflects the number of days from injury until the child follows commands. It is equivalent to the number of days on which the motor scale score of the Glasgow Coma Scale is below 6 and is clearly a useful index of severity. A severe injury is usually indicated when the duration of impaired consciousness exceeds 24 hours. Children who have overall Glasgow Coma Scale scores in the moderate range (9 to 12) but whose motor scale score on the Glasgow Coma Scale is below 6 for 24 hours (i.e., does not follow simple commands—see Table 1-3) most likely have injuries that should be classified as severe.

Another index of severity is the duration of posttraumatic amnesia. Although clinicians have estimated the duration of posttraumatic amnesia beginning with the onset of impaired consciousness and ending with return of memory for ongoing

TABLE 1-3. Glasgow Coma Scale

Function	Score	Criterion
Eye opening		
None	1	Not attributable to ocular swelling.
To pain	2	Pain stimulus is applied to chest or limbs.
To speech	3	Nonspecific response to speech or shout; does not imply the patient obeys command to open eyes.
Spontaneous	4	Eyes are open, but this does not imply intact awareness.
Motor response		
No response	1	Flaccid.
Extension	2	"Decerebrate": Adduction, internal rotation of shoulder, and pronation of forearm.
Abnormal flexion	3	"Decorticate": Abnormal flexion, adduction of the shoulder.
Withdrawal	4	Normal flexor response; withdraws from pain stimulus with abduction of the shoulder.
Localizes pain	5	Pain stimulus applied to supraocular region or fingertip causes limb to remove it.
Obeys commands	6	Follows simple commands.
Verbal response		
No response	1	Self-explanatory.
Incomprehensible	2	Moaning and groaning but no recognizable words.
Inappropriate	3	Intelligible speech (e.g., shouting or swearing) but no sustained or coherent conversation.
Confused	4	Patient responds to questions in a conversational manner, but the responses indicate varying degrees of disorientation and confusion.
Oriented	5	Normal orientation to time, place, and person.
Summed Glasgow Coma Scale Score (E + M + V) = 3 to 15		

Source: From Teasdale & Jennett, 1974.

events, recently developed bedside tests have focused on evaluating disorientation and amnesia (Ewing-Cobbs, et al., 1990). The duration of posttraumatic amnesia, which is distinguished herein from coma, represents the amount of time necessary for the child to move from recovery of consciousness (i.e., following commands) to complete temporal and spatial orientation, with return of episodic memory. Length of posttraumatic amnesia is often estimated retrospectively by asking caretakers, but it should be measured formally with an instrument such as the Children's Orientation and Amnesia Test (COAT) (Ewing-Cobbs et al., 1990). McDonald et al. (1993) found that the COAT score and the number of days to reach a Glasgow Coma Scale score of 15 were the best predictors in a case-control study examining multiple early predictors of 1-year outcomes. Although retrospective reports of posttraumatic amnesia are of questionable reliability, they are often used as an index of severity in studies of pediatric TBI.

How and when injury severity is measured accounts for variability in results across studies. The British studies, for example, relied on retrospective assessments of posttraumatic amnesia (Shaffer, this volume). The Galveston-Houston studies used the emergency room and the lowest postresuscitation Glasgow Coma Scale score, length of impaired consciousness, and length of posttraumatic amnesia (Levin et al., this volume). The Los Angeles studies used only the initial Glasgow Coma Scale score (Asarnow et al., this volume). Although these measures are correlated, children will be classified differently depending on how the indices of severity are used. It goes without saying that studies that do not use these established indices of injury severity will be difficult to interpret. This may be a problem for many of the older studies of outcome after pediatric TBI (Klonoff et al., 1993; Klonoff et al., this volume). A study with well-characterized injury variables from a tertiary-care trauma center will have a different subject population than a study with subjects drawn from a rehabilitation facility or a subdivision hospital emergency room. The inability to compare injury characteristics across studies from different sites is a major problem in interpreting the variability in outcomes after pediatric TBI.

   3. *Pathophysiological effects on the brain.* The advent of contemporary neuroimaging shows considerable variation in the response of the brain to TBI. Although it has been common to conceptualize TBI after closed head injury due to blunt trauma as a "diffuse" insult, magnetic resonance imaging shows focal areas of abnormal signal in over 50% of severely injured children, with a particular predilection for the frontal lobes (see Levin et al., this volume). It is becoming increasingly important to have neuroimaging studies at the time of injury and after the subacute phase of recovery to adequately understand the pattern of changes in the brain produced by the injury. Neuroimaging variables are related to outcome depending on how the neuroimaging data are treated and how outcome is assessed (Aldrich et al., 1992).

Conclusions: Injury Sources of Variability

How and when injury severity is assessed is a major source of variability in outcomes, particularly when the results of various studies from different sites are compared. Although it is apparent that a variety of methods should be used to assess severity, inclusion of a subset of measures that are uniform across studies is recommended. Such assessments should also include reports of neuroimaging studies, neurological status, and mechanisms of injury. If this basic descriptive information is not reported, the results of different studies of outcome will be difficult to compare.

   Assessments of injury severity should be made prospectively from the time of injury. If the only information available is retrospective, all information should be gathered from chart review, since caregiver reports may not be reliable. The best retrospective information concerning severity is probably the Glasgow Coma Scale and the duration of impaired consciousness defined as the number of days to follow commands. Nurses' notes should also be studied for this assessment. Whenever possible, the results of neuroimaging studies should be independently reviewed for the purposes of a research study.

Environmental Sources of Variability

There are at least three major sources of variability in outcome that can be loosely characterized as environmental: (1) premorbid characteristics of the child and family; (2) the postinjury environment; and (3) various interventions.

1. *Premorbid characteristics.* In contrast to adult studies (see Grafman and Salazar, this volume), little is known about the relationship of environmental variables characterizing the child and family prior to TBI and outcome. There are many presumptions. For example, it is presumed that children who were functioning at a higher intellectual level or who come from high socioeconomic levels have better outcomes, which is apparent in adults (Grafman and Salazar, this volume). Similarly, it is presumed that injured children whose families were intact at the time of injury have better outcomes. A child who did not have a preexisting learning disability or behavior disorder is presumed to have a better prognosis. Unfortunately, other than the British studies (Shaffer, this volume), there are virtually no studies addressing this source of variability, although there are studies now in progress (see Taylor et al., this volume). All of these presumptions about premorbid characteristics are hypotheses awaiting evaluation.

2. *Postinjury environment.* The British studies provide convincing evidence for relationships of the postinjury environment and outcome (Brown et al., 1981; Rutter, 1981; Shaffer, this volume). These studies showed that severely injured children who recovered under conditions of psychosocial adversity were three times more likely to develop a new psychiatric disorder than severely injured children who recovered in environments that were not characterized as adverse. It is not clear what mechanisms enhance or retard outcomes. To understand these mechanisms, it is necessary to assess the family's material and psychological resources as well as the effects of the injury on the family, including parents and siblings (Perrot et al., 1991). The important point is that such factors account for variability in outcome that is not explained by injury variables.

There is also a major need to replicate the British studies. Brown and coworkers (1981) reported that injury severity and the postinjury environment *interacted* in producing behavioral adjustment problems (also see Rutter, 1981). This study is one of the few investigations showing that the effects of brain injury and the environment are not simply additive (see review by St. James-Roberts, 1979). Studies of children with other forms of brain injury, such as spina bifida and cerebral palsy, have not found evidence for an interaction effect. Rather, these studies demonstrate a main effect for the injury and for the environment (Breslau, 1990; Wallander et al., 1988). The results of these studies may reflect the need to more carefully define the nature of the brain injury in children with spina bifida and cerebral palsy, since investigations may not have dealt adequately with the heterogeneity of these children. In addition, children with spina bifida and cerebral palsy are injured very early in development, whereas TBI can occur at any age. This characteristic of TBI may make an interaction of injury severity and the environment more likely. If the postinjury environment does interact with severity, it may be possible to identify environmental modifications that will enhance recovery and reduce some of the morbidity associated with TBI.

    3. *Interventions.* The neurosurgical literature outlines many characteristics of treatment, particularly in the acute phase of TBI, that influence survival. There is still considerable variability across centers in how children are evaluated, triaged, and treated. The effect of acute-care interventions on morbidity is unclear. Treatment factors that influence mortality may be different from those that influence morbidity (Bruce, this volume).

    The effects of interventions after the subacute phase of injury are largely unknown. Most children with TBI return to home and school, with only the most severely injured receiving intensive inpatient and rehabilitation interventions. There is wide variation in receipt of services. Presumably these services vary in their appropriateness for the child and in their overall quality. The effects of rehabilitation, somatic interventions such as medications for alertness, educational placements, and parent training and education have not been studied. There is a major need for intervention studies specifically designed for children with TBI.

Conclusions: Predictors of Outcomes

Studies of prognosis after pediatric TBI often attempt to predict outcomes on the basis of injury and environmental characteristics. Few studies simultaneously examine both injury and environmental factors. Indices of injury severity are significant predictors of mortality and cognitive morbidity. However, injury variables do not robustly predict behavioral adjustment and adaptive functioning, which may be influenced by environmental factors both before and after the accident (Perrot et al., 1991). Further research is clearly needed on the role of environmental factors in outcome. In addition, studies that examine the joint and potentially interactive effects of injury and environmental variables on outcomes should be completed. How outcomes are assessed may also determine what factors emerge as predictive in a particular analysis.

Measurement of Change

This brief review lists a number of factors that account for the variability in outcomes after TBI. These factors include how outcomes are assessed and a host of injury and environmental variables. It is important to recognize that the assessment of outcome is a measurement problem at the level of the injury and the environment. Comprehensive models of outcomes require an attempt to measure variables in all of these domains. Equally important, however, is the approach taken to assess outcome. This issue extends beyond the nature of the outcome measure and requires consideration of the underlying model of change or recovery.

    Many of the methods used to assess the relationships of injury variables and the environment to outcomes are based on models of qualitative change or simply treat outcome as a static end point. Qualitative models are quite appropriate for outcomes that are clearly noncontinuous, such as survival. However, the appropriateness of such models for outcomes that are quantitative or continuous is questionable. This is particularly true for children, who are developing organisms who change over time (Fletcher et al., 1989).

The change in performance that occurs over time following TBI is often addressed by comparing a child's performance to normative data that change with age. Such an approach will address the child's outcome relative to age-matched peers at a particular age or time, but it provides little information on the child's future (or past) course of development. This approach to outcome assessment fails to predict future performance because it fails to explicitly model behavior as a function of time. Under this approach, change in performance over time is masked by the ever-changing baseline of "normal" performance given the child's age.

To a certain extent, the tendency to treat outcomes after pediatric TBI as static processes reflects the imposition of adult models onto children (Dennis, 1988; Fletcher & Taylor, 1984). Adult models can certainly be heuristic, but they often lead to the wrong set of questions. For example, it may be interesting to compare outcomes after adult and child TBI. When an adult, for whom recovery is gauged in terms of to an established baseline, is compared to a child, whose recovery is based on a changing baseline, a major characteristic of pediatric TBI is not addressed: the fact that children are changing. Development and recovery are inherently processes of change. To fully appreciate recovery after pediatric TBI, it may be necessary to use conceptual models and designs that permit assessments of outcome from a developmental perspective. The age of the child is clearly a factor in outcome (Levin et al., 1984). However, age is not the explanatory factor; rather, it is the processes of development marked by age and reflecting change that are most important (Fletcher & Taylor, 1984).

Individual Growth Approaches to Change

Children are evolving organisms for whom a static conceptualization of outcome may misconstrue the effects of TBI. This misconstrual stems from the failure to view performance as a time-dependent function. It is possible and desirable to model explicitly the processes whereby the child is developing. The process view evaluates change as a continuing process that underlies a child's ability to perform and adapt in the environment. When outcome is viewed as a static end point or change is viewed as incremental, heterogeneity in change is treated as error variability that hinders the measurement of outcome. If change is viewed as a process, this "error" becomes the end point of interest. Hence, a major source of variability in outcome after pediatric TBI—implicit throughout this chapter—is the view of change underlying the assessment of outcome. The explanation of outcomes involves how change is measured at the level of the instrument as well as how change is conceptualized and modeled.

There are models that permit the investigation of developmental change (Burchinal & Applebaum, 1991; Fletcher et al., 1991; Francis et al., 1991). These models, which have been developed largely in the biological and educational literature, permit the analysis of individual differences and rates of change separately for each child and collectively for groups of children. Intraindividual change can be characterized as an individual growth curve that quantifies the rate at which development is proceeding (rate) as well as the overall level (end point) of the outcome. The use of these models represents a shift from measurements of an expected end point only to one in which the end point becomes the entire growth curve.

Models of individual change begin with a within-subjects component in which a growth curve is estimated for each subject. The parameters of these curves can then be explored to identify predictors of intraindividual change in a between-subjects component. For example, if growth is estimated on a particular attribute, such as intelligence, it is possible to measure characteristics of an injury and environment and to use these characteristics as predictors of change. When this process view of change is adopted, growth is estimated at the level of the individual. Issues involving the relationships of injury, the environment, and outcome are reformulated in terms of their influences on growth and development. Of particular interest is the fact that the determinants of intraindividual change can be addressed at the level of the single case (Bryk & Raudenbush, 1987).

It is obvious that these methods require multiple time points. In order to evaluate processes that are not linear, at least four assessments of outcome must be made. The advantages of these models include the focus on individual change, the incorporation of both categorical and continuous determinants of change, and the capacity to model processes of change that are not linear. These approaches permit more flexibility because they accommodate staggered time points. Since the growth curve is weighted according to the number of time points available for each subject, missing data (so long as they are random) are not a major problem for these methods. Such models can also be used to study qualitative change (see Fletcher et al., 1991).

To illustrate how such models can be applied to the study of recovery after pediatric TBI, we completed a study utilizing individual change models (Thompson et al., 1994). Traditional assessments of the relationships of injury characteristics and outcome typically account for approximately 30% of the variability in outcome (Levin et al., 1982). Thompson and colleagues (1994) provided an initial application of individual change methods to recovery from pediatric TBI in 49 children followed prospectively for up to 5 years postinjury. Each child received up to seven psychometric assessments of motor, visual-spatial, and somatosensory skills. Hence, the outcomes were measured on a quantitative, continuous scale. An obvious problem for static end-point methods is to determine the time point at which to measure outcome. In contrast, individual change models utilize all of the longitudinal data.

The application of individual growth curves by Thompson and coworkers (1994) demonstrated systematic nonlinear change after injury. The variability among individual growth patterns was strongly related to injury predictor variables. In contrast to traditional assessments of incremental change with only a single end point, Thompson and coworkers (1994) were able to account for up to 93% of the true parameter variance underlying the relationship of specific injury variables to motor, visual-spatial, and somatosensory performance. These methods did not require artificial truncation of the neuropsychological measures.

Figure 1-3 illustrates the end result such an analysis would provide. In this figure, individual growth curves for each subject on the Beery Test of Visual-Motor Integration, a measure of perceptual-motor skills, are displayed as a function of age at follow-up and injury severity (Glasgow Coma Scale ≤ 8 = severe; > 8 = mild-moderate). The growth curves are the result of the within-subjects process, in which the parameters of change are estimated for each child and reconstructed into the estimated growth curves in each of the four panels in Figure 1-3. For the between-subjects phase, age at injury, severity, and pupillary abnormalities were used to predict the absolute level of performance averaged over time (i.e., intercept) as well as differences in the rate of change (i.e., slope of the curves). The severity variable is a composite of the Glasgow Coma Scale score, duration of impaired consciousness, and duration of posttraumatic amnesia, which were highly correlated. Age at testing indicates the time points at which the child was tested. The influence of age at injury can be assessed because the follow-up interval represents the actual age of the child.

For the intercept, there was a significant age × severity interaction. This can be seen in Figure 1-3 by comparing the two left-hand panels (mild to moderate injury) with the two right-hand panels (severe injury). Note that the growth curves for children with mild/moderate injuries tend to be higher on the plot than for severe injuries and that this effect is more apparent for severely injured children who were evaluated at younger ages. There was also an age × severity interaction for the slopes. This effect is most obvious when the lower two panels of Figure 1-3 are compared. For children with mild/moderate injuries, the growth curves are steep and in an upward direction. In contrast, the curves for severely injured children cluster together and are relatively flat, particularly for children evaluated at young ages (before age 10). Older severely injured children also show steeper curves, implying that children severely injured at a younger age show less recovery. Finally, pupillary abnormalities were not related to the absolute level of performance or to the variability in slopes, so that the panels in Figure 1-3 for normal/abnormal pupils are not obviously different within each severity group.

Conclusions

Models of intraindividual change may have considerable promise for understanding relationships of injury and environmental characteristics to outcome after pediatric TBI. To account for the variability in outcomes, the characteristics of the injury and the environment must be carefully measured. In addition, procedures for assessing outcome must be conceptualized in terms of what aspect of outcome is being measured and the underlying model of change.

It may be possible to account for more of the variability in outcomes by evalu-

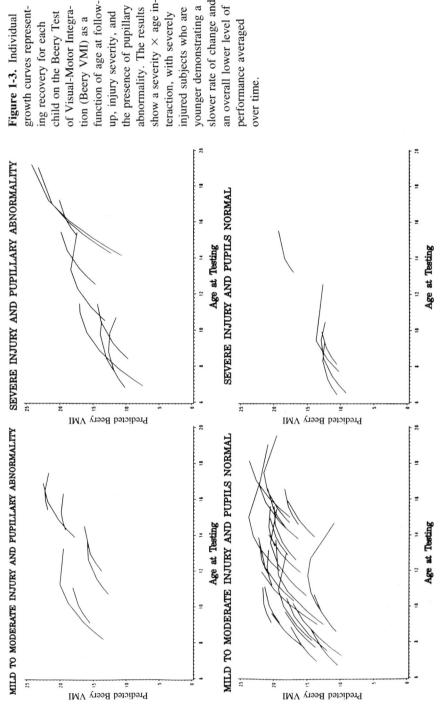

Figure 1-3. Individual growth curves representing recovery for each child on the Beery Test of Visual-Motor Integration (Beery VMI) as a function of age at follow-up, injury severity, and the presence of pupillary abnormality. The results show a severity × age interaction, with severely injured subjects who are younger demonstrating a slower rate of change and an overall lower level of performance averaged over time.

ating individual change. Such approaches are particularly useful for evaluating quantitative change. Since many of the outcome measures commonly employed in studies of pediatric TBI are quantitative measures, the application of these models should be carefully considered. It may be possible to enhance clinical trials research and the more general question of outcomes by adapting statistical methods to outcomes as opposed to the more traditional method of modifying the outcome assessment to fit the statistical model.

Any approach to the assessment of outcomes in children should incorporate a developmental perspective. In the absence of this perspective, which includes an emphasis on change, the unique characteristics of pediatric investigations is lost. Future investigations of outcome after pediatric TBI should be based on conceptual models that explicitly incorporate change in order to account for the variability in outcomes.

Acknowledgments

This work was supported in part by NICHD grant HD 27597, Neuropsychological Sequelae of Pediatric Head Injury, and NINDS grant NS 25368, Neurobehavioral Outcomes After Pediatric Head Injury. The assistance of Linda Kimbrough with manuscript preparation, Amy Boudousquie with data collection, and Kimberly Copeland with data analysis is gratefully acknowledged.

References

Achenbach, T. M. (1991). *Manual for the Child Behavior Checklist 4-18 and 1991 Profile*. Burlington, VT: Department of Psychiatry, University of Vermont.

Aldrich, E. F., Eisenberg, H. M., Saydjari, C., Leversen, T. G., Foulkes, M. A., Jane, J. A., Marshall, L. F., Marmarou, A., & Young, H. F. (1992). Diffuse brain swelling in severely head injured children. *J. Neurosurg.*, 76, 450–454.

Annegers, J. F. (1983). The epidemiology of head trauma in children. In K. Shapiro (Ed.), *Pediatric head trauma* (pp. 1–10). Mount Kisco, NY: Futura.

Breslau, N. (1990). Does brain dysfunction increase children's vulnerability to environment stress? *Arch. Gen. Psychiatry, 47,* 15–20.

Brown, G., Chadwick, O., Shaffer, D., Rutter, M., & Traub, M. (1981). A prospective study of children with head injuries: III. Psychiatric sequelae. *Psychol. Med., 11,* 63–78.

Bryk, A. S., & Raudenbush, S. W. (1987). Application of hierarchical linear models to assessing change. *Psychol. Bull., 101,* 147–158.

Burchinal, M., & Appelbaum, M. I. (1991). Estimating individual developmental functions: Methods and their assumptions. *Child Dev., 62,* 23–43.

Dennis, M. (1988). Language in the young damaged brain. In T. Boll & B. K. Bryant (Eds.), *Clinical neuropsychology and brain function: Research measurement and practice* (pp. 85–123). Washington, DC, American Psychological Association.

DiScala, C., Osberg, J. S., Gans, B. M., Chin, L. J., & Grant, C. C. (1991). Children with traumatic head injury: Morbidity and postacute treatment. *Arch. Phys. Med. Rehabil., 72,* 662–666.

Ewing-Cobbs, L., Iovino, I., Fletcher, J. M., Miner, M. E., and Levin, H. S. (1991). Academic achievement following traumatic brain injury in children and adolescents. *J. Clin. Exp. Neuropsychol., 13,* 93 (abstract).

Ewing-Cobbs, L., Levin, H. S., Fletcher, J. M., Miner, M. E., & Eisenberg, H. M. (1990). The Children's Orientation and Amnesia Test: Relationship to severity of acute head injury and recovery of memory. *Neurosurgery, 27,* 683–691.

Ewing-Cobbs, L., Miner, M. E., Fletcher, J. M., & Levin, H. S. (1989). Intellectual, motor, and language sequelae following closed head injury in infants and preschoolers. *J. Pediatr. Psychol., 14,* 531–547.

Fletcher, J. M., Ewing-Cobbs, L., Miner, M. E., Levin, H. S., & Eisenberg, H. M. (1990). Behavioral changes after closed head injury in children. *J. Consult. Clin. Psychol., 58,* 93–98.

Fletcher, J. M., Francis, D. J., Pequegnat, W., Raudenbush, S. W., Bornstein, M. H., Schmitt, F., Brouwers, P., & Stover, E. (1991). Neurobehavioral outcome in diseases of childhood: Individual change models for pediatric human immunodeficiency viruses. *Am. Psychol., 46,* 1267–1277.

Fletcher, J. M., & Levin, H. S. (1988). Neurobehavioral effects of brain injury in children. In D. Routh (Ed.), *Handbook of pediatric psychology* (pp. 258–295). New York: Guilford Press.

Fletcher, J. M., Levin, H. S., Lachar, D., Kusnerik, L., Harward, H., Mendelsohn, D., & Lilly, M. A. (submitted). Behavioral adjustment after pediatric closed head injury: Relationships with age, severity, and lesion size.

Fletcher, J. M., Miner, M., & Ewing-Cobbs, L. (1989). Age and recovery from head injury in children: Developmental issues. In H. S. Levin, H. Eisenberg, & J. Grafman (Eds.), *Neurobehavioral recovery from head injury* (pp. 279–291). New York: Oxford University Press.

Fletcher, J. M., & Taylor, H. G. (1984). Neuropsychological approaches to children: Towards a developmental neuropsychology. *J. Clin. Neuropsychol., 6,* 39–56.

Francis, D. J., Fletcher, J. M., Stuebing, K. K., Davidson, K. C., & Thompson, N. M. (1991). Analysis of change: Modeling individual growth. *J. Consult Clin. Psychol., 59,* 27–37.

Jellinger, K. (1983). The neuropathology of pediatric head injury. In K. Shapiro (Ed.), *Pediatric head trauma* (pp. 87–115). Mount Kisco, NY: Futura.

Jennett, B., & Bond, M. (1975). Assessment of outcome after severe brain damage: A practical scale. *Lancet, 1,* 480–484.

Klonoff, H., Clark, C., & Klonoff, P. S. (1993). Long-term outcome of head injuries: A 23-year follow-up study of children with head injuries. *J. Neurol. Neurosurg. Psychiatry, 56,* 410–415.

Lachar, D. (1982). *Personality Inventory for Children (PIC): Revised format supplement.* Los Angeles, CA: Western Psychological Services.

Lachar, D. (1993). Symptom checklists and personality inventories. In T. R. Kratochwill & R. J. Morris (Eds.), *Handbook of psychotherapy for children and adolescents* (pp. 38–57). New York: Allyn & Bacon.

Langfitt, T. W. (1978). Measuring the outcome from head injuries. *J. Neurosurg., 48,* 673–678.

Levin, H. S., Benton, A. L. & Grossman, R. G. (1982). *Neurobehavioral consequences of closed head injury.* New York: Oxford University Press.

Levin, H. S., Ewing-Cobbs, L., & Benton, A. L. (1984). Age and recovery from brain damage: A review of clinical studies. In S. W. Scheff (Ed.), *Aging and recovery of function in the central nervous system* (pp. 233–240). New York: Plenum.

McDonald, C. M., Jaffe, K. M., Fay, G. C., Polissar, N. L., & Liao, S. (1993). A comparison of indices of traumatic brain injury severity as predictors of neurobehavioral outcome in children. *Soc. Neurosci.,* p. 78 (abstract).

Miner, M. E., Fletcher, J. M., & Ewing-Cobbs, L. (1986). Recovery versus outcome after head injury in children. In M. E. Miner & K. A. Wagner (Eds.), *Neural trauma: Treatment, monitoring and rehabilitation issues* (pp. 233–240). Stoneham, MA: Butterworth.

Perrot, S. B., Taylor, H. G., & Montes, J. L. (1991). Neuropsychological sequelae, familial stress, and environmental adaptation following pediatric head injury. *Dev. Neuropsychol., 7,* 69–86.

Rappoport, M., Hall, K. M., Hopkins, K., Belleza, T., & Cope, D. N. (1982). Disability rating scale for severe head traumas: Coma to community. *Arch. Phys. Med. Rehabil., 63,* 118–125.

Rutter, M. (1981). Psychological sequelae of brain damage in children. *Am. J. Psychiatry, 138,* 1533–1544.

St. James-Roberts, I. (1979). Neurological plasticity, recovery from brain insult, and child development. In H. W. Reese (Ed.), *Advances in child development and behavior* (Vol. 14; pp. 253–319). New York: Academic Press.

Sattler, J. M. (1992). *Assessment of children* (3rd ed.). San Diego, CA: Jerome M. Sattler Publishers.

Sparrow, S. S., Balla, D. A., & Cicchetti, D. (1984). *Vineland Adaptive Behavior Scales.* Circle Pines, MN: American Guidance Service.

Teasdale, G., & Jennett, B. (1974). Assessment of coma and impaired consciousness: A practical scale. *Lancet, 2,* 81–84.

Thompson, N. M., Francis, D. J., Stuebing, K. K., Fletcher, J. M., Ewing-Cobbs, L., Miner, M. E., Levin, H. S., & Eisenberg, H. (1994). Motor, visual-spatial, and somatosensory skills after closed head injury in children and adolescents: A study of change. *Neuropsychology, 8,* 333–342.

Wallander, J. L., Varni, J. W., Babani, L., Banis, H. T., & Wilcox, K. T. (1988). Children with chronic physical disorders: Maternal reports of their psychological adjustment. *J. Pediatr. Psychol., 13,* 197–212.

Wechsler, D. (1974). *Wechsler Intelligence Scales for Children-Revised.* New York: Psychological Corporation.

Wirt, R. D., Lachar, D., Klinedinst, J. K., & Seat, P. D. (1990). *Multidimensional description of child personality. A manual for the Personality Inventory for Children.* Los Angeles, CA: Western Psychological Service.

2

Epidemiological Features of Brain Injury in Children: Occurrence, Children at Risk, Causes and Manner of Injury, Severity, and Outcomes

JESS F. KRAUS

This chapter synthesizes information from a number of research reports on child brain and head injury published in the English language in the last 20 years. To derive a numerical value for some parameters, it was necessary to approximate a number from printed figures or interpolate from tabular materials in the published documents. Since there is a general lack of uniformity among the various studies in case definitions, data sources, case-finding techniques, and the manner in which certain descriptive variables are reported, the reader should exercise a degree of caution in interpreting the findings discussed in this chapter. Even the term "brain injury," for example, is defined in different ways. (Table 2-1). A reading of the papers reviewed suggests that the authors generally intended to study damage to the brain, yet some used the term "head injury"; thus, it is quite possible that the inclusion criteria may have encompassed damage to soft tissues of the head or fracture of the skull without concurrent injury to the brain.

Case inclusion criteria vary from study to study. Study groups may have been restricted to injured children who were referred to neurological intensive care units or children treated in emergency departments and released for outpatient observation. Some studies exclude children who died at the scene or on arrival at the emergency department, but others may include such cases. There are differences in age criteria among the studies as well.

It is important to recognize that the findings cited here may not necessarily be applicable to all countries and regions in the world. The actual rate of occurrence, injury-reporting practices, medical care institution admission policies, and levels of risk in the populations may vary widely. While the findings discussed in this chapter may be broadly generalizable and therefore of some use for regional purposes, the best approach in estimating the occurrence and characteristics of brain injury in a population is to conduct surveillance in the local region with attention to case definition, case finding, factor specification, and data-collecting practices.

The general purpose of this chapter is to analyze the published literature on the occurrence (both incidence and mortality) of brain injury in populations. Population groups at high risk are described as well as the external causes or manner of injury. The type and severity of injury are presented, including outcome following injury, and a method to estimate community prevalence of disability from brain trauma is provided. The final section addresses future needs and directions in the epidemiology of pediatric brain injury.

The Occurrence of Brain Injury

Incidence

A number of reports provide incidence rates of child brain injury in the population or allow estimates to be made from the data. In this chapter "incidence" means the number of new cases in the population of children at risk of injury in a defined period of time. As seen in Figure 2-1, the age ranges of the study populations shown vary from 0 to 19 in Norway (Nestvold et al., 1988) to 0 to 7 in Israel (Horowitz et al., 1983). Most investigators, however, have defined childhood as the age range from birth through age 14. There are vast differences in reported incidence in the nine studies charted in Figure 2-1. The average incidence rate in the studies is approximately 180 per 100,000 children per year. This rate encompasses all levels of severity and includes reports where the children were admitted to a hospital with confirmed medical diagnoses of brain injury.

Mortality and Mortality Rates

In 1991, over 9000 children in the United States under the age of 15 died from acute traumatic injuries (Hoyert & Hudson, 1993). Some 40% to 50% had a diagnosis of brain injury. Findings from Oklahoma (Oklahoma State Department of Health, 1991) and France (Tiret et al., 1990) show similar findings, namely, from 40% to 50% of all acute traumatic injury deaths involve damage to the brain.

Figure 2-2 shows the association of brain injury deaths, hospital discharges, and medically attended cases among U.S. children for 1991. The ratio of deaths to hospital discharges and reported medically attended instances is approximately 1:32:152; in other words, for each brain injury death there are about 32 hospital discharges and 152 reported episodes of medically attended cases.

TABLE 2-1.   Brain Injury Case Definition and Severity Scoring Criteria, Selected
Studies

Study Location (source)	Study Years	Case Definition	Severity Scoring Criteria
Olmsted County, Minnesota (Annegers et al., 1980)	1965–1974	Head injury with evidence of presumed brain involvement, i.e., concussion with LOC, PTA, or neurological signs of brain injury, skull fracture.	*Fatal* (<28 days). *Severe:* Intracranial hematoma, contusion, or LOC>24 hours, or PTA>24 hours. *Moderate:* LOC or PTA 30 minutes to 24 hours, skull fracture, or both. *Mild:* LOC or PTA<30 minutes without skull fracture.
Rhode Island (Fife et al., 1986)	1979–1980	Presence of ICD codes 800–801.9, 803–804.9, and 850–854.9 (head injuries).	Not determined.
Kfar-Sava, Israel (Horowitz et al., 1983)	1970–1976	Chart diagnoses of cerebral contusion, concussion, or other head injury.	Not determined.
Central Virginia (Jagger et al., 1984)	Oct. 1977–June 1979	CNS referral patients with significant head injury admitted to neurosurgical service.	GCS (*severe* = ≤8, *moderate* = 9–12, *mild* = 13–15).
San Diego County, California (Kraus et al., 1984)	1981	Physician-diagnosed physical damage from acute mechanical energy exchange resulting in concussion, hemorrhage, contusion, or laceration of brain.	Modified GCS (*severe* = ≤8; *moderate* = 9–15 *plus* hospital stay of 4–8 hours *and* brain surgery, or abnormal CT, or GCS 9–12; *mild* = all others, GCS 13–15).
Maryland (MacKenzie et al., 1989)	1986	ICD codes 800, 801, 803, 804, 850–854.	ICDMAP computer program to convert ICD codes to

(continued)

Children at High Risk of Injury

Sex-Specific Rates

Data from San Diego County, California (Kraus et al., 1984), show a male-to-female incidence rate ratio of 1.8 to 1. In Israel, Horowitz and coworkers (1983) report a rate ratio of 1.5 to 1 for children aged 0 to 7 years. Hayes and Jackson (1989), using nonfatal brain injury information from England and Wales, reports for those under age 5 a male-to-female hospital admissions ratio of 1.3 to 1. For children aged 5 to 14, occurrence of injury is 2.2 times more common in males

TABLE 2-1.   (*continued*)

Study Location (source)	Study Years	Case Definition	Severity Scoring Criteria
			abbreviated injury severity scores.
Ahershus County, Norway (Nestvold et al., 1988)	1974–1975	Trauma to face, head, or neck with one or more of the following: unconsciousness, retroamnesia, PTA, skull/neck fracture, or trauma with headache, nausea, or vomiting. First day postinjury date.	Length of PTA (mild to severe): 0 = No PTA 1 = PTA < 5 hours 2 = PTA 5–6 hours 3 = PTA 6–24 hours 4 = PTA 1–2 days 5 = PTA 3–7 days 6 = PTA > 1 week (for children < 10 years use length of impaired consciousness)
Oklahoma (Oklahoma State Department of Health, 1991)	1989	Discharged with one (or more) ICD (9) codes 800.0–801.9, 803.0–804.9, 850.0–854.9, 905.0, 907.0 *or* died in emergency room with diagnosis of brain injury.	*Minor* = AIS 1 *Moderate* = AIS 2 *Severe* = AIS 3–5
Aquitaine, France (Tiret et al., 1990)	1986	Contusion, laceration, skull fracture, brain injury, and/or LOC after a relevant event. Facial fractures without LOC were excluded.	*Severe* = LOC > 6 hours. *Moderate* = skull fracture without brain injury or LOC > 15 minutes < 6 hours *mild* = contusion with no LOC or LOC < 15 minutes.

Abbreviations: LOC, loss of consciousness; PTA, posttraumatic amnesia; ICD, International Classification of Diseases; CNS, central nervous system; GCS, Glasgow Coma Scale; AIS, Abbreviated Injury Scale; CT, computed tomography.

than in females. It would appear that male children are more likely than female children to incur brain injury.

Age

The incidence of hospital-attended brain injury in children is not uniform across all ages. In one study (Kraus et al., 1986) that reported age-specific rates, children through ages 1 to 5 years have a similar incidence—namely, about 160 injuries per 100,000 population. At age 5, the incidence increases at a higher rate in males. Brain injury rates increase for males but decline for females in late childhood and adolescence (Figure 2-3).

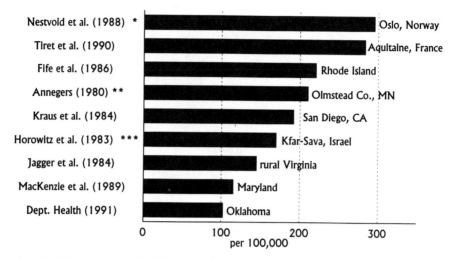

Ages 0 - 14, except * ages 0 - 19, ** ages 0 - 16, *** ages 0 - 7

Figure 2-1. Incidence of pediatric brain injury—selected studies. Ages 0–14, except *-0–19, **-0–16, ***-0–7.

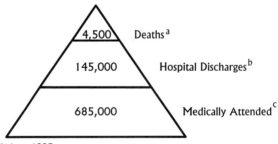

a. Source: Hoyert & Hudson, 1993.

b. Source: Graves, 1994. Includes any listed diagnoses of ICD(9-CM) codes 800, 801, 803, 804, 850-854, 907, ages 0 - 15.

c. Source: Collins, 1990. Includes 1985-87 average data adjusted to 1991 U.S. population of 55,130,000 children under age 18, and encompasses ICD(9-CM) codes 800-804, 850-854.

Figure 2-2. Fatalities, hospital discharges, and medically attended head injuries among U.S. children, 1991. (a) From Hoyert & Hudson, 1993. (b) From Graves, 1994. Includes any listed diagnoses of ICD(9-CM) codes 800, 801, 803, 850–854, 907; ages 0–15. (c) From Collins, 1990. Includes 1985–1987 average data adjusted to 1991 U.S. population of 55,130,000 children under age 18 and encompasses ICD(9-CM) codes 800–804, 850–854.

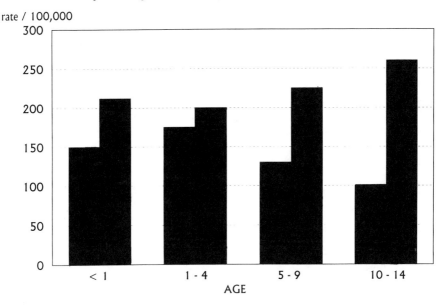

Figure 2-3. Incidence of pediatric head injury by age; female on left in each case (San Diego County, CA).

Race, Ethnicity, and Socioeconomic Status

There is little information in the published population-based epidemiological liter-ature on brain injury that addresses the questions of differential risk by race, eth-nicity, or socioeconomic gradient. One study (Kraus et al., 1990) from San Diego County showed that brain injury incidence rates for children were related to me-dian family income as determined from census tract data. This finding did not change when age and/or race/ethnicity were controlled. Data are needed to explore the environmental and/or socioeconomic bases for differential brain injury occur-rence by race, ethnicity, and socioeconomic status. The findings above, however, were ecological in nature and not based upon characteristics of the individual.

External Cause

The type of external cause provides information as to the mechanism or exposure that resulted in brain injury to the child. Many reports in the published literature provide data on this important descriptive parameter. Unfortunately, there is lack of consistency in the inclusiveness of the categories reported. For example, in some reports, "sports and recreation" sometimes includes bicycles and at other times does not. Crash or transport-related brain injuries include motor vehicle crashes, but occasionally the investigator has also included injuries to riders of bicycles or mopeds, pedestrians, or even passengers on trains. Note that there is wide variance in the definition of the study base, the study population, the ages included, severity of injuries, and date of the study (Table 2-1). Despite these inconsistencies in categorization of external cause, it is possible to summarize the basic findings from 10 studies (Table 2-2). The most common cause noted in five studies is transport, while falls are the most common exposure in the remaining five studies. Transport and falls account for approximately three-quarters to four-fifths of all brain injuries in the studies. The high proportion of transport-related brain injuries in the Salt Lake report (Mayer et al., 1981) and the low proportion of transport-related crashes in the study of three medical institutions in the eastern United States (Duhaime et al., 1992) suggest that referral patterns (among other factors) may have influenced the distribution of brain injury by external cause.

TABLE 2-2.   Percent of Child Brain Injury by External Cause: Selected International Studies

Study Location (reference)	Transport	Fall	Assault/Abuse	Sport/ Recreation	Other
San Diego County (Kraus et al., 1990)[a]	37	24	10	21	8
San Diego County (Kraus et al., 1986)[b]	28	35	6	27	4
Salt Lake (Mayer et al., 1981)[c]	88	2	6	NR	4
Atlanta (Henry et al., 1992)[d]	57	23	6	9	6
United States (Levin et al., 1992)[e]	67	16	6	8	3
England (Sharples et al., 1990)[f]	77	13	2	NR	8
Three U.S. medical institutions (Duhaime et al., 1992)[g]	9	73	2	NR	16
Chicago (Hahn & McLone, 1993)[h]	20	65	4	NR	11
Haifa, Israel (Levi et al., 1991)[i]	25	69	3	1	2
Kfar-Sava, Israel (Horowitz et al., 1983)[j]	19	72	NR	NR	9

NR = not reported.

[a] Age 0–19.

[b] Age 0–14.

[c] Severe pediatric trauma, age 0–16.

[d] Defined as "closed head injury," age 0–14.

[e] From the Traumatic Coma Data Bank, age 0–15.

[f] Fatal accidents involving head injury, age 0–15.

[g] Age 0–2.

[h] "Minor head injury," age 0–16.

[i] Includes all hospital admitted referrals, age 0–14.

[j] Age 0–7.

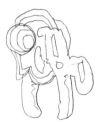

While the data in Table 2-2 show the wide variation in percent distribution by external cause, investigators interested in exposure information on a regional or local basis are urged to determine local occurrence by cause.

Severity

Level of severity of injury has been measured a number of different ways, including the Abbreviated Injury Scale (AIS) (Association for Advancement of Automotive Medicine, 1990) and the Glasgow Coma Scale (GCS) (Jennett & Teasdale, 1981). The AIS requires a specific injury diagnosis to determine severity. The GCS is derived from physiological assessment postinjury by assigning scores to the child's level of eye opening, verbal performance, and motor response. The total score ranges from 3 (which is no response to stimulus), to 15, which indicates no abnormalities in the three areas of assessment (Table 2-3). Seven reports have used the GCS to assess level of brain injury severity either during emergency department evaluation or upon admission to the hospital. The reader should be cautious in assessing the distributions in Table 2-4 because the GCS has been administered at varying times postinjury. In some cases, many hours elapsed before the GCS was determined; in other cases, following a time delay, there may have been some improvement in the status of the patient, hence the improvement in the GCS. It is noteworthy that for some children the verbal response may be inappropriate because of their very young age or limited verbal skills. In addition, assessment of eye opening may not be possible because of facial swelling. Data in Table 2-4 show, for most children seen in an emergency department or admitted to a hospital, GCS in the mild category. The report from Haifa, Israel (Levi et al., 1991), combined severe and moderate into one category, i.e., the severe GCS is 12 or less and mild is 13 to 15. The reports from Atlanta (Henry et al., 1992) and Birmingham, UK (Wagstyl et al., 1987) indicate that the referral patterns in the institutional catchment areas may include patients transferred from smaller institutions. The reports that are generally comparable in methods [San Diego, California (Kraus et al., 1986), United States Coma Data Bank (Luerssen et al., 1980), and the National Pediatric Trauma Registry (Lescohier & DiScala, 1993)] show severity ranges between 80% to 90% for mild, 7% to 8% for moderate, and 5% to 8% for severe brain injury categories. These studies excluded children who were dead on arrival but included those who may have died following admission to the hospital.

Early Outcomes following Brain Injury

The most severe result of a brain injury is death, and one measure that is routinely reported in the literature is the case fatality rate (the number of in-hospital deaths among persons admitted to the hospital alive with the injury). As can be seen in Figure 2-4, there is a wide range in reported case fatality rates, from about 2 to 3 per

TABLE 2-3. Glasgow Coma Scale

Eye opening	
Spontaneous	E4
To speech	3
To pain	2
Nil	1
Best Motor response	
Obeys	M6
Localizes	5
Withdraws	4
Abnormal flexion	3
Extensor response	2
Nil	1
Verbal response	
Orientated	V5
Confused conversation	4
Inappropriate words	3
Incomprehensible sounds	2
Nil	1
Coma Score $(E + M + V) = 3$ to 15	

Source: From Jennett & Teasdale, 1991.

TABLE 2-4. Severity in Brain Injured Children: Selected Studies

Study Location (reference)	Severity (%) (Glasgow Coma Scale)		
	Severe (3–8)	Moderate (9–12)	Mild (13–15)
San Diego County (Kraus et al., 1986)	5	7	89
United States Coma Data Bank (Luerssen et al., 1988)	6	8	84
Atlanta (Henry et al., 1992)	26	17	56
National Pediatric Trauma Registry (Lescohier & DiScala, 1993)[a]	13	10	76
Birmingham (UK) (Wagstyl et al., 1987)[b]	21	18	61
Haifa, Israel (Levi et al., 1991)[c]	(41 combined for both categories)		59
Oklahoma (Oklahoma State Department of Health, 1991)[d]	30	63	6

[a] Includes "head injury" only and "head injury plus extracranial injury."

[b] Severe = 3–7; moderate 8–10; mild = 11–15.

[c] Severe = <12; mild = ≥12.

[d] Discharged alive with traumatic brain injury; percentage excludes 131 in-hospital deaths.

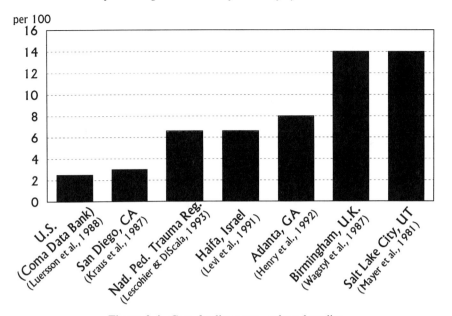

Figure 2-4. Case fatality rates—selected studies.

100 in the U.S. National Coma Data Bank (Luerssen et al., 1988) and San Diego County, California (Kraus et al., 1987) studies, to a high of 14 per 100 admitted patients from Birmingham, UK (Wagstyl et al., 1987), and the Salt Lake reports (Henry et al., 1992). The range of 3 to 14 in case fatality rates is not unusual considering the wide variation in hospital admission referral patterns as well as the nature of injuries sustained. For example, in the Oklahoma report (Oklahoma State Department of Health, 1991), the case fatality rate was highest among gunshot injuries (91 per 100) and lowest in persons injured in motor vehicle crashes, including pedestrians and motorcyclists. Thus, generalizations from one case fatality rate to other populations or institutions must consider the hospital admission practices, referral patterns, and base of external causes that result in brain injury.

In five reports, it is possible to determine case fatality rates according to severity of injury (Table 2-5). All reports show the highest case fatality rates among those with severe brain injuries as defined by a Glasgow Coma Scale score of 8 or less. Only one report shows any deaths among children with a mild brain injury, and in only three reports are there any deaths among those with moderate brain injury [Atlanta (Henry et al., 1992), Birmingham, UK (Wagstyl et al., 1987), and the U.S. Coma Data Bank (Luerssen et al., 1988)].

Other Outcome Measures: Glasgow Outcome Score

In an attempt to determine level of disability or outcome at time of hospital discharge, Jennett and Teasdale (1981) introduced the Glasgow Outcome Scale

TABLE 2–5.   Case Fatality Rate per 100 Hospital-Admitted Patients by Severity of Brain Injury: Selected Studies

Study Location (reference)	Case Fatality Rate (%)		
	Severe	Moderate	Mild
San Diego County (Kraus et al., 1987)	59	0	0
U.S. Coma Data Bank (Luerssen et al., 1988)	28	1	0
Atlanta (Henry et al., 1992)	12	4	0
Birmingham, UK (Wagstyl et al., 1987)[a]	62	4	1
Salt Lake (Mayer et al., 1981)[b]	45	0	0

[a]Computed from tabular data in original report.

[b]Generally equivalent to severe and nonsevere categories.

(GOS) in 1975. This scale has categories of death, persistent vegetative state, severe disability, moderate disability, and "good recovery." It is a qualitative scale and few reports have been consistent in its application. For example, some investigators have used the GOS at the time of patient discharge from the hospital or intervals of months or years postdischarge. The data in Table 2-6 show that between 75% and 95% of all children admitted to the hospital alive are discharged with "good recovery." Jennett and Teasdale note that "good recovery" was not intended to mean complete recovery, and a substantial portion of these children may have mild, transient, or permanent levels of cognitive, memory, or physical deficits or impairments. Generally, less than 1% of all children admitted to the hospital sustain a persistent vegetative state and from 1% to 3% will have severe disability. The values reported by Michaud and coworkers (1992) reflect the severe level of initial brain injury in the study group.

Long-Term Outcomes following Brain Injury

A number of outcome measures have been used to assess qualitative as well as quantitative results of brain injury. Table 2-7 shows findings on seven reports that provide measures of severity and outcome assessment. While it is not possible to evaluate the results of the outcome measures effectively because of the vast differences in patient inclusion criteria, it is noteworthy that several reports have shown a significant relationship between brain injury and the outcome measure proposed. For example, Chadwick and colleagues (1981) found that the severity of head injury as determined by the length of posttraumatic amnesia (PTA) is associated with impaired reading ability. That is, those with severe injury and a PTA of more than 1 week have the greatest cognitive impairment, but impairment did improve

TABLE 2-6. Percent Outcome following Brain Injury in Children: The Glasgow Outcome Scale

Study Location (reference)	Death	Persistent Vegative State	Severe Disability	Moderate Disability	Good Recovery
Haifa, Israel (Levi et al., 1991)	6.6	NR	2.3		90
Birmingham, UK (Wagstyl et al., 1987)	14		(2 combined for both categories)		84
Salt Lake (Mayer et al., 1981)	14	0.6	NR	11	74
San Diego (Kraus et al., 1990)[a]	2.5	0.5	1.3	1.4	94
Seattle (Michaud et al., 1992)[b]	33	5	19	12	31

NR = not reported.

[a] Age 0–19.

[b] Two years postinjury, age ≤ 16, with severe nonpenetrating injury.

TABLE 2-7. Measure of Severity and Outcome Assessment in Children with Brain Injury: Selected Studies

Study Location (reference)	Severity Measure	Outcome Assessment
England (Chadwick et al., 1981)	Length of PTA	Cognitive functions impaired
Galveston (Ewing-Cobbs et al., 1987)	GCS	Language performance declined and other deficits
Houston-Galveston (Fletcher et al., 1990)	GCS, CT Duration of unconsciousness	Poor behavior scores with more severe injury
Houston-Galveston (Levin et al., 1993)	GCS, MRI	Cognitive performance impaired
Seattle (Michaud et al., 1993)	Any head injury	Odds of enrollment in special education higher
The Netherlands (Ruijs et al., 1990)	Coma duration	Functional impairment of behavior, also cognitive and motor skills
Vancouver, Canada (Klonoff et al., 1993)	Length of unconsciousness, skull fracture, and PTA	Psychosocial measures, educational lag, current psychological problems, unemployment, and troubled family relationships

Abbreviations: PTA, posttraumatic amnesia; GCS, Glasgow Coma Scale; CT, computed tomography; MRI, magnetic resonance imaging.

over time. Ewing-Cobbs and coworkers (1987) determined that closed head injury causes language and neurological impairment and that severe closed injury causes a higher degree of impairment than mild closed head injury. Fletcher and associates (1990) evaluated the relationship between behavioral disorders and severity of injury measured by the GCS, by computed tomography (CT) and by duration of unconsciousness. Although children with mild and moderate levels of brain injury improved between 6 and 12 months postinjury, the severely brain injured child worsened. Ruijs and colleagues (1990) followed 70 patients longitudinally for 2 years after brain injury for evidence of behavioral change. The investigators used duration of coma as the indicator of severity. Their findings showed that children with longer duration of coma had more behavioral changes, more school problems, and more neurological deficits than those with shorter duration of coma. Unfortunately, no patients without brain injury were followed for evidence of similar outcomes.

One of the longest follow-up studies of children was by Klonoff and associates (1993), who followed 159 children for 23 years postinjury (see Klonoff, this volume). They found that severity of injury had the greatest impact on the "reconstitution process," but the investigators acknowledged that intervening events over 23 years may also have had an impact on outcome. It is possible that many of the outcome events were confounded by other factors that could have had a role in final outcome assessment and hence could not be properly evaluated.

Cognitive sequelae may be a product of morbid factors prior to the head injury and not due to the head injury itself. For example, Michaud and associates (1993) wished to determine if there was an association between traumatic head injury and subsequent behavioral disorders for which special education services are often provided. This was a case-control design which compared the occurrence of prior head injury in children receiving special education to similar occurrences in children in regular education. The chance of a history of brain injury among children with behavioral disorders was more than three times that of controls. A history of head injuries sustained during the preschool years was almost eight times more frequent in children in special education than in children in the comparison group. Again, results from studies summarized above are not strictly comparable, but the evidence accumulated thus far strongly suggests that children who have had brain injury of any severity should be followed to determine the presence, nature, degree, and type of cognitive, memory, or physical impairment that may develop following the head injury. Because of the longitudinal nature of the studies required to assess these parameters, collaborative epidemiological studies across institutions may be the most cost-efficient and effective way to determine the exact nature of and amount of brain injury and may also point to ways in which interventions can be developed.

Estimating Disability from Brain Injury in the Population

It is possible to estimate the annual number of neurologically disabled children in the population, but this must begin with several assumptions and a body of incidence and mortality rate data. For purposes of discussion, assume the following:

An annual overall rate of 160 per 100,000 children in the community
A population base (e.g., the United States, 1991, of 55.130 million)
A prehospital brain injury death rate of 20 per 100,000 per year

Then: $160 \div 100,000 \times 55,130,000 = 88,000$ new cases per year in the United States. Of this number, about 5000 die before reaching the hospital. Thus, 83,000 children are admitted alive.

The next set of assumptions is about the severity distribution. Assume 85% are mild, 8% moderate, and 7% are severe. Then

$0.85 \times 83,000 = 70,550$ mild severity cases
$0.08 \times 83,000 = 6640$ moderate severity cases
$0.07 \times 83,000 = 5810$ severe cases

The next step requires information on the case fatality rate. Let us assume (using average data presented in this chapter) that:

For mildly brain injured children, there is a zero case fatality rate (CFR)
For moderately brain injured, children the CFR is 4 per 100
For severely brain injured children, the CFR is 40 per 100

Using these findings, we can calculate how many children are discharged alive following brain injury hospitalization. Thus

Of 70,550 mild cases, all are discharged alive
Of 6640 moderately severe brain injured children, 96% are discharged alive, or $1 - 0.04 \times 6640 = 6374$
Of 5810 severely brain injured children, 60% are discharged alive or $1 - 0.40 \times 5810 = 3486$

The final step requires assumptions about disability rates by severity class. Precise measures of this factor are not available, but let us assume that 10% of children with mild brain injury have some level of residual neurological impairment or deficit in the year postinjury. Assume also that 67% of children with moderately severe and 100% of children with severe brain injury have residual neurological deficits. Thus, the total number of new brain injured disabled children is:

$70,550 \times 0.10 = 7,055$ (mild)
$6,374 \times 0.67 = 4,271$ (moderate)
$5,810 \times 1.0 = \underline{5,810}$ (severe)
$17,136$ per year

These are the new cases to be added to the existing prevalence level in the community.

As has been demonstrated, it is possible to estimate the new case load in the community but knowledge of incidence, mortality rate, case fatality rate, and severity distribution is essential. The disability rate for each severity level must be assumed for now.

Future Needs and Prospects in Brain Injury Epidemiology

Surveillance

As mentioned previously in this chapter, it is essential to develop mechanisms at the regional or local level to measure the amount, characteristics, and treatment needs with regard to brain injury in the population. The application of findings from broad descriptive studies as summarized in this chapter may not be applicable to the local level, and if the outcomes following brain injury are essential to the community's preparation and implementation of immediate and long-care follow-up, then a precise estimate of occurrence, characteristics of severity, and immediate and long-term sequelae is needed.

Whereas most outcomes following severe brain injury in children are well established, outcome features following mild and moderate injury are less well known. The literature is provocative in terms of cognitive changes months or years postinjury. Better organized cross-center longitudinal follow-up of representative samples of children with such injuries is essential before questions regarding the nature, type, and full impact of mild brain injury are understood.

Prehospital Information

Most data on brain injury are collected beginning in the emergency department, but there is little consistent and standardized information on prehospital management. For example, treatment at the scene—whether it is oxygenation, fluid administration, intubation, or drug administration—has not been scientifically studied, and knowledge of the role of these prehospital factors is essential in determining the most favorable outcome strategies to be employed in a complete system of secondary and tertiary prevention.

Pharmacological or Therapeutic Interventions

Opportunities to enhance favorable outcome following brain injury are being explored with a number of clinically based randomized trials. For example, tirilazad, a synthetic inhibitor of lipid peroxidation, and antagonists of NMDA (*N*-methyl D-aspartate) are evaluated, but only for use in adults. Are such drugs useful in pediatric populations? If so, at what age should an intervention be planned?

Factor Interactions

Many of the factors described in this chapter have been studied without regard to the combination of effects from several factors. For example, consider the interaction between gender and exposure. Strong male/female differences appear not only in the taking of risky behaviors but also in underlying convictions about the components of risk and the consequences of certain actions as well as in societal expectations and personal attitudes about injury prevention. These may be important in placing a given child at risk of injury. Boys are often overrepresented in hospital trauma samples, probably because of several such factors at work simultaneously. These kinds of data can best come from multiple center-based studies of large populations of children with varying severities of brain injury.

Preventive Countermeasures

This chapter does not address preventive measures. There is ample evidence in the literature that for certain exposures, such as bicycle riders or passengers on motorcycles or mopeds, brain injuries can be prevented. However, for a variety of recreational and sporting activities—such as horseback riding, hockey, soccer, and baseball—the injury prevention potential has yet to be fully realized or evaluated. The evidence on effectiveness of child restraint systems, seat belts, and air bags in automobiles is very promising, but many segments of the pediatric population do not have the benefit of these countermeasures.

Although epidemiological studies have provided much information on pediatric head injury, more rigidly designed and implemented studies are needed to address the questions outlined above.

Acknowledgments

This work was supported by The Southern California Injury Prevention Research Center through CDC Center Award CCR903622. Support was also provided by the UCLA Brain Injury Research Center, P50 NS 30308.

Contributions to this work by David L. McArthur (graphic design) and Madhangi Jayaramanan (review of relevant literature) are gratefully acknowledged.

References

Annegers, J. F., Grabow, J. D., Kurland, L. T., & Laws, E. R. (1980). The incidence, causes, and secular trends of head trauma in Olmsted County, Minnesota, 1935–1974. *Neurology, 30,* 912–919.

Association for Advancement of Automotive Medicine. (1990). *Abbreviated Injury Scale.* Des Plaines, IL.

Chadwick, O., Rutter, M., Brown, G., Shaffer, D., & Traub, M. U. (1981). A prospective study of children with head injuries: II. Cognitive sequelae. *Psychol. Med., 11,* 49–61.

Collins, J. G. (1990). Types of injuries by selected characteristics. U.S. 1985–87. DHHS, Pub. No. (PHS) 91-1503, Series 10: *Data for the National Health Survey.* No. 175.

Duhaime, A. C., Alario, A. J., Lewander, W. J., Schut, L., Sutton, L. N, Seidl, T., Nudelman, S., Budenz, D., Hertle, R., Tsiaras, W., & Loporchio, S. (1992). Head injury in very young children: Mechanisms, injury types, and ophthalmologic findings in 100 hospitalized patients younger than 2 years of age. *Pediatrics, 90,* 179–185.

Ewing-Cobbs, L., Levin, H. S., Eisenberg, H. M., & Fletcher, J. M. (1987). Language functions following closed-head injury in children and adolescents. *J. Clin. Exp. Neuropsychol., 9,* 575–592.

Fife, D., Faich, G., Hollinshead, W., & Boynton, W. (1986). Incidence and outcome of hospital-treated head injury in Rhode Island. *Am. J. Public Health, 76,* 773–778.

Fletcher, J. M., Ewing-Cobbs, L., Miner, M. E., Levin, H. S., & Eisenberg, H. M. (1990). Behavioral changes after closed head injury in children. *J. Consult. Clin. Psychol., 58,* 93–98.

Graves, E. (1994). *Detailed diagnoses and procedures, National Hospital Discharge Survey, 1991.* DHHS, Pub. No. (PHS) 94-1776, Series 13, No. 115, Feb.

Hahn, Y. S., & McLone, D. G. (1993). Risk factors in the outcome of children with minor head injury. *Pediatr. Neurosurg., 19,* 135–142.

Hayes, H. R. M., & Jackson, R. H. (1989). The incidence and prevention of head injuries. In D. A. Johnson, D. Uttley, & M. A. Wyke (Eds.), *Children's head injury: Who cares?* London: Taylor and Francis.

Henry, P. C., Hauber, R. P., & Rice M. (1992). Factors associated with closed head injury in a pediatric population. *J. Neurosci. Nurs., 24,* 311–316.

Horowitz, I., Costeff, H., Sadan, N., Abraham, E., Geyer, S., & Najenson, T. (1983). Childhood head injuries in Israel: Epidemiology and outcome. *Int. Rehabil. Med., 5,* 32–36.

Hoyert, D. L., & Hudson, B. L. (1993). Advance report of final mortality statistics, 1991. *Monthly vital statistics and report.* Vol. 42, No. 2, supplement. National Center for Health Statistics. Hyattsville, MD: Public Health Service.

Jagger, J., Levine, J. I., Jane, J. A., & Rimel, R. W. (1984). Epidemiologic features of head injury in a predominantly rural population. *J. Trauma, 24,* 40–44.

Jennett, B., & Teasdale G. (1981). *Management of head injuries* (p. 78). Philadelphia, PA: F. A. Davis Co.

Klonoff, H., Clark, C., & Klonoff, P. S. (1993). Long-term outcome of head injuries: A 23-year follow-up study of children with head injuries. *J. Neurol. Neurosurg. Psychiatry, 56,* 410–415.

Kraus, J. F., Black, M. A., Hessol, N., Ley, P., Rokaw, W., Sullivan, C., & Bowers, S. (1984). The incidence of acute brain injury and serious impairment in a defined population. *Am. J. Epidemiol., 119,* 186–201.

Kraus, J. F., Fife, D., & Conroy, C. (1987). Pediatric brain injuries: The nature, clinical course, and deadly outcomes in a defined United States population. *Pediatrics, 79,* 501–507.

Kraus, J. F., Fife, D., Cox, P., Ramstein, K., & Conroy, C. (1986). Incidence, severity, and external causes of pediatric brain injury. *Am. J. Dis. Child., 140,* 687–693.

Kraus, J. F., Rock, A., & Hemyari, P. (1990). Brain injuries among infants, children, adolescents, and young adults. *Am. J. Dis. Child., 144,* 684–691.

Lescohier, I., & DiScala, C. (1993). Blunt trauma in children: Causes and outcomes of head versus extracranial injury. *Pediatrics, 91,* 721–725.

Levi, L., Guilburd, J. N., Linn, S., & Feinsod, M. (1991). The association between skull fracture, intracranial pathology and outcome in pediatric head injury. *Br. J. Neurosurg. 5*, 617–625.

Levin, H. S., Aldrich, E. F., Saydjari, C., Eisenberg, H. M., Foulkes, M. A., Bellefleur, M., Leurssen, T., Jane, J. A., Marmarou, A., Marshall, L., & Young, H. F. (1992). Severe head injury in children: Experience of the traumatic coma data bank. *Neurosurgery, 31*, 435–444.

Levin, H. S., Culhane, K. A., Mendelsohn, D., Lilly, M. A., Bruce, D., Fletcher, J., Chapman, S., Harward, H., & Eisenberg, H. M. (1993). Cognition in relation to magnetic resonance imaging in head-injured children and adolescents. *Arch. Neurol., 50*, 897–905.

Luerssen, T. G., Klauber, M. R., & Marshall, L. F. (1988). Outcome from head injury related to patient's age: A longitudinal prospective study of adult and pediatric head injury. *J. Neurosurg., 68*, 409–416.

MacKenzie, E. J., Edelstein, S. L., & Flynn, J. P. (1989). Hospitalized head-injured patients in Maryland: Incidence and severity of injuries. *Maryland Med. J., 38*, 725–732.

Mayer, T., Walker, M. L., Johnson, D. G., & Matlak, M. E. (1981). Causes of morbidity and mortality in severe pediatric trauma. *J.A.M.A., 245*, 719–721.

Michaud, L. J., Rivara, F. P., Grady, M. S., & Reay, D. T. (1992). Predictors of survival and severity of disability after severe brain injury in children. *Neurosurgery, 31*, 254–264.

Michaud, L. J., Rivara, F. P., Jaffe, K. M., Fay, G., & Dailey, J. L. (1993). Traumatic brain injury as a risk factor for behavioral disorders in children. *Arch. Phys. Med. Rehabil., 74*, 368–375.

Nestvold, K., Lundar, T., & Blikra, G. (1988). Head injuries during one year in a central hospital in Norway: A prospective study. *Neuroepidemiology, 7*, 134–144.

Oklahoma State Department of Health. (1991). *Traumatic brain injuries, Oklahoma, 1989.* Injury Epidemiology Division, Epidemiology Service, Oklahoma State Department of Health.

Ruijs, M. B. M., Keyser, A., & Gabreels, F. J. M. (1990). Long-term sequelae of brain damage from closed head injury in children and adolescents. *Clin. Neurol. Neurosurg., 92*, 323–328.

Sharples, P. M., Storey, A., Aynsley-Green, A., & Eyre, J. A. (1990). Causes of fatal childhood accidents involving head injury in Northern region, 1979–86. *Br. Med. J., 301*, 1193–1197.

Tiret, L., Hausherr, E., Thicoipe, M., Garros, B., Maurette, P., Castel, J. P., & Hatton, F. (1990). The epidemiology of head trauma in Aquitaine (France), 1986: A community-based study of hospital admissions and deaths. *Int. J. Epidemiol., 19*, 133–140.

Wagstyl, J., Sutcliffe, A. J., & Alpar, E. K. (1987). Early prediction of outcome following head injury in children. *J. Pediatr. Surg., 22*, 127–129.

3

Pathophysiological Responses of the Child's Brain Following Trauma

DEREK A. BRUCE

A great deal of information on head injuries in children has been reported in recent years. Much of this has come from the clinical use of computed tomography (CT) and magnetic resonance imaging (MRI), which have permitted a longitudinal, anatomical view of head injuries in children who died and in those who survived. Studies of intracranial pressure (ICP), cerebral blood flow (CBF), and metabolism have added to our understanding of the physiological changes that occur. In addition, autopsy studies have increased our knowledge of the neuropathology, and cognitive follow-up studies have allowed the comparison of anatomic injury to later intellectual function. Now physiological measures—single-photon emission tomography (SPECT) and positron emission tomography (PET)—are being used after recovery to try to explain why there is not a better correlation between anatomic injury and cognitive dysfunction.

The problems that complicate studies of the effects of head trauma in children differ from those of adult studies. The most pertinent difference may be the fact that the brain is continuously changing in its anatomy, chemistry, and physiology through the years of childhood. In addition, the skull reacts differently to trauma when the bone is thin and the sutures and fontanelle open than after they have closed and fused. Thus, the same traumatic injury is likely to produce a different spectrum of injury to the brain at different ages of infancy and childhood, making comparison very difficult and possibly leading to erroneous conclusions if data from children of different ages are pooled. If pooled data are not used, however, the actual numbers of head-injured children that fall into any given age group and mechanism of injury in one center are usually too small to permit meaningful conclusions.

As in adults, the mechanisms of injury vary widely and tend to be different in each age range of childhood, again making the collection of meaningful data difficult. To these problems one must add the variation in time from injury to any therapy; the type and extent of in-field resuscitation; the therapy after hospitalization; and the extent and intensity of rehabilitation—physical, cognitive, and psychosocial. Unfortunately, we have more information on the pathology associated with death than we do on that which is present in the children who recover. The belief that children who survive simply have a lesser degree of the same pathological insult that those who die had received is probably not valid; it is likely that the causes of residual cognitive disability will turn out to be more subtle changes in chemistry, anatomy, and physiology (Oppenheimer 1968: Povlishock et al., 1983) These less devastating injuries may be amenable to therapies that do not increase survival or affect the dramatic pathology responsible for death and major disability.

Evaluation of Degree of Injury

If the outcome after head injury can be altered by therapy, then it is imperative to have tools for evaluating as accurately as possible the extent of injury. Only then can similar injuries be compared and therapies evaluated. The problems of different causes of trauma and different ages of children is compounded by not having an accurate clinical tool to evaluate and record the degree of clinical trauma that the brain has sustained. With any scoring system, there is the question of how well the measured degree of brain dysfunction reflects the intensity of the underlying brain injury. Concussion—which is a transient, reversible period of cerebral dysfunction—may be associated at its onset with an examination that suggests brain death (fixed, dilated pupils, flaccid muscle tone, and apnea). Yet seconds later, there may be an entirely normal clinical neurological exam, incompatible with significant brain injury. We know that such a short, reversible event can leave evidence of disturbed higher cognitive functions—especially of short-term memory—for weeks in the absence of gross clinical or neuroimaging abnormality. Thus, any clinical neurological scoring system will be limited in its ability to accurately reflect the degree of cerebral trauma because of the variation that occurs with time.

The Glasgow Coma Score (GCS) was developed as a clinical tool to measure the intensity of gross neurological function compared over time, so that alterations in level of function could be identified with minimal interexaminer variation (Teasdale & Jennett, 1974). In large studies of adult head injuries, there was a strong correlation between the actual GCS and ultimate neurological recovery. The best correlation was obtained at 48 hours posttrauma. Indeed, the scoring system was not to be utilized until 6 hours after injury. It was hoped that this delay in scoring would allow transient neurological dysfunction (as after concussion, resuscitation, and drug administration) to wear off and would avoid categorizing the injury as more severe than it actually was. Because of the inclusion in the GCS of obeying commands and talking, the score had limited applicability to infants who had not yet developed verbal skills. Modifications to the scoring system were made and specific pediatric scores developed (Reilly et al., 1988). For example, the Adelaide score was tested for interobserver reproducibility, which was found to be good.

Currently, with the rapid response times to major head trauma, most patients have already entered treatment by 6 hours and often within 30 minutes of the injury. The early use of endotracheal intubation, usually associated with administration of muscle relaxants, sedatives, or anesthetic agents, makes the application of any scoring system difficult if not impossible (Marion et al., 1994). While the lack of standardization of the evaluation of injury by a clinical score may not seem a major problem in a routine setting, some of the dangers are as follows:

1. Children may get unnecessary therapy because of a presumed major injury that is not present.
2. Altered consciousness that is due to hypoxia, shock, seizures, or drugs may not be recognized even after resuscitation because the child is in medical coma; once again receiving greater intensity and length of therapy than is necessary.
3. If an effort is being made to compare results of therapy, the lack of a standardized, accurate clinical tool to evaluate the degree of trauma or the depth of coma will render any study uninterpretable. This is an area for further study that may not be solvable for the infant.

Causes of Trauma

Infants and children are exposed to different forms of trauma at different ages. Thus, the pathology that results is a joint function of the type of trauma and the age of the child. In infants and toddlers, the commonest cause of head trauma is a fall, and the resultant trauma to the brain is usually minor. The causes of severe head trauma are most frequently child abuse or automobile injury as a passenger. As children age, pedestrian and bicycle accidents that involve an automobile are the most frequent causes of severe head injury. Finally, in the teenage years, vehicular accidents (as the driver) and gun injuries become the most frequent causes of severe injury. The forces applied to the brain in these various settings are different and will result in somewhat different pathology. In addition, the extent of primary damage to the brain is likely to vary markedly; e.g., a bicycle/ automobile collision at 20 to 30 miles per hour versus an automobile hitting a tree at 70 to 80 miles per hour. Once consciousness is lost and an abnormal motor examination is present, the clinical examination becomes a poor tool for evaluating the extent of injury to the brain. Diffuse axonal injury, global cortical ischemia, and elevated intracranial pressure can all produce a similar neurological picture.

The degree of primary, irreversible, pathological damage to the brain cannot be defined by the initial clinical examination, but it can be overwhelming: 50% of childhood trauma deaths occur at the accident site. It is unlikely that anything other than preventing the head injury will modify the primary damage. The profiles of brain injury in children at different stages of childhood are known, and it is clear that prevention of many head injuries is possible with greater public efforts at education and producing a safer environment for children. Research in this area is being done, and results suggest that impressive reductions in the incidence of pediatric trauma are possible if it is a major societal goal (Bergman et al., 1991). Secondary damage from hypoxia or ischemia is common in children who die from their head injury; yet we cannot be certain either when that second injury occurs or what role it plays in the neurological examination. Research concerning injuries to the brain that occur subsequent to trauma (secondary injury) is also important. It is likely that the secondary injuries are preventable if we can define their causes and the time within which they arise (Bouma et al., 1992; Chestnut et al., 1993).

In all published series of pediatric head trauma, the outcome is worse for any given GCS if multiple trauma has occurred (Luerssen et al., 1988; Walker et al., 1985). This is a complex but surely fruitful area for research, since many questions present themselves: When does the worse outcome become established? With what type of multiple trauma? Does hypotension have to occur? Why do children admitted with a systolic blood pressure below 50 torr rarely have a good recovery? Studies of adult head trauma have shown a high incidence of hypoxia on arrival in the emergency room. Is this also true in children, and what are the relationships between multi-trauma, hypoxia, hypotension, and a poor outcome? Experimental delivery of catecholamines to animals with leaky blood-brain barriers results in increased cerebral metabolism and blood flow; this physiological pattern has been described in children after head trauma. Is there a relationship between catecholamines and cerebral physiology that could be clinically manipulated to improve outcome? In shock syndromes in both immature animals and children, excessive amounts of the chemical mediators of inflammation are released and seem to play a role in the high mortality that occurs. Is this mechanism operative after multiple trauma? After trauma, the brain also produces free radicals (Kontos et al., 1986), cytokines, heat shock protein, and other mediators of shock. Production of these compounds is seen in areas of blood-brain barrier disruption, but do they cause the damage or are they results of that damage? As it becomes possible to give drugs that could modify the results of these chemical events, further research to help us understand the cascade of chemical events following trauma is surely important (see Ward, this volume).

Another area of potential directed therapy to prevent second injury is that of excitotoxicity. Once again, experimental observations after status epilepticus, global and focal ischemia, and head injury have demonstrated that certain excitatory neurotransmitters—glutamate and aspartate—are released and their reuptake blocked such that increased receptor cell firing occurs, with resultant secondary cell death. Various compounds have been shown to block or modify this secondary cell death, and some of these agents are in clinical trials.

The need to understand the relationships between head injury, multiple trauma, hypoxia, hypotension, and the various secondary chemical releases is important also in trying to ensure the best possible prehospital care strategy for the injured child. Should endotracheal intubation in the field, with the use of muscle paralysis and sedative drugs, be encouraged? Is it better to spend time at the accident site to insert an intravenous line and give fluid resuscitation, or is it better to simply "scoop and run"? To some degree, this will depend on the proximity of the trauma center to the accident site, but these are important questions that could be answered, and the answers would affect any guidelines developed for pediatric trauma care.

Pathology

The current approach to the treatment of head injury is based on the belief that the primary head injury (the direct effects of the application of force to the brain) has already taken place prior to any medical therapy and that we currently do not understand the pathology adequately to modify this primary injury. Treatment is aimed at preventing the second head injury, which can occur minutes, hours, or days after the primary injury. The second injury has been presumed to result from systemic hypotension and shock, hypoxia, hypercarbia, and intracranial hypertension, all of which can be modified or prevented by currently available management that begins at the injury site. The role of neuroimaging done early after trauma is to identify any intracranial mass lesions that would lend themselves to surgical evacuation, to prevent cerebral herniation, and to identify as fully as possible the focal and diffuse aspects of the injury. Newer insights into the neurochemistry of brain injury have been reported and a new area of potential therapy to prevent second injury is opening up.

In children who die as a result of head trauma, the common pathological findings are brain swelling, areas of ischemia, cerebral herniation, contusions of the brain, diffuse white matter tears, subarachnoid hemorrhage, and, less frequently, subdural hematomas (Graham et al., 1989a, b). Except for the frequency of contusions, these findings correlate well with early CT findings after head injury, where diffuse brain swelling, subarachnoid hemorrhage, and areas of low density are frequent. There are often signs of increased intracranial pressure at autopsy and clinically elevated ICP is present in at least 50% and possibly as many as 95% of children with a GCS of 8 or less (Bruce et al., 1979). Thus, the pathology associated with a fatal outcome is fairly consistent.

A major question is whether the brain pathology associated with recovery is simply a lesser degree of similar injury or is in fact the result of different pathological processes that affect neuronal function. This remains unclear, but ongoing follow-up studies in children after head injury are trying to correlate specific neurocognitive outcomes with late pathological changes seen on MRI. These studies have demonstrated a high incidence—50%, of frontal and/or temporal contusions—in follow-up MRIs in children who recover from their injury (Levin et al., 1993; Mendelsohn et al., 1992), despite the absence of visible contusions on the acute CT. This suggests that contusions may be easily missed on the acute CT and shows a consistency with autopsy findings of frequent contusions. These same studies have found a low incidence of diffuse axonal injury; a general loss of cerebral bulk, especially frontally; and, in a few cases, progressive loss of white matter in the corpus callosum. Whether the loss of brain bulk is due to degeneration of gray matter or white matter is not yet clear. If it is due to white matter loss, this finding might favor the end result of diffuse axonal damage not visible on the follow-up MRI. If it is due to gray matter loss, results would favor a different pathology than that associated with death or the early phases after injury. The site of neuronal loss might support the neurotoxic transmitter hypothesis (Baker et al., 1993; Faden et al., 1989).

Finally, follow-up studies in children after moderate or severe head injury are demonstrating that decreased cognitive skills can be identified in the absence of MRI pathology (Levin et al., 1993). This raises the question of physiological dysfunction that does not have a gross anatomical substrate. Preliminary data suggests that decreased cerebral blood flow may correlate better with the results of the neuropsychological studies than do the MRI scans (Newton et al., 1992). What is the pathological lesion? In conclusion, much of the pathology that is encountered at autopsy is similar to that identified in the children who survive, with apparently less diffuse axonal injury and little evidence of multiple areas of post-ischemic infarction. It is not clear whether there are pathological processes that occur in the children who survive that are not present in those who die or that the processes are not developed enough to be identified when early death occurs.

Clinical Observations

The lack of accurate information on the normal values of many of the cerebral parameters that are treated during head injury limits the ability to interpret collected data. The normal ICP in the newborn with an open fontanelle is 3 to 5 mm Hg; the assumed normal ICP in teenagers is up to 15 mm Hg. In head injury, the upper level of ICP used to govern therapy for children of all ages is often assumed to be 15 mm Hg. Is this appropriate? In the absence of better information, it probably is after the fontanelle has closed. It cannot be assumed to be the appropriate value for the child with an open fontanelle. Mortality rates for similar GCS scores have been reported to be higher in the youngest children. There are a host of possible reasons, from the frequency of child abuse as a cause to the different structure of the brain in the first year of life. Another possible factor that may be present in younger children is a tolerance for ICP levels that may be too high. Certainly this is an important area for study.

Intracranial mass lesions, epidural hematomas, subdural hematomas, and intra-cerebral hematomas all occur after head injury in children, but only 20 percent of unconscious children will require a surgical operation, as compared with 50 percent of adults with head injury. Subdural hematomas are most frequently seen in the infant who sustains nonaccidental injury (child abuse); here the lesions are usually thin, along the falx, and do not need surgical intervention. Mass lesions are not a major contributing factor to death or disability produced by childhood head trauma.

Brain swelling is common after pediatric head trauma and is readily identified on CT by narrowed ventricles and compressed or absent mesencephalic and other basal cisterns (Aldrich et al., 1992; Bernardi et al., 1993; Bruce et al., 1981; Muizelaar et al., 1989; Yoshino et al., 1985). Swelling comes as two entities: (1) in association with normal brain density and a clear separation between gray and white matter and (2) with the brain of relatively low density and indistinct separation of the gray matter and white matter. The former is usually associated with good recovery and seems to be the result of cerebrovascular dilatation associated with a higher-than-expected cerebral blood flow (CBF) and blood volume (Barie et al., 1993; Bruce et al., 1981; Muizelaar et al., 1989). The latter is the result of prior or ongoing cerebral ischemia from either low blood pressure or high ICP and the prognosis for recovery is poor.

In this setting, the pattern of increased brain bulk may be due to increased water content (edema) of the cellular components of the brain (neurons, glia, and possibly myelin) as a result of inadequate metabolic substrate secondary to limited CBF. Diffuse swelling, due to increased blood volume (hyperemia), is different from cerebral edema, where the increase in brain bulk is due to increased water content. The potential detrimental effects of the hyperemia are as follows: (1) increased ICP; (2) increased tissue oxygenation, which in the face of free iron in the tissues from hemorrhage may increase free radical production; (3) increased end capillary pressure as a result of the vasodilatation, leading to vasogenic cerebral edema.

Brain metabolism has generally been shown to be decreased out of proportion to the increased CBF; but in at least one study, the metabolism was also increased early after the injury in the absence of any seizure activity. The ideal treatment of increased CBF depends on whether metabolism is increased and if so, why. Hyperventilation decreases $Paco_2$ and the CBF. If metabolism is high, then, in addition, sedative agents should be given to decrease the metabolic needs to match the reduced flow. It is possible that this clinical pattern is the result of excitotoxic neurotransmitters, and, as specific agents become available to block these responses, a fruitful area for therapeutic research will open up. After head injury in children, cerebrovascular autoregulation (Paulson et al., 1990) appears to be intact and disturbance of pressure autoregulation does not appear to be the cause of the increased CBF (Muizelaar et al., 1989).

Subarachnoid hemorrhage is common after severe head injury (50% to 75%), but the role it plays in the evolving pathophysiology is not clear. Potential effects of subarachnoid hemorrhage are (1) vasospasm which can occur and produce secondary ischemia; (2) obstruction of arachnoid villi, leading to an increase in cerebrospinal fluid outflow resistance and increased intracranial pressure; and (3) increased iron in the tissues and therefore increased free radical production. Does some of the early secondary ischemia occur as a result of acute vasospasm that is relieved by the time CBF studies are performed (Bouma et al., 1992)? Agents that scavenge free radicals may have a beneficial effect if given early after trauma, and this is currently being examined in adult head-injured patients. If the results are encouraging, similar studies need to be done in children.

As noted earlier, the intracranial pressure is above normal (< 15 mm Hg) in 75% to 95% of children with a GCS of 8 or less in whom ICP monitoring is done (Alberico et al., 1987). The cerebral perfusion pressure (CPP) is the driving force for cerebral blood flow and is clinically measured as CPP = MAP − ICP, where MAP is the mean arterial pressure and ICP the mean intracranial pressure. The cerebrovasculature exhibits pressure autoregulation such that despite a changing perfusion pressure, the CBF remains constant within certain limits. In adult humans and many animal models, the CBF remains constant until the CPP falls below 50 mm Hg. In adults following head injury, recent information suggests that at a CPP below 70 mm Hg, the CBF begins to fall (Chan et al., 1993). In many pediatric intensive care units the CPP that has been considered acceptable has also been 50 mm Hg. Unfortunately, there is very little information on the limits of autoregulation in children and no knowledge of how the autoregulatory curve varies with age during childhood. The arbitrary assumption that a CPP of 50 mm Hg is adequate must be questioned; research is required to establish appropriate parameters for ICP and CPP in head-injured children. The bedside use of transcranial Doppler is one technique that is readily applicable to children; while not giving an absolute value, it certainly gives qualitative information about changes in flow velocity that can be used to make inferences about the CBF.

Much of the therapeutic focus in head injury has been to control the intracranial pressure. There are a number of reasons for this. Elevated ICP was a common cause of death and is still a common accompaniment of death in head-injured children. It is technically easy to measure the ICP, and a variety of therapies are available to maintain a "normal" ICP at 15 to 20 mm Hg. This level is maintained by a dynamic balance between the volumes of the intracranial contents, i.e., cerebrospinal fluid (CSF), blood, and brain. After a severe head injury, this balance is disturbed because some increase in volume can occur in all of the intracranial components at the same time.

The CSF is affected by

1. Potential increased production as a result of increased blood flow
2. Interference with circulation as a result of
   a. Distortion of the ventricular system from mass effect
   b. Obstruction of the subarachnoid space from brain swelling, herniation, or subarachnoid blood
3. Increased pressure required for absorption due to plugging of the villi by red cells from subarachnoid hemorrhage

The cerebral blood volume can be increased by

1. Increased CBF
2. Increased cerebral venous blood due to increased ICP and venous compression at the sagittal sinus
3. Hypercarbia or hypoxia, both resulting in vasodilation

The brain volume is increased as a result of

1. Cerebral contusion
2. Intracerebral hemorrhage
3. Brain edema

Thus, the ability of one component to compensate for an increase in volume of another is limited and an elevation of the ICP is common. The deleterious effects of elevated ICP appear to be the result of either global ischemia due to decreased CPP and CBF or focal ischemia due to cerebral herniation. In most head-injured children, it is now possible to control the ICP in a reasonable range and prevent herniation or death (Alberico et al., 1987; Bruce et al., 1979). The children who die of head injury, however, usually have uncontrollably elevated ICP. It may be, since all current regimens to control ICP in this setting are ineffective, that the degree of cerebral insult is so great that the brain is irreversibly damaged and that death is due primarily to that damage. The increased ICP is the result of this damage rather than the cause. It seems certain that no further improvements in outcome of head injury are likely to occur as a result of improved ICP control, since current practice has probably maximized that aspect of therapy.

Nonaccidental Trauma: Child Abuse

In children under two years of age, a specific type of head injury occurs with a clinical course and pathological outcome that is unique. The assumed mechanism is a combination of shaking and impact that results in the exposure of the immature, unmyelinated brain to severe deceleration forces (Duhaime et al., 1987). At this age the CSF spaces are relatively more capacious than in the older child and the veins that bridge the space from the brain to the sagittal sinus relatively longer. At the moment of trauma there is a peak of elevated ICP, the bridging veins are torn with resultant interhemispheric subdural blood, shearing injuries occur to the cerebral tissue, and multiple cortical hemorrhages result. Unconsciousness usually follows such injuries, but because of guilt and fear, the injury is not reported and the children are usually placed in bed. Ventilation is often poor because of the coma, with resultant hypercarbia and hypoxia, resulting in a further increased ICP and brain hypoxic or ischemic injury. Medical attention is sought because, over time, there is no recovery and either seizure or respiratory arrest may occur. Clinical presentation is usually of a child in coma or in arrest with no good history for any precipitating event. There are usually retinal hemorrhages, a full bulging fontanelle, and poor respiratory exchange. The scalp is often normal and there is no apparent facial or cranial injury. At autopsy, however, there is evidence of impact injury to the scalp or skull. The CTs in these children usually show a combination of interhemispheric subdural hematomas plus low-density brain swelling, and the MRIs show multifocal cortical hemorrhages (Bruce et al., 1989). The infants usually develop increased ICP that may be impossible to control. Death often occurs with the intracranial and arterial pressure equal and no CBF.

If the abused children survive, the brain rapidly, over days, can develop calcifications and atrophy with extracerebral accumulation of CSF or subdural fluid. The calcifications may resolve, but the cerebral atrophy is permanent. The outcome for those infants presenting with altered mental state is dreadful: one-third will die, one-third will be left severely disabled, and only one-third will make a moderate or good recovery. The present understanding of this form of traumatic injury is that there is a combination of traumatic plus ischemic damage and that a lot of secondary damage has already occurred before the children come to medical attention. Once again, the only real solution is to prevent this type of injury. For such prevention to become a priority, changes in the public health and legal systems will be required. The person who commits the injury must be convinced to seek medical care for the baby immediately without fear of repercussions. This unique injury is an important area for further research.

Conclusion

Much new information has been gathered about the anatomic pathology of head injury in the last few years. In children, there is still a paucity of physiological and metabolic information about both the acute injury and the recovery process. Control of the ICP has become possible in most children, as has the ability to rapidly establish normal systemic physiological parameters. Mortality is uncommon in all but the most severely injured children unless multiple trauma has occurred. We still do not understand the detrimental effects of multiple trauma on the brain injury or how to modify them. As specific chemical therapies become available to control free radical production and the excitotoxic neurotransmitters, it will be difficult to determine whether an improvement in outcome is occurring unless we have more precise tools to define the severity of the injury and a better understanding of the alterations in physiology and micropathology.

References

Alberico, A. M., Ward, J. D., Choi, S. C., Marmarou, A., & Young, H. F. (1987). Outcome after severe head injury, relationship to mass lesions, diffuse injury and ICP course in pediatric and adult patients. *J. Neurosurg., 67,* 648.

Aldrich, E. F., Eisenberg, H. M., Saydjari, C., Luerssen, T. G., Foulkes, M. A., Jane, J. A., Marshall, L. F., Marmarou, A., & Young, H. F. (1992). Diffuse brain swelling in severely head-injured children. *J. Neurosurg., 76,* 450.

Baker, A. J., Moulton, R. J., MacMillan, V. H., & Shedden, P. M. (1993). Excitatory amino acids in cerebrospinal fluid following traumatic brain injury. *J. Neurosurg., 79,* 369.

Barie, P. S., Ghajar, J. B., Firlik, A. D., Chang, V. A., & Hariri, R. J. (1993). Contribution of increased cerebral blood volume to post-traumatic intracranial hypertension. *J. Trauma 35,* 88.

Bergman, A. B., & Rivara, F. P. (1991). Sweden's experience in reducing childhood injuries. *Pediatrics, 88,* 69.

Bernardi, B., Zimmerman, R. A., & Bilaniuk, L. T. (1993). Neuroradiological evaluation of pediatric craniocerebral trauma. *Topics MRI, 5,* 161.

Bruce, D. A., Alavi, A., Bilaniuk, L., Dolinskas, C., Obrist, W., & Uzzell, B. (1981). Diffuse brain swelling following head injury in children: The syndrome of "malignant brain edema." *J. Neurosurg., 54,* 170.

Bruce, D. A., Raphaely, R. C., Goldberg, A. I., Zimmerman, R. A., Bilaniuk, L. T., Schut, L., & Kuhl, D. E. (1979). Pathophysiology, treatment and outcome following severe head injury in children. *Childs Brain 5,* 174.

Bruce, D. A., & Zimmerman, R. A. (1989). Shaken impact syndrome. *Pediatr. Ann., 18,* 482.

Bouma, G. J., Muizelaar, J. P., Stringer, W. A., Choi, S. C., Fatouros, P., & Young, H. F. (1992). Ultra-early evaluation of regional cerebral blood flow in severely head-injured patients using Xenon-enhanced computerized tomography. *J. Neurosurg., 77,* 350.

Chan, K. H., Dearden, N. M., Miller, J. D., Andrews, P. J., & Midgley, S. (1993). Multimodality monitoring as a guide to treatment of intracranial hypertension after severe brain injury. *Neurosurgery, 32,* 547.

Chestnut, R. M., Marshall, L. F., Klauber, M. R., Blunt, B. A., Baldwin, N., Eisenberg, H. M., Jane, J. A., Marmarou, A., & Foulkes, M. A. (1993). The role of secondary injury in determining outcome from severe head injury. *J. Trauma, 34,* 216.

Duhaime, A. C., Gennarelli, T. A., Thibault, I. E., Bruce, D. A., Margulies, S., & Wiser, R. (1987). The shaken baby syndrome: A clinical, pathological and biomechanical study. *J. Neurosurg., 66,* 409.

Faden, A. I., Demediuk, P., Panter, S. S., & Vink, R. (1989). The role of excitatory amino acids and NMDA receptors in traumatic brain injury. *Science 244,* 798.

Graham, D. I., Ford, I., Adams, J. H., Doyle, D., Lawrence, A. E., McLellan D. R., & Ng, H. K. (1989a). Fatal head injury in children. *Clin. Pathol., 42,* 18.

Graham, D. I., Ford, I., Adams, J. H., Doyle, D., Teasdale, G. M., Lawrence, A. E., & McLellan D. R. (1989b). Ischemic brain damage is still common in fatal, non-missile head injury. *J. Neurol. Neurosurg. Psychiatry, 52,* 346.

Kontos, H. A., & Wei, E. P. (1986. Superoxide production in experimental brain injury. *J. Neurosurg., 64,* 803–807.

Levin, H. S., Culhane, K. A., Mendelsohn, D., Lilly, M. A., Bruce, D., Fletcher, J. M., Chapman, S. B., Harward, H., & Eisenberg, H. M. (1993). Cognition in relation to magnetic resonance imaging in head injured children and adolescents. *Arch. Neurol., 50,* 897.

Luerssen, T. G., Klauber, M. R., & Marshall, L. F. (1986). Outcome from head injury related to patients age. *J. Neurosurg., 68,* 409.

Marion, D. W., & Carlier, P. M. (1994). Problems with initial Glasgow Coma Scale assessment caused by prehospital treatment of patients with head injuries: results of a national survey. *J. Trauma 36,* 89.

Mendelsohn, D., Levin, H. S., Bruce, D., Lilly, M., Harward, H., Culhane, K. A., & Eisenberg, H. M. (1992). Late MRI after head injury in children: Relationship to clinical features and outcome. *Childs Nerv. Syst., 8,* 445.

Muizelaar, J. P., Marmarou, A., DeSalles, A. A., Ward, J. D., Zimmerman, R. S., Li, A., Choi, S. C., & Young, H. F. (1989). Cerebral blood flow and metabolism in severely head-injured children: Part I. Relationship with GCS, outcome, ICP and PVI. Part II. Autoregulation. *J. Neurosurg., 71,* 63.

Newton, M. R., Greenwood, R. J., Britton, K. E., Charlesworth, M., Nimmon, C. C., Carroll, M. J. & Dolke, G. (1992). A study comparing SPECT with CT and MRI after closed head injury. *J. Neurol. Neurosurg. Psychiatry, 55,* 92.

Oppenheimer, D. R. (1968). Microscopic lesions in the brain following head injury. *J. Neurol. Neurosurg. Psychiatry, 31,* 299.

Paulson, O. B., Strandgaard, S., & Edvinsson, L. (1990). Cerebral autoregulation. *Cerebrovasc. Brain Metab. Rev., 2,* 161.

Povlishock, J. T., Becker, D. P., Cheng, C. L., & Vaughan, G. W. (1983). Axonal changes in minor head injury. *J. Neuropathol. Exp. Neurol., 42,* 225.

Reilly, P. L., Simpson, D. A., Sprod, R., & Thomas, L. (1988). Assessing the conscious level in infants and young children: A pediatric version of the Glasgow coma scale. *Childs Nerv. Syst., 4,* 30.

Teasdale, G., & Jennett, B. (1974). Assessment of coma and impaired consciousness: A practical scale. *Lancet 2,* 81.

Walker, M. L., Mayer, T. A., Storrs, B. B., & Hylton, P. D. (1985). Pediatric head injury: Factors which influence outcome. *Concepts Pediatr. Neurosurg., 6,* 84.

Yoshino, E., Yamaki, T., Higuchi, T., Horikawa, Y., & Hirakawa, K. (1985). Acute brain edema in fatal head injury: An analysis by dynamic CT scanning. *J. Neurosurg., 63,* 830.

II

THE DATA

4

Behavioral Sequelae of Serious Head Injury in Children and Adolescents: The British Studies

DAVID SHAFFER

The relationship between central nervous system (CNS) damage and psychiatric disorder in children was well demonstrated in an epidemiological study undertaken nearly 30 years ago on the Isle of Wight in the United Kingdom (Rutter et al., 1970). In this study, a representative sample of physically healthy children and a total population of children with a wide variety of physical disorders were studied; similar criteria for psychiatric disorder and assessment procedures were used in both groups. The study avoided the assignment bias that can occur in a treated sample and which generally has the effect of exaggerating the incidence of psychiatric disorder. The findings were that the prevalence of psychiatric disorder among children with CNS disorders such as seizures and cerebral palsy was more than twice as high as in children with other forms of chronic illness, including those with major sensory handicaps (see Table 4-1) that would generally be thought to be more handicapping. Children with epilepsy—which, in most instances, was well controlled and interfered little with everyday life or schooling—were more likely to have an associated psychiatric disorder than were children with peripheral deafness or blindness or a chronic illness that could pose a threat to life and result in a far greater disturbance of social and educational routine. These findings have since been confirmed in larger populations of children with chronic physical illness (Breslau, 1985; Breslau & Marshall, 1985; Weiland et al., 1992).

Although the strength of the relationship between CNS damage and psychiatric disorder in children had been demonstrated, a number of theoretically and clinically important questions remained. As with most studies that target physically handicapped or physically ill children, even though the Isle of Wight study avoided the pitfalls of assignment bias, it could only demonstrate an association between the two conditions. It could not demonstrate a temporal sequence—important for establishing causality—in which brain injury preceded the psychiatric disorder. Second, the

TABLE 4-1.   Psychiatric Disorder and Physical
Illness in an Unselected Population

General population	6.7%
Chronic non-CNS illness	12%
Peripheral sensory deficits (deaf/blind)	18%
Idiopathic epilepsy	28%
Structural brain damage	35%
Structural brain damage with epilepsy	54%

Source: From Rutter et al., 1970.

study only identified individuals with evidence of gross neurological disorder, such as seizures or motor abnormalities. The association between brain damage and psychiatric disorder might be different in children who had CNS injury without gross clinical manifestations. Other questions that remained unanswered were whether psychiatric complications are a function of age at injury or location or magnitude of injury; whether there are any specific behavioral or emotional symptoms that are characteristic of brain injury; and whether there is a threshold of severity of injury below which behavioral sequelae do not occur. Finally, does brain injury interact with other risk factors to increase vulnerability to psychiatric disorder, or does it have an effect that is independent of social circumstances? These questions became the focus of a series of studies by British child psychiatrists and psychologists in the middle to late 1970s (Brown et al., 1981; Chadwick et al., 1981; Rutter et al., 1980; Shaffer et al., 1975; Shaffer et al., 1980).

Methodological Considerations

The requirements and possibilities for describing the neurological aspects of brain injury are beyond the scope of this chapter but have clearly advanced a good deal since the British studies were conducted. There have also been improvements in techniques for measuring posttraumatic amnesia in children (Ewing-Cobbs et al., 1990), a key indicator in one of the studies described here. By contrast, design considerations and the methods available for examining the psychiatric correlates have changed little. The following design issues are among those we considered:

1. Because emotional and behavioral problems occur commonly throughout childhood with high rates of onset and offset, it is important that investigations include a *comparison group*.

2. Injuries do not occur at random. There is good evidence that children who suffer accidents are different from the noninjured population. They have higher rates of preexisting behavior difficulties (Craft et al., 1973; Donders, 1992; see also Asarnow et al., this volume) and are exposed to a number of risk factors that are similar to those for psychiatric disorder. These include temperamental differences (Manheimer & Mellinger, 1967) and family difficulties (Rune, 1970). In the most comprehensive examination of this issue, Bijur and her colleagues (1990;

see also Bijur & Haslum, this volume) studied longitudinal, prospectively collected records of a British birth cohort of 13,000 children to determine the sequelae of mild head injuries. It was possible to compare pretrauma scores on the behavior ratings that were collected regularly during the follow-up of children who had had a head injury and/or other types of injury with the noninjured cohort. The children who would be injured had higher aggression and hyperactivity scores before their injury, and their mothers had higher depression scores than those of the noninjured cohort. These risk factors could plausibly have increased vulnerability to injury through a reduction of supervision and/or an increase in exploratory or impetuous behavior.

Regardless of mechanism, the confounding of risk factors for injury and psychiatric disorder requires that the *child's behavioral status prior to the injury* be evaluated and taken into account in any study of this kind. This is not always feasible, especially if the evaluation is being done some time after the injury. The seemingly attractive strategy (Asarnow et al., 1991) of confining study subjects to those without any preexisting psychiatric disorder may, by limiting the population available for study, make the research more difficult and could preclude the possibility of examining interactions between preexisting behavior problems and brain injury.

3. The confounding of risk factors for injury and psychiatric disorder requires that research assessments should anticipate that accident victims will likely differ from nonaccident controls on psychosocial measures as well as on history of brain damage. In the case of children, this requires that a determination of psychosocial correlates of disorder—such as quality of marriage, parental psychiatric state, and the child's caretaking experiences—be made.

4. There is a tendency for patients to try to understand their own or their child's problems by linking them to signal events. This tendency, which may introduce a recall bias, with symptoms becoming artificially tethered to the traumatic incident, can be minimized by collecting baseline data as soon after the injury as possible.

5. Because of the importance of early evaluation, subjects are almost invariably enrolled from a treatment center rather than from household or school surveys. One treatment center may differ from another, and the resultant "assignment bias" may make for unrepresentative samples. This problem can be reduced by drawing subjects from a centralized trauma or coma center that treats patients with certain levels of severity from a broad geographic area, although this may introduce its own form of bias. A preferable alternative is to draw from many different treatment centers, ideally covering all those that serve the same defined geographic area.

6. It is possible to minimize recall biases and biases particular to the circumstances of injury, such as parental remorse and/or involvement in litigation, by using structured or semi-structured *assessment procedures* that require a full definition of the symptoms of interest.

7. A causal relationship can be assumed if (1) there is a dose-response relationship between injury and subsequent psychiatric disorder; (2) there is prospective evidence that the psychiatric disorder appeared after the occurrence of the

injury; (3) the injured group show pathognomonic behaviors that occur only or predominantly in individuals with a head injury. Opportunities for examining these parameters can be anticipated and can be built into the design.

These methodological considerations figured strongly in the design of the two studies described below.

Study 1: Localization and Age at Injury

Method

The purpose of this study (Shaffer et al., 1975) was to determine whether age at injury or locus of injury was related to the rate and type of psychiatric disorder. The original intention had been to study a population with cerebral abscess. However, a close examination of an abscess population indicated that most had developed their infection secondary to another chronic illness, most commonly congenital cardiac malformations. Anticipating that it would be difficult to disentangle the psychiatric consequences of the predisposing chronic illness from the effects of localized destruction of brain matter, a localized head injury population was selected instead.

The target injury was a unilateral compound depressed fracture of the skull with associated dural tear, in which gross damage to the underlying brain substance had been confirmed at operation where and there had been no clinical evidence of *contrecoup* effects. In order to collect data from observers other than the parent, subjects were to be of school age at the time of the examination. To exclude short-term adjustment reactions to trauma, hospitalization, and separation, the injury had to have occurred at least 2 years prior to the examination. A total of 118 children meeting these criteria were identified by a systematic search of admission and discharge registers of 12 regional neurosurgical units throughout the United Kingdom. During the course of this enumeration, it became apparent that this injury affected mainly children under age 6; this led to selective oversampling of children in middle childhood. Of the 118 eligible children found, 98 were examined.

The mental and psychiatric state of the child and parents and an evaluation of home and family circumstances were assessed with standardized interviews of known reliability (Brown & Rutter, 1966; Graham & Rutter, 1968; Quinton et al., 1976; Rutter & Brown, 1966; Rutter & Graham, 1968). Interrater reliability was assessed in approximately half of the children and was satisfactory. A Rutter Teacher Questionnaire (Rutter, 1975) was completed on each subject and on the next child of the same sex and age on the class register.

Findings

The sex difference in the number of children injured was trivial before age 4, but there was a strong male predominance after age 6. About half (48%) of the children did not lose consciousness and a further 15% were reported to have been unconscious for less than 30 minutes. Duration of coma was unrelated to age at injury or sex. Nine children had seizures within 1 week of the injury and a further 12 had a first convulsion some time after that, several at the time of cranioplasty (which was carried out on 27% of all children and in over 60% of the older children). Four children had a residual handicapping hemiplegia. Nine children had a mild or moderate aphasia. There were strong confounds between age and activity at injury and locus of injury, which could have implications for interpreting the relationship between locus of injury and psychiatric sequelae. The confound was that children injured before age 6 were significantly more likely to be injured at home or on the road and less likely to be injured during sport, recreation, or at school. Frontal injuries were significantly less frequent in accidents in which the child was a pedestrian and significantly more frequent in sporting and recreational injuries.

Psychiatric Disorder. Teacher questionnaire scores were significantly higher for the group with brain injuries than for controls, and twice as many children with head injury scored in the deviant range. Based on child and parent interview, two-thirds of the injured children had evidence of at least a mild psychiatric disturbance.

Correlates of Psychiatric Disorder

Localization of Injury. After taking account of psychosocial correlates, no significant localization difference was observed. There was a trend for nondominant hemisphere injuries to be associated with mood symptoms.

Age. Again, after correction for psychosocial differences, psychiatric outcome did not differ by age at injury.

Severity of Injury. No significant association was noted between prevalence of psychiatric disorder and coma duration. There was a tendency for psychiatric disorder to be more common in children who had had a seizure, being highest in those with late-onset epilepsy. These differences fell short of statistical significance. Despite this, cranioplasty was not associated with a higher rate of disorder.

Some of the strengths of this study were that it examined a total population of children who had experienced a specific and relatively unusual type of injury and that it employed a standardized assessment procedure. Its limitations were that it was retrospective, that it did not ascertain information about premorbid state, and that the methods used to determine localization were not as refined as is now possible. No other reports of the psychiatric sequelae of localized head injury associated with compound depressed fracture have been published since this study.

Study 2: A Prospective Controlled Study of Mild and Severe Head Injury

Design Considerations

The first study had been designed to determine lateralization of injury and age at injury effects; it had failed to find either. It was apparent, however, that while neurological morbidity was slight, psychiatric morbidity was considerable, regardless of how it was measured. While fewer than 5% of the children had persistent motor impairment, psychiatric problems were present in more than half.

The study provided numerous examples of small children who had been standing in the roadway and had sustained a penetrating head injury from a protuberance on a passing automobile, bicycle, or other vehicle. Were these children being properly looked after at the time or did they have a temperament that was difficult to control? Similar questions could have been asked of the older children, some of whom had been injured by darts or gun pellets, others while playing on rooftops or up high trees. The absence of baseline information on behavior was a significant limitation, but the wealth of psychosocial environment data that had been collected proved to be invaluable in showing that apparently significant laterality and age at injury effects could be accounted for by social environmental differences. The absence of such data in the classroom controls made it very difficult to know whether the elevated rate in the injured group was a function of the injury or of the traumatized children's psychosocial risk profile.

A second study was designed to correct some of these problems (Brown et al., 1981; Chadwick et al., 1981; Rutter et al., 1980). It resembled the first in examining an *unreferred* group defined by their injuries rather than any behavior problems, but it addressed several of the drawbacks of the first study:

1. It examined the behavioral effects of closed head injury, a *more common type of injury.*
2. It obtained a good account of *premorbid behavior* from the parent as soon as the child's survival had been assured.
3. It examined the *course of behavior change* over time with a longitudinal design.
4. It determined whether there was any *threshold* effect of severity of injury by studying children with both severe and mild head injuries. The "serious" group ($n=31$) was defined as having posttraumatic amnesia (PTA) of at least 7 days. The "mild" group ($n=29$) had PTA of more than 1 hour but less than 1 week.
5. It included a *comparison group* of children ($n=28$) who had received inpatient hospital care for accidental orthopedic injuries that did not involve damage to the central nervous system. This made it possible to differentiate change due to recovery from the effects of repeated testing, to control for family or personality factors, and to take account of the nonspecific effects

of being involved in an accident—hospitalization, physical incapacity, missing school, etc.

6. Psychosocial as well as behavioral data were collected from the *comparison* group to control for social environmental differences that escaped the matching procedure.

Method

Sample. As in the first study, the sample was restricted to children who would be expected to attend school throughout the course of the study. A preliminary investigation indicated that most children with at least 7 days of PTA were admitted to regional neurosurgical units. Six such units were used as the sampling frame.

The *"severe"* head injury group comprised 23 children with a PTA of 1 to 4 weeks and 8 with a PTA of 1 to 3 months. Children whose injuries were so severe that psychological assessment could not be undertaken within 3 months of injury were excluded, as were the only 2 children whose recovery was complicated by the development of an extradural hematoma. Of the total, 19 had no fracture, 8 had a linear fracture, and 4 had depressed fractures, all without dural tears. The *"mild"* head injury group comprised 19 patients with a PTA of 1 to 24 hours and 10 with a PTA of 1 to 7 days. Among these, 6 children had a linear and 1 a compound depressed fracture with dural tear. Some 40% of the severe and 13% of the mild injuries were treated for raised intracranial pressure. The non-CNS orthopedically injured controls included 12 who had suffered a fracture of the leg, 5 with a fracture of the arm, 2 with a dislocated elbow, and 9 with other forms of injury. The rate of refusal and loss from follow-up was low.

Accident and treatment history differed in the two head injury groups. The severe injury group was just as likely as the mild to have had a surgical intervention, but the length of stay in hospital was significantly longer and they were twice as likely to have suffered an associated orthopedic injury. The non-head-injured controls were intermediate with respect to the duration of hospitalization, but more than twice as many had received some form of surgical intervention.

Most severe injury victims were pedestrians in a road traffic accident. In 90% of cases, the child was unaccompanied by an adult at the time of the injury. In contrast, only a third of the mild injuries resulted from pedestrian road traffic accidents, and most took place during play. Children in the mild head injury group were more than twice as likely as the severe group to have been engaging in some prohibited activity at the time of the accident. The severe head injury and non-CNS orthopedic injury groups were similar in age, sex, social class, person-to-room ratio, sibship size, and psychosocial adversity score. The mild head injury group, selected from local hospitals, included a higher proportion of boys, more children from a socially disadvantaged background, and substantially more who had shown school achievement or behavior problems (or both) before the accident. These differences were taken into account in interpreting all analyses.

Assessment of Severity. Posttraumatic amnesia rather than coma duration was adopted as the index of severity because it allows at least an approximate quantification along a single continuum for both the mild and severe injuries; it correlates well with coma duration (Jennett et al., 1977) and has been reported to be a reasonably good predictor of long-term mental and physical recovery (Jennett, 1976). The length of PTA—the interval between injury and the point at which the memory for ongoing events of daily life became continuous—was ascertained by interview with the parent.

Psychiatric Assessment

Contact with the subjects was made after survival seemed likely. At this time information was obtained from parents and schoolteachers about psychiatric symptoms and school achievement *prior* to the accident. The interview measures were similar to those used in the first study, described above. A limitation of the study was that the principal interviewer was not blind to subject status or prior evaluations. Blind ratings made of clinical summaries, however, showed very high levels of interrater agreement on the presence or absence and severity of disorder. In addition, parents completed a self-administered rating form (Conners, 1973) and teachers completed a standardized behavior problem inventory (Rutter, 1967). At the final follow-up of the severe head injury group, the children's teachers were interviewed personally. Follow-up examinations were held at 4, 12, and 24 months after the accident.

Findings

Psychiatric Disorder. The premorbid rate of psychiatric disorder was highest among children with mild head injuries (see Table 4-2) and was similar in the severe head injury and the orthopedic injury groups. New cases of disorder developed in all groups during the course of the follow-up, but the increase was greatest among those with a severe head injury, such that by the end of the follow-up period their rate was more than twice that of the control group.

TABLE 4-2.   Psychiatric Disorder in Head Injury
Groups and Controls (Parent Interview)

		Head Injuries	
	Controls ($N = 28$)	Severe ($N = 28$)	Mild ($N = 29$)
Initial	10.7	14.3	31.0
4 months	14.3	53.6[a]	20.7
1 year	22.2	50.0	17.2
2½ years	24.0	60.7[a]	24.1

Source: From Brown et al., 1981.

[a]$p < 0.01$.

The excess of psychiatric disorder in the severe injury group was replicated by the blind rater, and there were broadly similar increases on teacher and parent questionnaire measures. By the end of the 2-year follow-up, the severe head injury group was also much more likely to have been referred for a psychiatric/psychological evaluation.

Instances of new disorders (i.e., disorders that were not present before the injury, Table 4-3) occurred in all three groups, but the rate was much higher in the severe group, where about half of the children developed new psychiatric disorders—more than triple the rate in the controls. The rates of increase in the mild head injury and the orthopedic injury groups were lower and similar to each other and were significantly different from those of the severe head injury group.

There appeared to be a threshold effect and a modified dose-response effect of severity. Among the mild head injury group, children with less than 7 days of PTA had rates similar to those with less than 24 hours. In the severe injury group, children who had PTA for longer than 22 days had a higher rate of new disorder than those who had PTA of 7 to 21 days.

Predictors of New Disorder. The appearance of new disorders seemed to be unrelated to sex or to age at injury. New disorders were somewhat more common among children with persistent *neurological abnormalities* and among children with *initial intellectual impairment,* defined as an initial Performance IQ score on the Wechsler Intelligence Scale for Children (WISC) of more than 24 points below an assessment 1 year after the injury (Wechsler, 1949). Intellectual impairment was associated most strongly with psychiatric disorder that appeared shortly after the injury and was less important for disorders that appeared late. Most importantly, the rate of disorder among children with severe head injury *without* neurological abnormality and *without* intellectual impairment was well above that in the control group. Brown et al. (1981) concluded that this finding—coupled with the rather modest dose-response relationship between severity and disorder—meant that not all of the increase in psychiatric disorder was a direct consequence of neurological damage and that *indirect* as well as direct mechanisms were at play, especially in disorders that first appeared some time after the injury. While this was supported by analyses of interaction with preinjury behavior, one must recognize that, in comparison with modern imaging techniques, manifest neurological and gross cognitive impairment may be relatively insensitive indices of structural damage.

Preinjury Behavior. Preinjury behavior was a powerful predictor of later problems in all groups. All of the children with a clinically significant disorder before injury continued to have behavioral and emotional symptoms. Over half of the children with only a doubtful disorder prior to the injury developed a definite disorder at the 1-year follow-up, and *none* were without symptoms. By contrast, half of the children who had had no evidence of previous emotional or behavioral problems would be entirely symptom-free at 12 months.

TABLE 4-3.   The Development of New Psychiatric Disorders after the Accident
According to Parental Interview (% disorder)

	Controls ($N=22$)	Severes ($N=21$)	Significance Controls vs. Severes[a]	Milds ($N=20$)	Significance Controls vs. Milds[a]
4 months	4.5	47.6	$p=0.0028$	15.0	NS
1 year	13.6	47.6	$p=0.034$	10.0	NS
2½ years	13.6	61.9	$p=0.0026$	20.0	NS

Source: From Brown et al., 1981.

[a]Fisher's exact probability test.

Psychosocial Adversity. The relationship of emergent psychiatric disturbance to
psychosocial adversities or stresses was examined, as it had been in the study of
localized injury (Shaffer et al., 1975). An index comprising items known to relate
to psychiatric disorder—including family integrity and size, use of welfare services, parental psychiatric illness and criminality, and low socioeconomic status—
was used for this purpose. The association between disorder and psychosocial
adversity was similar in the severe head injury group and the controls. The rate
of appearance of new disorders was significantly greater in children who experienced the combination of a severe head injury and psychosocial adversity.

Pathognomonic Syndromes. In order to determine whether there were specific
syndromes that could be attributed to head injury, it was first necessary to define
what was an attributable disorder. The following criteria were adopted: (1) that
PTA had lasted at least 7 days; (2) that the disorder had arisen *after* the head
injury; and (3) that there was no evidence of psychiatric disorder before the injury.
This was a conservative approach, because it is always possible that some of the
new disorders in the mild group were attributable. Twelve children met these
criteria, 10 by the 1-year follow-up. For the purposes of comparison, a group of
disorders were judged as not attributable to head injury. These included all disorders in the orthopedic control group and all disorders that were present in the
head-injured groups *before* injury.*

   The pattern of "disinhibited" behavior affected 5 children and appeared to be
attributable to injury. All 5 cases had had a PTA exceeding 3 weeks; 3 of the
children showed persistent and 2 showed transient intellectual impairment. Typical
behaviors included being unduly outspoken, making frequent personal remarks
or asking embarrassing questions, and getting undressed in inappropriate social
situations. Brown et al. (1981) quote a 9-year-old who frequently made loud com-
ments to his mother about other people on the bus: e.g., "You've got a nig-nog
sitting next to you" or "I don't like that lady, she smells," and a 13-year-old who

---

*Brown also included three cases of new disorders in the mild injury group. Exclusion of these did
not alter the findings.

woke repeatedly at about 5 A.M. and wandered around the house without his clothes. Other behaviors in this group included forgetfulness, loquaciousness, carelessness in personal hygiene and dress, and impulsivity. Some of these behaviors resemble those reported in the so-called frontal lobe syndromes seen in brain-injured adults (Lishman, 1978). Others are reminiscent of attention-deficit hyperactivity disorder (ADHD), and it is of interest that 2 of the 5 disinhibited children were diagnosed as ADHD at the 2-year follow-up. In general, however, restlessness and overactivity were significantly *less* frequent in the disorders attributable to head injury. The behaviors are also reminiscent of hypomanic states. A child who was not among the 5 disinhibited subjects had an acute—and brief—psychotic breakdown about 2 years after her head injury. She became agitated, had flight of ideas and ideas of reference, giggled in a silly way, changed the intonation of her speech, and expressed bizarre ideas. There was also a trend for a number of specific symptoms to be attributable to head injury. These included overeating, overtalkativeness, bed-wetting, general slowness, and stuttering.

Conclusions

The British studies carried out or published in the 1970s established that neurological damage is a potent risk factor for psychiatric disorder in children. The causal nature of the relationship could be inferred by the dose-response relationship and by the temporal sequencing of exposure to injury and subsequent psychiatric morbidity. The studies suggested that there is a threshold for risk and that only injuries of a certain magnitude resulting in motor or cognitive impairment, epilepsy, or PTA of at least 1 week's duration enhance the risk for psychiatric disorder. The studies failed to demonstrate an effect of age at injury or locus of injury. Although the number of children who had been injured when they were infants or toddlers was small, the absence of an age effect is compatible with the findings in a much larger sample studied by Bijur (1990). The methods available for studying localization were poorly developed by current standards. More recent studies using magnetic resonance imaging (Mendelsohn et al., 1992) indicate that frontal lobe damage is especially likely to be associated with residual social and behavioral disability. The studies also suggested that traumatic brain injury may not have an all-or-nothing effect, and that its effect on psychiatric morbidity is potentiated by preexisting psychiatric symptoms and by a stressful or suboptimal psychosocial environment.

In recent years, a number of authorities (Boll & Barth, 1983; Kraus et al., 1986) have dismissed the notion of a high threshold for psychiatric complications and have suggested that clinically mild injuries can lead to degenerative changes and, through these, to permanent behavioral sequelae. These assertions draw some indirect support from computed tomography studies showing persistent structural abnormalities in spite of apparent clinical neurological recovery (Rivara et al., 1987; Zimmerman & Ilaniuk, 1981). As Bijur et al. (1990) have pointed out, however, some of the behavioral studies that are quoted to support this view are uncontrolled (Casey et al., 1986) and, in some instances (Farmer et al., 1987), include transient conditions. Others included adults and, in some instances, patients with severe head injuries. Still others do not differentiate between new and preexisting disorders.

To what extent do the British studies address the question of whether or not a minor head injury can lead to psychiatric complications? The epidemiological study on the Isle of Wight is clearly not helpful here, because it identified only gross manifestations of neurological damage (i.e. motor handicap and seizures). It did not and could not address latent or occult neurological disorder. Although the main thrust of the prospective longitudinal study is that there is a high severity threshold, the findings are, in some respects, consistent with the mild injury argument. Attributable psychiatric disturbance did occur in children without clinically observable neurological complications or cognitive deficits. It must also be remembered that sample numbers, as Szatmari (1985) has pointed out, were too small to rule out a type II error. On the other hand, the study does not stand alone in identifying a threshold effect. Other studies have noted a relationship between duration of coma and enduring cognitive impairment (Levin & Eisenberg, 1979), and return to school (Ruff et al., 1993), albeit the threshold noted in these studies was less than 1 week.

The findings from the prospective study suggest that some severe head injuries give rise to a distinctive clinical syndrome of disinhibited, socially inappropriate behavior. There was also a tendency for head-injured children to overeat after the injury. The disinhibited behaviors resemble those found in the frontal lobe syndrome. Social disinhibition, however, is also characteristic of many children with ADHD, and it was of interest that the clinical picture in 2 of the disinhibited children evolved to a picture of ADHD by the second year. These findings have some parallels in the literature. Early studies of children recovered from encephalitis (Blau, 1936; Strecker & Ebaugh, 1924) noted restlessness, hyperactivity, impulsiveness, and resistance to discipline. In an uncontrolled prospective study of children admitted to hospital for complicated head injuries, Black et al. (1970) identified a posttraumatic syndrome characterized by emotional lability, headache, eating problems, hyperactivity, and impaired attention. Theories about the role of frontal lobe functioning in the genesis of ADHD are well established (Benson, 1991), and recent studies using magnetic resonance imaging (Giedd et al., 1994) have noted abnormalities that are consistent with frontal lobe dysfunction. There is also evidence from psychological test performance (Shue & Douglas, 1992) of frontal lobe dysfunction among children with ADHD, although its significance has been disputed (Barkley et al., 1992). Most recently, Bijur et al. (1990) found a small but statistically significant excess of hyperactivity in a unique study of a large cohort of children who had experienced a minor head injury. That study was a powerful one because systematic behavioral data had been collected both before and after injury, the sample was very large and representative, and it was possible to undertake extensive controls for group differences. Children with a minor head injury were compared with non-head-injured controls after taking account of a variety of psychosocial risk factors and the base rate of hyperactivity. However the magnitude of increase in hyperactivity (0.4 of a standard deviation) was of marginal clinical significance.

Implications

It is clear both from these studies and from abundant research (which has used more modern methods of visualizing CNS structure and function) that psychiatric disorder may arise as a result of brain injury without motor abnormality or seizures. Although the British studies suggested that prolonged PTA was a good indicator of severity, other indicators may prove to be more sensitive than coma and PTA length as we learn more about the structural effects of injury. Not all of the methodological cautions in this chapter have been learned and research reports of uncontrolled samples or studies in which procedures have not been adopted to distinguish between old and new disorders continue to be published and contribute to an often confusing literature.

Both studies showed that psychiatric morbidity is common in the head-injured population. It appears to arise both through the direct effects of brain injury and by increasing vulnerability in children who, as a group, already carry a number of risk factors for psychiatric disorder. Behavioral complications are probably the most prevalent complications of head injury. Similarly, CNS damage or abnormality is probably the single most powerful risk factor for psychiatric disorder in children. Despite this, these factors are only infrequently translated into service provisions. Neurological assessment is far from routine in psychiatric services and few neurological or head injury clinics provide facilities for behavioral assessment and treatment.

Acknowledgments

This work was supported by NIMH Research Training Grant MH16434, and NIMH Center Grant MH43878 to The Center to Study Youth Depression, Anxiety and Suicide.

References

Asarnow, R. F., Satz, P., & Light, R. (1991). Behavior problems and adaptive functioning in children with mild and severe closed head injury. *J. Pediatr. Psychol., 16,* 543–555.

Barkley, R. A., Grodzinsky, G., & DuPaul G. J. (1992). Frontal lobe functions in attention deficit disorder with and without hyperactivity: A review and research report. *J. Abnorm. Child Psychol., 20,* 163–88.

Benson, D. F. (1991). The role of frontal dysfunction in attention deficit hyperactivity disorder. *J. Child Neurol., 6*(suppl.), S9–12.

Bijur, P., Haslum, M., & Golding, J. (1990). Cognitive and behavioral sequelae of mild head injury in children. *Pediatrics, 86,* 337–344.

Black, P., Slumer, D., Wellner, A. M., & Walker, A. E. (1970). The head-injured child: Time-course of recovery with implications for rehabilitation. In *Proceedings of an International Symposium on Head Injury* (pp. 131–137). Edinburgh and Madrid: Williams & Wilkins, 1970.

Blau, A. (1936). Mental changes following head trauma in children. *Arch. Neurol. Psychiatry, 35,* 723–769.

Boll, T. J., & Barth, J. (1983). Mild head injury. *Psychiatr. Dev., 1,* 263–276.

Breslau, N. (1985). Psychiatric disorder in children with physical disabilities. *J. Am. Acad. Child Adolesc. Psychiatry, 24,* 87–94.

Breslau, N., & Marshall, I. (1985). Psychological disturbance in children with physical disabilities: Continuity and change in a 5-year follow-up. *J. Abnorm. Child Psychol., 13,* 199–215.

Brown, G., Chadwick, O., Shaffer, D., Rutter, M., & Traub, M. (1981). A prospective study of children with head injuries: III. Psychiatric sequelae. *Psychol. Med., 11,* 63–78.

Brown, G. W., & Rutter, M. (1966). The measurement of family activities and relationships: A methodological study. *Hum. Rel., 19,* 241–263.

Casey, R., Ludwig, S., & McCormick, M. C. (1986). Morbidity following minor head trauma in children. *Pediatrics, 78,* 497–502.

Chadwick, O., Rutter, M., Brown, G., Shaffer, D., & Traub, M. (1981). A prospective study of children with head injuries: II. Cognitive sequelae. *Psychol. Med., 11,* 49–61.

Conners, C. (1973). Rating scales for use in drug studies in children. In *Pharmacotherapy of Children* (pp. 24–84). *Psychophamacol. Bull.,* special suppl. to vol. 9.

Craft, A. W., Shaw, D. A., & Cartlidge, N. E. F. (1973). Bicycle injuries in children. *Br. Med. J., 4,* 146–147.

Donders, J. (1992). Premorbid behavioral and psychosocial adjustment of children with traumatic brain injury. *J. Abnorm. Child Psychol., 20,* 233–246.

Ewing-Cobbs, L., Levin, H. S., Fletcher, J. M., Miner, M. E., & Eisenberg, H. M. (1990). The Children's Orientation & Amnesia Test: Relationship to severity of injury and to recovery of memory. *Neurosurgery, 27,* 683–691.

Farmer, M. Y., Singer, H. S., Mellits, E. D., Hall, D., & Charney, E. (1987). Neurobehavioral sequelae of minor head injuries in children. *Pediatr. Neurosci., 13,* 304–308.

Giedd, J. N., Castellanos, F. X., Casey, B. J., Kozuch, P., King, A. C., Hamburger, S. D., & Rapoport, J. L. (1994). Quantitative morphology of the corpus callosum in attention deficit hyperactivity disorder. *Am. J. Psychiatry, 151,* 665–669.

Graham, P., & Rutter, M. (1968). The reliability of the psychiatric assessment of the child: II. Interview with the parent. *Br. J. Psychiatry, 114,* 581–592.

Jennett, B. (1976). Assessment of severity of head injury. *J. Neurol. Neurosurg. Psychiatry, 39,* 647–655.

Jennett, B., Teasdale, G., Galbraith, S., Pickard, J., Grant, H., Braakman, R., Avezaat, C., Maas, A., Minderhoud, J., Vecht, C. J., Heiden, J., Small, R., Caton, W., & Kurze, T. (1977). Severe head injuries in three countries. *J. Neurol. Neurosurg. Psychiatry, 40,* 291.

Kraus, J. F., Fife, D., Cox, P., Ramstein, K., & Conroy, C. (1986). Incidence, severity and external causes of pediatric brain injury. *Am. J. Dis. Child., 140,* 687–693.

Levin, H. S., & Eisenberg, H. M. (1979). Neuropsychological outcome of closed head injury in children and adolescents. *Childs Brain, 5,* 281–292.

Lishman, W. A. (1978). *Organic Psychiatry* (Chap. 5). Oxford: Blackwell Scientific.

Manheimer, D. I., & Mellinger, G. D. (1967). Personality characteristics of the child accident repeater. *Child Dev., 38,* 491–513.

Mendelsohn, D., Levin, H. S., Bruce, D., Lilly, M., Harward, H., Culhane, K. A., & Eisenberg, H. M. (1992). Late MRI after head injury in children: Relationship to clinical features and outcome. *Childs Nerv. Syst., 8,* 445–452.

Quinton, D., Rutter, M., & Rowlands, O. (1976). An evaluation of an interview assessment of marriage. *Psychol. Med., 6,* 577–586.

Rivara, F., Tanaguchi, D., Parish, R. A., Stimac, G., & Mueller, B. (1987). Poor prediction of positive computed tomographic scans by clinical criteria in symptomatic pediatric head trauma. *Pediatrics, 80,* 579–584.

Ruff, R. M., Marshall, L. F., Crouch, J., Klauber, M. R., Levin, H. S., Barth, J., Kreutzer, J., Blunt, B. A., Foulkes, M. A., Eisenberg, H. M., Jane, J. A., & Marmarou, A. (1993). Predictors of outcome following severe head trauma: follow-up data from the Traumatic Coma Data Bank. *Brain Injury, 7,* 101–111.

Rune, V. Acute head injuries in children. (1970). *Acta Paediatr. Scand.,* suppl. 209.

Rutter, M. (1967). A children's behavior questionnaire for completion by teachers: Preliminary findings. *J. Child Psychol. Psychiatry, 8,* 1–11.

Rutter, M., & Brown, G. W. (1966). The reliability and validity of measures of family life and relationships in families containing a psychiatric patient. *Soc. Psychiatry, 1,* 38–53.

Rutter, M., Chadwick, O., Shaffer, D., & Brown, G. (1980). A prospective study of children with head injuries: I. Design and methods. *Psychol. Med., 10,* 633–646.

Rutter, M., & Graham, P. (1968). The reliability and validity of the psychiatric assessment of the child: I. Interview with the child. *Br. J. Psychiatry, 114,* 563.

Rutter, M., Graham, P., & Yule, W. (1970). *A neuropsychiatric study in childhood.* London: SIMP/Heinemann Medical.

Shaffer, D., Bijur, P., Chadwick, O., & Rutter, M. (1980). Head injury and later reading disability. *J. Am. Acad. Child Psychiatry, 19,* 592–610.

Shaffer, D., Chadwick, O., & Rutter, M. (1975). *Psychiatric outcome of localized head injury in children.* Amsterdam: Excerpta Medica.

Shue, K. L., & Douglas, V. I. (1992). Attention deficit hyperactivity disorder and the frontal lobe syndrome. *Brain Cogn., 20,* 104–124.

Strecker, E. A., & Ebaugh, F. G. (1924). Neuropsychiatric sequelae of cerebral trauma in children. *Arch. Neurol. Psychiatry, 12,* 443–453.

Szatmari, P. (1985). Some methodologic criteria for studies in developmental neuropsychiatry. *Psychiatr. Dev., 3,* 153–170.

Wechsler, D. (1949). *Wechsler Intelligence Scale for Children (Manual).* New York: Psychological Corporation.

Weiland, S. K., Pless, I. B., & Roghmann, K. J. (1992). Chronic illness and mental health problems in pediatric practice: Results from a survey of primary care providers. *Pediatrics, 89,* 445–449.

Zimmerman, R. A., & Ilaniuk L. T. (1981). Computed tomography in pediatric head trauma. *J. Neuroradiol., 8,* 257–271.

5

Neurobehavioral Outcome of Pediatric Closed Head Injury

HARVEY S. LEVIN, LINDA EWING-COBBS, ∫
and HOWARD M. EISENBERG

Before our research began in the 1970s, recovery from pediatric closed head injury (CHI) was studied primarily by assessing global outcome. The pioneering neurosurgical outcome studies of severe pediatric CHI by Bruce and coworkers (1979, 1980) at the Children's Hospital of Philadelphia (see Chapter 3) disclosed a low mortality rate (about 6%). Further, Bruce and his colleagues documented that 90% of the sample were either moderately disabled or had a good recovery, according to the Glasgow Outcome Scale (GOS) of Jennett and Bond (1975), at 6 months postinjury. These findings were interpreted as support for the view that children are more resilient to the effects of CHI than adults. Using the Glasgow Coma Scale (GCS) of Teasdale and Jennett (1974) and computed tomography (CT) to characterize the pathophysiology of acute CHI, Bruce and his coworkers elucidated the relationship between acute head injury severity and outcome in children. From a neurobehavioral perspective, however, these important studies were limited chiefly by their dependence on global measures of outcome and lack of cognitive and behavioral measures.

During the 1970s, major neurobehavioral studies were initiated by Michael Rutter (Rutter et al., 1980) and his group in England (see Chapter 4). These investigators made methodological refinements by their use of cognitive and psychiatric outcome measures, repeated assessments over time, and screening for preinjury developmental problems. But their research was completed before the development of the GCS and the CT scan, thus limiting the characterization of acute injury severity.

70

The Texas Studies: 1979–1990

Global Outcome of Severe Pediatric Head Injury—The Traumatic Coma Data Bank

The Galveston group's participation in the Traumatic Coma Data Bank provided an opportunity to prospectively study the global outcome of severe pediatric head injury for patients whose acute injury data, intensive care management, and CT scans were recorded on uniform research forms at four centers. After excluding patients who sustained gunshot wounds or were brain dead in the emergency room, Levin and coworkers (1992) studied the outcome of 103 children and adolescents at the time of hospital discharge, at 6 months ($n = 92$), and at 1 year ($n = 82$) postinjury. As depicted by the survival curves shown in Figure 5-1, the slope for the probability of survival is steeper and persists over 3 months in the 0-to 4-year-old group. The infants and preschoolers had a 62% mortality rate by the close of the first year, while the 5- to 10-year-old group obtained the most favorable outcome (two-thirds had a good recovery by 1 year postinjury). The outcome for adolescents approximated the distribution obtained by adults in the Traumatic Coma Data Bank.

The lowest postresuscitation GCS score and pupillary reactivity were predictive of 6-month outcome in the pediatric component of the Traumatic Coma Data Bank,

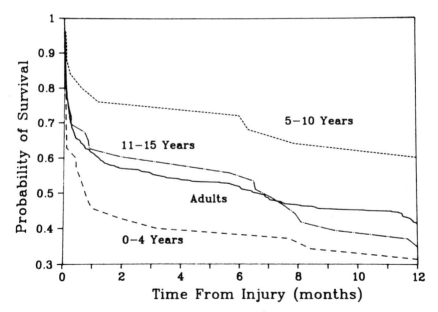

Figure 5-1. Estimated probability of survival over the first year following severe head injury, plotted for each age group of pediatric patients and for adults who were also studies in the Traumatic Coma Data Bank. (From Levin et al., 1992, with permission.)

as was the interaction of these injury indices (i.e., a low GCS score was more predictive of a poor outcome in the presence of unilateral or bilateral pupillary nonreac-
tivity). Distinctive pathophysiological features of the 0- to 4-year-old group included a high rate of acute subdural hematomas (20%) and hypotension (32%).
Analysis of the CT scan diagnosis within 24 hours of injury revealed that diffuse
brain swelling (i.e., obliteration of the cisterns) was related to sustained elevation of
intracranial pressure within the first 72 hours and a higher risk of devastated outcome
at 6 months postinjury (Figure 5-2). In contrast, normal CT scans were associated
with at least a 50% rate of good recovery by 6 months postinjury.

Neurobehavioral Outcome Studies. Neurobehavioral investigation of pediatric
head injury involved recruitment of prospective patients admitted to the neurosurgery services of the University of Texas, Galveston and Houston. The GCS score,
neurological examination, and CT scan were used to characterize the severity and
type of head injury, whereas school records and developmental history were employed to screen for preexisting neuropsychiatric disorder, mental deficiency, and
learning disability necessitating placement in special resource classes prior to the
injury. Although these criteria excluded about 10% of hospital admissions for
head injury, interpretation of the outcome data was not complicated by including
children with confounders.

Assessment of Posttraumatic Amnesia. The duration of impaired consciousness is
often regarded as an indicator of the severity of closed head injury. Russell and
Smith (1961) defined posttraumatic amnesia (PTA) as the period during which a
patient is unable to store and recall ongoing events. Levin and colleagues (1979)
developed the Galveston Orientation and Amnesia Test to assess objectively the
duration of PTA in adults. However, the assessment of PTA in children was based
on subjective estimates. Consequently, we devised and normed the Children's
Orientation and Amnesia Test (COAT) to assess orientation and memory objectively in children and adolescents during the early stage of recovery from traumatic brain injury. The COAT (see appendix to this chapter) consisted of 16
items evaluating (1) general orientation to person and place, recall of biographical
information; (2) temporal orientation; and (3) memory (immediate, short-term,
and remote). Normative data were obtained on 146 neurologically intact children
aged 3 to 15. Ewing-Cobbs and colleagues (1990) studied the validity of the
COAT in 37 children and adolescents between 4 and 15 years of age who sustained CHI. The COAT was administered daily at bedside to verbally responsive
patients. The duration of PTA was defined as the number of days following resolution of coma that a child's COAT scores were at least 2 standard deviations below
the age-corrected mean obtained from the normative sample. The clinical sample
was divided into three groups based on duration of posttraumatic amnesia as defined by serial COAT scores: group 1 had PTA ≤ 7 days, group 2 had PTA
persisting from 8 to 14 days, and group 3 had PTA for more than 14 days. Verbal
and nonverbal selective reminding procedures were employed prospectively after
resolution of PTA as well as 6 and 12 months after injury to assess verbal and

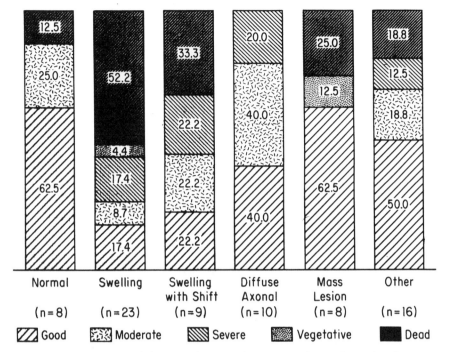

Figure 5-2. Distribution of Glasgow Outcome Scale categories at 6 months after severe head injury in children for each diagnostic group, defined by the initial computed tomography (CT) scan performed within 24 hours of injury. (From Levin et al., 1992, with permission.)

nonverbal memory functions. The consistent long-term retrieval scores, which reflect the amount of information recalled consistently over several trials from each of the selective reminding tests, were converted into standard scores with a mean of 10 and a standard deviation of 3. As depicted in Figure 5-3A and B, the duration of PTA as assessed by the COAT was significantly related to memory performance. Both verbal and nonverbal memory scores were significantly more impaired at 6 and 12 months after the injury in patients with PTA that persisted for at least 3 weeks than in patients whose disorientation, confusion, and gross amnesia resolved within 1 week. The verbal memory scores of children who were in PTA for less than 1 week recovered to the average range by 6 months following the injury. In contrast, children who had PTA for at least 1 week continued to exhibit a reduction in verbal memory functions. Nonverbal memory scores were significantly lower at follow-up in patients with PTA persisting for at least 2 weeks than in those with shorter PTA durations. The duration of PTA as estimated by COAT scores was more strongly related than the GCS score to memory scores obtained at follow-up. These findings supported the validity of the COAT as a measure of PTA duration in children and adolescents as well as its prognostic usefulness in predicting residual memory impairment.

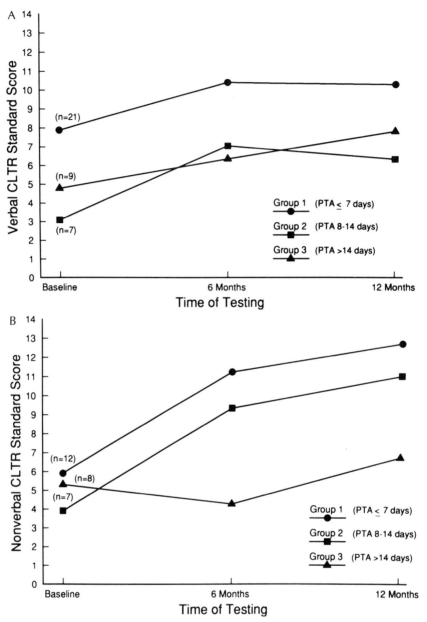

Figure 5-3. A. The mean verbal consistent long-term retrieval scores obtained at baseline and follow-up evaluations for children and adolescents with posttraumatic amnesia of varying duration. Posttraumatic amnesia persisting for at least 2 weeks was associated with significantly lower scores on verbal memory measures than postttraumatic amnesia persisting for less than 1 week. **B.** The mean nonverbal consistent long-term retrieval scores plotted against the time of testing. Patients with posttraumatic amnesia persisting for at least 2 weeks had significantly lower nonverbal memory scores and showed less recovery during the first year after injury than patients with posttraumatic amnesia of shorter duration.

Pattern of Deficits across Neurobehavioral Domains. Levin and Eisenberg (1979a, b) analyzed composite scores for the neuropsychological domains of memory, language, visuospatial ability, somatosensory performance, and motor function for 64 pediatric patients tested 3 to 4 weeks after injury (provided that their posttraumatic amnesia had substantially resolved). The presence of a neuropsychological deficit was defined by a deficient score on at least one test within the domain (i.e., a test score which fell at least two standard deviations below the mean score for normal children of similar age). The severity of head injury as judged by persistence of coma was graded I to III. Grade I included children who were awake and responsive to commands on admission; momentary loss of consciousness at the time of impact was not considered to be inconsistent with grade I provided that no neurological deficit was present at the time of hospital admission. Grade II included children whose coma did not exceed 24 hours or who were conscious but had a neurological deficit, implying cerebral injury (e.g., hemiparesis). Head injury producing a coma that lasted more than 24 hours was classified as grade III.

As depicted in Table 5-1, memory was the most frequently impaired neuropsychological domain, affecting nearly one-half of the sample. The Selective Reminding Test (Buschke, 1974) was used to evaluate verbal memory, whereas visual memory was assessed by the Continuous Recognition Memory Test (Hannay, Levin, & Grossman, 1979). Assuming that words correctly recalled on at least two consecutive trials had entered long-term memory storage, Levin and Eisenberg (1979b) interpreted the proportion of stored words that was consistently retrieved as an index of retrieval efficiency. Utilizing this index, the investigators found that the efficiency of retrieval relative to storage of information was reduced in the head-injured patients as compared to normal controls. Approximately one-fourth to one-third of the patients had deficits in each of the other neuropsychological domains (Table 5-1). The proportion of patients whose performance was defective was directly related to the severity of injury, which Levin and Eisenberg defined according to the duration of impaired consciousness.

TABLE 5-1.   Composite Neuropsychological Impairment According to Grade of Injury and Age[a]

Composite Function	6–12 Years			13–18 Years			Total
	I	II	III	I	II	III	
Language	1/8	1/2	3/4	3/12	1/5	5/9	14/40 (35%)
Visuospatial[c]	2/8	0/2	4/4	1/13	3/5	4/8	14/40 (35%)
Memory[b]	—	—	—	1/10	4/5	6/7	11/22 (50%)
Somatosensory	3/6	0/1	4/4	3/12	0/5	1/7	11/35 (31%)
Motor speed	1/5	0/1	4/4	3/7	2/5	1/3	11/25 (44%)

Source: From Levin and Eisenberg, 1979b, with permission.

[a]Memory data were unavailable in the 6- to 12-year group.

[b]$p < 0.05$ (significant effect of grade of injury on performance).

[c]$p < 0.01$.

Figure 5-4 depicts the relationship between the lowest postresuscitation GCS score recorded during the hospitalization and the proportion of children exhibiting a deficit in the respective domains. The percentage of children with defective visuospatial performance was significantly related to the lowest postresuscitation verbal and motor scores on the GCS. Although the percentage of children with defective memory was related to the verbal component of the GCS, this relationship was not significant for the motor component of the GCS. The investigators postulated that the reversal of an otherwise monotonic function for the motor response (see "None") could have been due to insufficient stimulation applied by the examiner, resulting in an erroneous recording of no extremity movement (i.e., a motor score of 1). In contrast, the composite functions of language, somatosensory ability, and motor speed were not significantly related to the GCS score. Neuropsychological deficits were also confirmed in a subgroup of children who had sustained relatively mild injuries, a finding that may reflect the relatively short

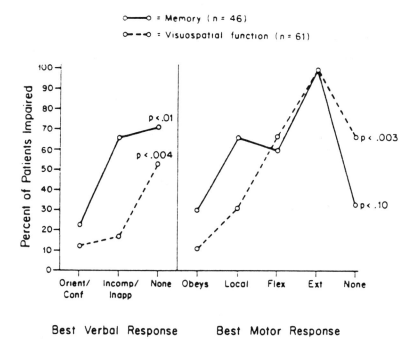

Figure 5-4. Percent of head-injured children performing within the impaired range on tests in the memory and visual/spatial domains, plotted for the verbal and motor responses of the Glasgow Coma Scale (GCS). The GCS scores were selected to reflect the most severe impairment of consciousness following hospital admission. Abbreviations: Orient = oriented; Conf = confused speech; Incomp = incomprehensible; Inapp = inappropriate; Obeys = obeys commands; Local = localizes source of painful stimulus; Flex = flexor response to stimulus; Ext = extensor posturing in response to stimulus. (From Levin & Eisenberg, 1979a, with permission.)

interval between injury and assessment. Analysis of the CT scan findings revealed a relationship between the presence of a left hemisphere mass lesion and impaired verbal memory (as measured by the Selective Reminding Test). Intellectual function, measured by the Wechsler Scale at least 6 months postinjury, was unequivocally impaired (i.e., IQ below 70) in a subgroup of the most severely injured patients, whereas no child having sustained a mild to moderate injury exhibited intellectual deficit at 6 months or longer after injury. However, this early study was limited by a single assessment during the first 6 months postinjury.

As reflected in the more recent studies described below, serial assessment has disclosed recovery functions that differ according to the severity of injury and the child's age.

Age at Injury in Relation to Recovery of Memory and Intellectual Function. To investigate the relationship between age at injury and neurobehavioral outcome, Levin and coworkers (1982) studied groups of head-injured children and adolescents with similar distributions of injury severity and type (e.g., focal brain lesion) as reflected by the GCS score and CT findings. In this initial comparison of neurobehavioral outcome in children versus adolescents, the proportion of cases with defective scores was compared for each age group, using as a reference the distribution of test scores in normal controls of similar age. Levin and coworkers (1982) found that the proportion of patients with defective scores on verbal selective reminding and visual continuous recognition memory was comparable in the children and adolescents. However, 5 (one-third) of the 15 severely injured children had residual intellectual deficit (i.e., IQ below 80) at the time of follow-up, whereas all 14 severely injured adolescents recovered to a higher level, according to the Wechsler Scale of Intelligence. The significant difference in the proportions of children versus adolescents with intellectual impairment was interpreted as evidence for more deleterious effects of diffuse cerebral insult on the young brain.

In 1988, Levin and colleagues expanded the analysis of age effects on memory by studying 58 pediatric CHI admissions sampled from three age ranges (6–8, 9–12, and 13–15 years) and tested at baseline and 1 year follow-up, using the Verbal Selective Reminding and Visual Recognition Memory Tests. The memory test data for patients sustaining mild to moderate head injury (i.e., GCS scores in the 9–15 range) were grouped together and compared to both the severely injured patients and the normal controls. To compare the memory scores of the three age groups directly, their data were transformed to standard scores using the distributions of raw scores of normal children and adolescents as a reference group (mean = 100, standard deviation = 15). As depicted in Figure 5-5A, severity of injury was related to the level of recognition memory at baseline and follow-up in the children and adolescents. There was no evidence for differential recognition memory deficit related to the age at injury.

In contrast, the transformed verbal memory scores of head-injured adolescents at baseline fell below the level of the children's performance (Figure 5-5B). However, the trend of lower verbal memory scores in the adolescents than in the children was not significant at follow-up. Plotting the transformed verbal memory

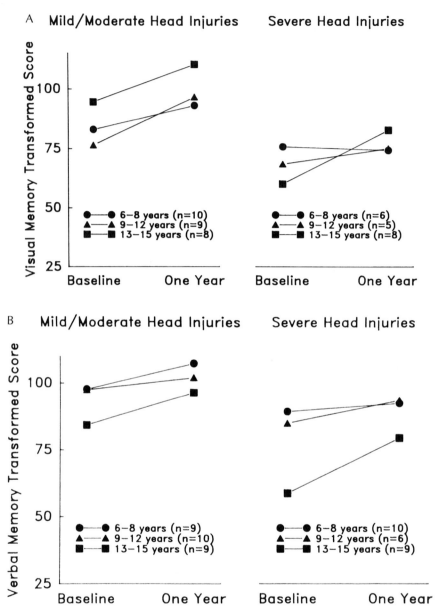

Figure 5-5. A. Visual recognition memory transformed scores plotted for children and adolescents at baseline (i.e., after resolution of posttraumatic amnesia and at 1 year postinjury). The transformed scores were based on the distribution of visual memory recognition test scores in uninjured children and adolescents. The mean transformed score for each age range is 100, with a stqndard deviation of 15. The visual recognition memory scores are shown separately for mild/moderate and severe head injuries. (From Levin et al., 1988, with permission.) **B.** Verbal memory (Selective Reminding Test) transformed scores plotted for children and adolescents at baseline (i.e., after resolution of posttraumatic amnesia and

scores against trials revealed a lag in word acquisition in the severely injured adolescents; a parallel pattern was not evident in the children. Levin and colleagues postulated that the late maturation of semantic organization as a mnemonic strategy contributed to the vulnerability of the adolescents and mitigated the impairment exhibited by children. According to this interpretation, it is anticipated that the severely injured children will have difficulty developing semantic organizational skills as they enter adolescence.

Neurobehavioral Sequelae in Infants and Preschoolers. Few studies have included children younger than 5 years of age at the time of injury. Ewing-Cobbs and associates (1989) prospectively studied 21 infants and preschoolers, including 13 severe and 8 mild to moderate injuries, using age-appropriate measures of cognition, motor function, and expressive and receptive language during the initial hospitalization and at least 6 months (mean was 8.3 months) postinjury. Analysis of standard scores adjusted for age allowed the investigators to combine the data of the infants and preschoolers. As depicted in Figure 5-6A, intellectual level improved over time. Despite the trend toward a steeper recovery in the more severely injured patients (the interaction of severity with occasions was nearly significant), the intellectual level of mild to moderate CHI children was higher than that of the severely injured children at follow-up. Collapsing the data across severity groups disclosed that motor function (Figure 5-6A) was impaired in relation to intellectual level. The investigators postulated that the topographic organization of motor functions may have limited the potential for recovery, whereas the greater recovery of intellectual ability may have been due to its more flexible, associative organization. Moreover, involvement of the subcortical white matter may affect motor skills to a greater extent than intellectual ability.

Recovery of expressive and receptive language is depicted in Figure 5-6B, which shows the parallel functions for the mild to moderate and severe CHI groups in the study of infants and preschoolers. Severely injured children demonstrated impaired expressive and receptive language, relative to the mild to moderate head injury group, on both the initial and follow-up examinations. Expressive language scores were below receptive language scores at baseline, whereas no significant difference surfaced at follow-up. Consistent with the impression in Figure 5-6B of a steeper recovery for expressive language than for receptive skills, the interaction between the language domain and occasion approached significance. This pattern of language recovery in infants and preschoolers parallels the findings in school-aged children, which reflect greater vulnerability of expressive than receptive language (Ewing-Cobbs et al., 1987). Ewing-Cobbs and coworkers also interpreted this disparity as consistent with the vulnerability of more rapidly

---

at 1 year postinjury). the transformed scores were based on the distribution of verbal memory test scores in uninjured children and adolescents. The mean transformed scores for each age range is 100, with a standard deviation of 15. The verbal memory scores are shown separately for mild/moderate and severe head injuries. (From Levin et al., 1988, with permission.).

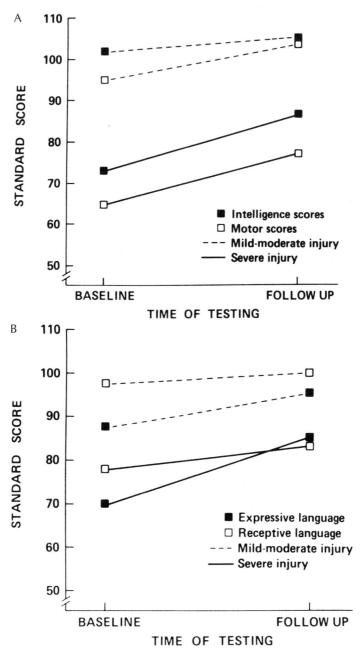

Figure 5-6. A. Intelligence and motor scores obtained on standardized tests, plotted for infants and preschool children according to severity of head injury. Test scores are shown for baseline and follow-up (mean follow-up interval, 8 months). (From Ewing-Cobbs et al., 1989, with permission.) **B.** Expressive and receptive language scores obtained on standardized tests, plotted for infants and preschool children according to severity of head injuury. Test scores are shown for baseline and follow-up (mean follow-up interval, 8 months). (From Ewing-Cobbs et al., 1989, with permission.)

developing skills (i.e., expressive language), as compared to the firmly established receptive abilities.

To evaluate the relationship between age at injury and neurobehavioral sequelae, Ewing-Cobbs and colleagues divided the patient sample according to whether their age was older or younger than 31 months. Comparison of the language performance (using standard scores) by the age-defined subgroups revealed that expressive language was lower in the younger group than in the older patients at both baseline and follow-up. Although receptive skills were also lower in the younger group on the initial examination, there was no age effect at follow-up.

Linguistic Deficits in Children and Adolescents. Hecaen (1976) documented nonfluent aphasia after CHI in children, including sequelae of dyscalculia, dysgraphia, and difficulty with spelling. To investigate the presence of specific linguistic disturbance in head-injured children who were not obviously aphasic on clinical examination, Ewing-Cobbs and coworkers (1987) administered the Neurosensory Center Comprehensive Examination for Aphasia (NCCEA) (Spreen & Benton, 1969) to 23 children (5 to 10 years of age) and 33 adolescents (11 to 15 years of age) who had sustained CHI of varying severity. The median injury test interval was about 1 month in both age groups. As shown in Figure 5-7A, the NCCEA variables were grouped into four composites of expressive and receptive language. The pattern of findings depicted in Figure 5-7A reflects a direct relationship between the severity of CHI and the percentage of patients who had impaired performance on the NCCEA measures. Expressive functions were more sensitive to severity of head injury than the receptive measures, as indicated by the significant effects of severity (according to the GCS score) on visual naming, sentence repetition, word fluency, and writing to dictation. In contrast, there were no differences between the moderate/severe and mild head injury groups on the receptive language measures.

To compare the findings on children and adolescents, the scores were transformed to age-adjusted centiles, which revealed that writing to dictation was impaired in the children relative to the adolescents (Figure 5-7B). Ewing-Cobbs and coworkers (1987) interpreted the disproportionate impairment of written language in children as consistent with the view that rapidly emerging linguistic skills are more vulnerable to disruption by head injury than are abilities more firmly established at the time of injury, such as comprehension of aural language. In this connection, the investigators noted that written language develops most rapidly between the ages of 6 and 8 years, reflecting a later maturation than with other linguistic skills, such as naming and repetition. The finding that writing to copy did not differ across the children and adolescents suggests that the disturbance in writing to dictation was not attributable entirely to visual-motor impairment. This study indicates that linguistic deficits frequently persist after severe head injury in children who are not aphasic according to clinical examination. The linguist sequelae documented by Ewing-Cobbs and coworkers have important implications for the academic performance of head-injured children. It is conceivable that even

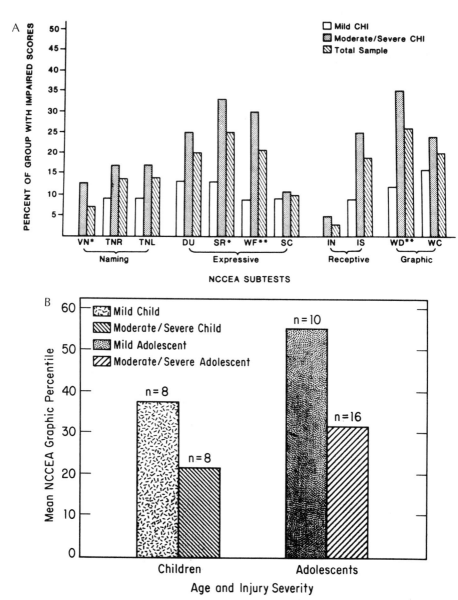

Figure 5-7. A. Percentage of children and adolescents with language test scores in the impaired range, plotted according to the severity of head injury and for various language domains. The scores were obtained from subtests of the Neurosensory Center Comprehensive Examination for Aphasia (NCCEA). Abbreviations: VN = visual naming; TNR = tactile naming for objects placed in the right hand; TNL = tactile naming for objects placed in the left hand; DU = description of use; SR = sentence repetition; WF = word fluency; SC = sentence construction; IN = identification by name; IS = identification by sentence; WD = writing to dictation; WC = writing to copy. (From Ewing-Cobbs et al., 1987 with permission.) **B.** Age-transformed standard scores for writing to dictation and copying on the writing subtests of the NCCEA. There was a disproportionate effect of severity of injury in the younger children relative to adolescents.

mild language impairment may disrupt the scholastic achievement of children who have sustained a head injury.

Attention after Head Injury. Recent conceptualizations (Baddeley, 1992) of working memory emphasize the coordination of resources by a central executive that integrates memory, attention, and perception. Although Chadwick and colleagues (1981) found that attention was impaired in children at 4 months after CHI (Stroop test, continuous performance test), these sequelae resolved over a 2-year follow-up period. To further investigate the effects of CHI severity on attention, Kaufmann and associates (1993) administered a computer-based adaptive-rate continuous performance test to groups with mild, moderate, and severe CHI who were studied at about 6 months postinjury. Children were instructed to press a response key as quickly as possible to the onset of the target (i.e., an airplane) while withholding response to distractors presented on the video screen. By increasing the rate of video presentation of targets and distractors after correct responses on a keyboard and slowing the input after incorrect or late responses, Kaufmann and coworkers obtained the mean interstimulus interval for each of four trial blocks. In this context, the interstimulus interval is an index of attentional efficiency, as the production of accurate short-latency responses caused the computer to reduce the interval. By analyzing age-adjusted standard scores (mean = 100, standard deviation = 15), the investigators were able to combine the data of various age subgroups.

Figure 5-8A shows that severely injured children exhibited attentional deficit across the four trial blocks, whereas the scores were collapsed to obtain a single overall attention score in Figure 5-8B. Consistent with the impression that young, severely injured children had the greatest impairment on the continuous performance test, the interaction of injury severity and age was significant. In contrast, no relationship of injury severity to performance surfaced on the Wechsler Digit Span, a subtest frequently interpreted by clinicians as a measure of attention.

Age and Neurobehavioral Outcome following Gunshot Wounds to the Brain in Children and Adolescents. This section is included for comparative purposes, to contrast the neurobehavioral outcome of gunshot wounds to closed head injury. However, we acknowledge the difference in injury mechanism. Ewing-Cobbs, Thompson, Miner, and Fletcher (1994) completed a prospective 3-year longitudinal follow-up of a consecutive case series of 13 children and adolescents with craniocerebral gunshot wounds to evaluate (1) whether developmental level at the time of injury was associated with differences in late outcome and (2) the type and magnitude of neuropsychological deficits. The younger group contained 7 children ages 1.5 to 4 years, while the older group was composed of 6 children ranging in age from 5 to 14. Outcome measures included the GOS as well as neuropsychological assessment of intelligence, language, motor skills, memory, attention, academic achievement, and adaptive behavior. At discharge from the hospital, GOS scores revealed moderate disabilities in 69% and severe disabilities in 23% of the sample. By 3 years after the injury, 85% had moderate disabilities

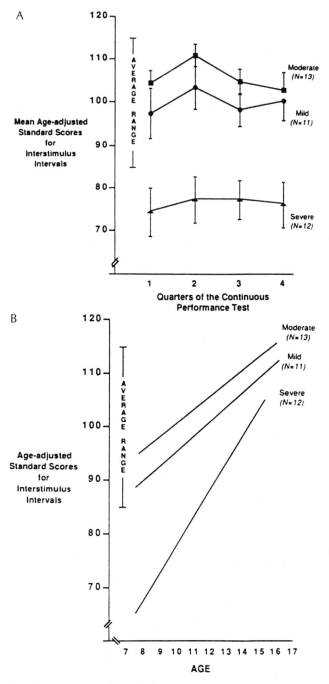

Figure 5-8. A. Mean age-adjusted standard scores for interstimulus intervals, plotted against the phase of the continuous performance test according to severity of head injury in children. The interstimulus interval reflects the child's performance as the time between stimuli was increased when the child responded late or inaccurately, whereas the interstimulus was reduced (i.e., there was a faster rate of presentation) after a series of accurate responses prior to the time limit. (Reproduced from Kaufmann et al., 1993, with permission.) **B.** Age-adjusted

and only 8% of the sample had a severe disability. The level of morbidity in our sample appeared to be comparable to that reported in other civilian series of patients evaluated using the GOS score.

Neuropsychological test results identified significant and persistent deficits that varied with the child's developmental level at the time of injury. Intellectual functioning was clearly more impaired in children less than 5 years of age at injury than in older children. Disability in the younger group was most closely related to cognitive and motor factors. In addition to a severe reduction in IQ test scores, young children exhibited significant deficiencies on measures of expressive language and gross motor functioning. These findings were very similar to those of our studies of infants and preschoolers who sustained severe closed head injuries (Ewing-Cobbs et al., 1989). In contrast, disability in older children and adolescents was primarily associated with impaired attention, adaptive behavior deficits, and behavioral disturbance. In the older group, median adaptive behavior scores were in the low average range on estimates of preinjury adaptive behavior. However, at the 3-year follow-up, all patients had adaptive behavior scores in the deficient range. In contrast to the high rate of behavioral disturbance, the median intelligence, language, memory, reading, and spelling scores improved to the average to low-average range at follow-up.

The disabilities identified following craniocerebral gunshot wounds were at least as severe as in our previous studies of deficits in patients sustaining severe pediatric CHI. In comparison with children with severe CHI, our group of younger children sustaining gunshot wounds had slightly lower IQ scores and similar receptive language, expressive language, and gross motor scores. However, the older gunshot wound patients scored significantly lower than patients with severe CHI on indices of adaptive behavior and attention. The findings were interpreted as suggesting that early brain injury may not be associated with a more favorable prognosis than comparable injuries in older children. Moreover, the types of deficits observed varied with the child's developmental level at the time of injury such that younger children were more likely to have significant intellectual impairment, while older children and adolescents had primary difficulties on measures of attention and adaptive behavior at long-term follow-up.

Contribution of Magnetic Resonance Imaging to Neurobehavioral Studies

Initial Magnetic Resonance Imaging Study

To investigate the contribution of focal brain lesions to the neurobehavioral outcome of pediatric head injury, Levin and colleagues (1989) completed an initial

---

standard score for interstimulus interval on the continuous performance test of attention, plotted against age according to severity of head injury. The degree of attentional deficit exhibited by severely injured patients was greater for the younger children than for the adolescents. (From Kaufmann et al. 1993, with permission.)

study of magnetic resonance imaging (MRI) in 21 children and adolescents who were at least 6 months postinjury. Of the 11 severely injured patients, 8 had areas of abnormal signal in the brain parenchyma; these included 4 children with lesions involving the frontal lobes, 3 cases of primarily parietal lesions, and a single patient with a lesion situated mainly in the temporal lobe. Five of the severely injured patients had lesions extending to the subcortical white matter and/or deep central gray. In contrast, none of the 10 children having sustained mild to moderate head injuries had areas of abnormal signal. Analysis of the relationship between the MRI findings and outcome disclosed that 7 of the 8 patients with an area of abnormal signal had a residual deficit (defined in terms of normative data) in at least one neurobehavioral domain. Three of the mildly injured patients had isolated neuropsychological defects.

Ongoing Project concerning Neurobehavioral Outcome of Head Injury in relation to Neuroimaging

In view of our preliminary MRI findings, a major goal of our current project is to study the relationship between the neuroanatomic localization of abnormal signal on MRI and the neurobehavioral sequelae of pediatric head injury. Considering the vulnerability of the frontal lobes to focal brain lesions after CHI, we employ cognitive measures of executive function in the current project. The project consists of two parallel studies, including a cross-sectional design to assess the long term outcome of previously injured children (3 years or longer since injury) and a longitudinal investigation of children prospectively recruited from acute neurosurgical admissions for head injury. Both studies address the effects of lesion localization (i.e., areas of abnormal signal) and age on neurobehavioral outcome measures.

To complete an initial study in the ongoing project, Levin and coworkers (1993) integrated data of 76 pediatric patients from the cross-sectional and longitudinal studies provided that MRI and neurobehavioral assessments were performed at 3 months postinjury or later. Forms designed for coding the MRI findings were completed by the neuroradiologist, independent of the neurobehavioral findings, and areas of abnormal signal were localized according to templates developed for MRI (Damasio, 1991). The number of children who had overlapping areas of abnormal signal is reflected by the degree of shading in Figure 5-9. Plotting the shaded areas of abnormal signal (Figure 5-9) revealed an anterocaudal gradient, reflecting a high frequency of children with lesions in the dorsolateral region (middle and superior frontal gyri), orbitofrontal region (i.e., orbital, rectal, and inferior frontal gyri), and frontal lobe white matter; a few areas of abnormal signal in the anterior temporal lobe; and isolated lesions in more posterior areas.

The neurobehavioral outcome measures (Table 5-2) encompass domains associated with frontal lobe functioning. In addition, three subtests of the Wechsler Intelligence Scale for Children—Revised (WISC-R) were given. Analysis of the neurobehavioral measures evaluated the effects of injury severity (GCS score ≤ 8, GCS score >8, controls) and age at the time of study (6–10 years, 11–16 years).

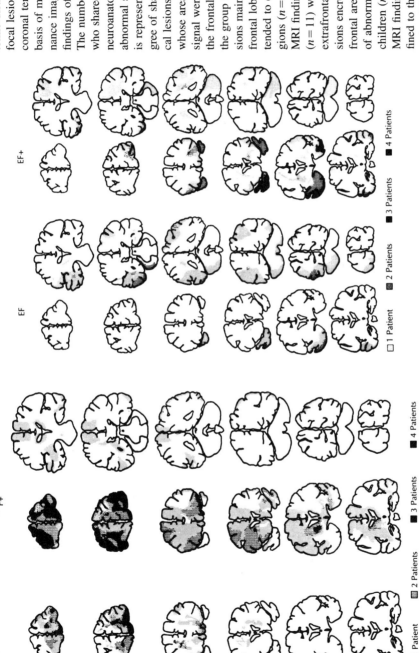

Figure 5-9. Neuroanatomic distribution of focal lesions plotted on coronal templates on the basis of magnetic resonance imaging (MRI) findings of 57 patients. The number of children who shared a common neuroanatomic region of abnormal signal on MRI is repressened by the degree of shading. Left-focal lesions of 20 patients whose areas of abnormal signal were restricted to the frontal lobes (F) and the group (F+) whose lesions mainly involved the frontal lobes but also extended to extrafrontal regions (n = 11). Right-MRI findings in children (n = 11) with essentially extrafrontal (EF+) lesions encroaching on the frontal area and on areas of abnormal signal for children (n = 15) whose MRI findings were confined to the extrafrontal region (EF). (From Levin et al., 1993, with permission.)

TABLE 5-2. Cognitive and Memory Procedures Organized According to Domain[a]

Domain	Procedure	Description	Measures
Concept formation—problem solving	20 Questions Test	Identify target picture on display by asking as few questions as possible; questions that eliminate >1 picture at a time (i.e., constraint) reflect sensitivity to semantic features; repeat for second target picture	% Constraint,[a] % identity, % pseudocon-straint, % redundant questions
	Wisconsin Card Sorting Test	Sort cards according to relevant dimension and shift strategy; computer-assisted administration	No. of categories used in sorting[a]; % perseverative errors
Planning	Tower of London	Plan and execute series of moves to rearrange 3 colored beads on rods to match model; 4 problems are given for each of 3 grades of difficulty, with simplest problems requiring 2 moves and most difficult problems requiring 5 moves	% Problems solved on first trial[a]; No. of broken rules
Verbal fluency	Controlled Oral Word Association	Generate as many words as possible beginning with specific letter in 60-sec time limit; repeat for 2 additional letters	No. correct words produced, summed over 3 letters[a]
Design fluency	Invention of Designs	Draw as many unique, abstract designs as possible with 3-min limit (free condition); repeat with additional constraint of using 4 lines in each design (fixed condition)	No. scorable designs created under fixed condition[a]; repeated for free condition
Memory	California Verbal Learning Test—Children's Version	Five recall trials of 15 words belonging to 3 semantic categories (i.e., fruit, clothing, toys); recall second 15-word list, then recognize and recall first list	% of responses that are clustered according to semantic category[a]
Response modulation	Go–No Go	Press computer key (Go) to onset of red light and withhold response (No Go) to blue light; test continued until child reaches criterion of 10 consecutive correct responses	No. of trials to criterion[a]

Source: From Levin et al., 1993, with permission.

[a] Most salient performance measures.

All measures were sensitive to the severity of injury and age, and these variables interacted on the Similarities subtest of the WISC-R, which is generally interpreted as a measure of verbal abstract reasoning.

To investigate the relationship of abnormal signal areas to cognitive outcome, multiple hierarchical regression was employed. This analysis addressed whether lesion volume could significantly increment the variance explained by the lowest postresuscitation GCS score in predicting performance on various cognitive measures. The results of the multiple regressions (Figure 5-10) indicate that the volume of left frontal lesion enhanced prediction of verbal fluency (Controlled Oral Word Association), performance on the Wisconsin Card Sorting Test, and inhibitory control (Go–No Go Test), while the volume of right frontal lesions incremented prediction of semantic clustering (California Verbal Learning Test), verbal fluency, and Go-No Go performance. Volume of extrafrontal lesion, however, failed to significantly enhance prediction of cognitive performance on any of the outcome measures. Pending replication as the project sample increases, these findings support the relationship between volume of frontal lobe lesion and cognitive sequelae of CHI, even after accounting for severity of injury by first entering the GCS score in the multiple regressions.

We interpret the relationship of focal areas of abnormal signal to the cognitive sequelae of pediatric head injury as evidence for the contribution of multifocal lesions to the effects of diffuse cerebral insult. As reported by Chapman (this volume), frontal lobe lesions are also associated with disorganized narrative discourse in which essential information contained in stories tends to be sparse. Consistent with recent cognitive neuroscience research in which neural networks have supplanted strict localization of lesion effects, we interpret our MRI and neurobehavioral findings as support for the involvement of frontal systems. Neurobehavioral consequences are likely to vary, however, depending on the region of the frontal lobe with abnormal signal, extension to the anterior temporal area, and involvement of the striatum. It is therefore plausible that functional brain imaging using activation tasks in children following severe CHI would demonstrate more extensive regions of cerebral dysfunction than would MRI. Utilization of functional brain imaging could also potentially elucidate the reorganization of function (e.g., recovery of language or problem-solving skills) over time and the impact of therapeutic interventions, such as cognitive modules in special resource classes or speech therapy.

Future Directions

Further refinements are needed in neuropsychological assessment. For example, traditional measures of academic achievement and behavioral functioning may not be sensitive to posttraumatic deficits. Ecologically valid measures of cognitive and behavioral functioning that reflect behaviors needed for successful functioning in school and social environments are lacking. Neuropsychological measures that more specifically evaluate brain-injured children's ability to attend to, process,

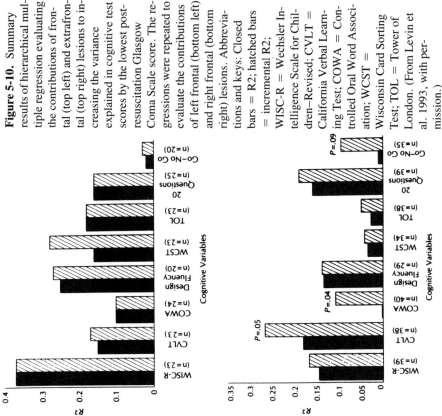

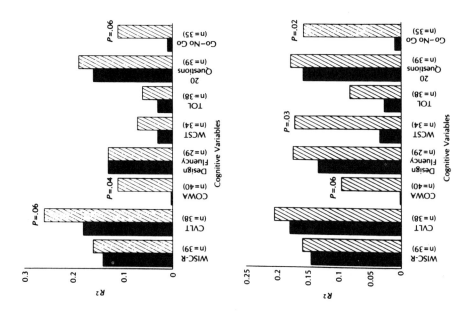

Figure 5-10. Summary results of hierarchical multiple regression evaluating the contributions of frontal (top left) and extrafrontal (top right) lesions to increasing the variance explained in cognitive test scores by the lowest postresuscitation Glasgow Coma Scale score. The regressions were repeated to evaluate the contributions of left frontal (bottom left) and right frontal (bottom right) lesions. Abbreviations and keys: Closed bars = R2; hatched bars = incremental R2; WISC-R = Wechsler Intelligence Scale for Children–Revised; CVLT = California Verbal Learning Test; COWA = Controlled Oral Word Association; WCST = Wisconsin Card Sorting Test; TOL = Tower of London. (From Levin et al. 1993, with permission.)

90

and organize information would likely be more sensitive to the types of cognitive deficits that seem to interfere with success in school and home environments. Given the importance of school functioning, future assessments should emphasize cognitive skills required for school success, such as reading larger segments of text, abstracting the gist, and organizing information logically, in addition to measures of attentional and executive functions.

Most studies of neurobehavioral and neuropsychological outcome to date have emphasized group trends. However, a sole focus on group data may obscure significant individual differences apparent in recovery curves of subtypes of patients. Statistical methods for modeling individual growth curves, such as those discussed by Fletcher and colleagues in this volume, may provide new approaches to studying recovery and individual change.

Neuropsychological studies often do not directly investigate the impact of moderator variables such as socioeconomic status and family environment on outcome measures. By carefully relating neurological, neuropsychological, and socioenvironmental data through a developmental model, the influence of moderator variables on outcome will be addressed more directly. It will be important to determine whether such variables make independent and additive contributions to behavioral outcome or whether specific interactions between biological and environmental variables best account for developmental outcomes.

Long-term follow-up of infants, preschoolers, and school-aged children is particularly needed to identify the presence of possible delayed deficits such as those identified in monkeys by Goldman on measures of executive function (Goldman, 1974). Since our research has identified differences in outcome attributable to a child's developmental level at the time of injury, it will be very important to track children longitudinally through adolescence to see if the symptom patterns evolve over time.

Multidisciplinary investigation is needed to develop a global measure of outcome suitable for a wide age range in the pediatric head injury population. Further investigation of the relationship of theoretically derived cognitive measures (e.g., Tower of London) to more conventional tests of intellectual function is indicated to determine their relative contributions to elucidating the relationship between the pathophysiology and outcome of CHI. Emerging technologies for minimally invasive functional brain imaging provide opportunities to investigate the substrate for the neurobehavioral sequelae of CHI in children, the process of functional reorganization, and the impact of rehabilitation on cognitive and psychosocial development of head-injured children.

Acknowledgments

Preparation of this chapter was supported by NIH Grant NS-21889. The authors are also indebted to Gail Ober for word processing assistance.

References

Baddeley, A. (1992). Working memory. *Science, 255,* 556–559.

Bruce, D. A., Raphaely, R. C., Goldberg, A. I., Zimmerman, R. A., Bilaniuk, L. T., Schut, L., & Kuhl, D. E. (1979). Pathophysiology, treatment and outcome following severe head injury in children. *Childs Brain, 2,* 174–191.

Bruce, D. A., Schut, L., Brown, L. A., Wood, J. H., & Sutton, L. N. (1980). Outcome following severe head injury in children. *J. Neurosurg., 97,* 721–727.

Buschke, H. (1974). Components of verbal learning in children: Analysis by selective reminding. *J. Exp. Child Psychol., 18,* 488–495.

Chadwick, O., Rutter, M., Shaffer, D., & Shrout, P. E. (1981). A prospective study of children with head injuries: IV. Specific cognitive deficits. *J. Clin. Neuropsychol. 3,* 101–120.

Damasio, H. (1991). Neuroanatomy of frontal lobe in vivo: A comment on methodology. In H. S. Levin, H. M. Eisenberg, & A. L. Benton (Eds.), *Frontal lobe function and dysfunction.* New York: Oxford University Press.

Ewing-Cobbs, L., Fletcher, J. M., & Levin, H. S. (1989). Intellectual, motor, and language sequelae following closed head injury in infants and preschoolers. *J. Pediatr. Psychol., 14,* 531–547.

Ewing-Cobbs, L., Levin, H. S., Eisenberg, H. M., & Fletcher, J. M. (1987). Language functions following closed-head injury in children and adolescents. *J. Clin. Exp. Neuropsychol., 9,* 575–592.

Ewing-Cobbs, L., Levin, H. S., Fletcher, J. M., Miner, M. E., & Eisenberg, H. M. (1990). The Children's Orientation and Amnesia Test: Relationship to severity of acute head injury and to recovery of memory. *Neurosurgery, 27,* 683–691.

Ewing-Cobbs, L., Thompson, N. M., Miner, M. E., & Fletcher, J. M. (1994). Gunshot wounds to the brain in children and adolescents: Age and neurobehavioral development. *Neurosurgery, 35,* 225–233.

Goldman, P. S. (1974). An alternative to developmental plasticity: Heterology of CNS structures in infants and adults. In D. G. Stein, J. R. Rosen, & N. Butters (Eds.), *Plasticity and recovery of function in the central nervous system* (pp. 149–174). New York: Academic Press.

Hannay, H. J., Levin, H. S., & Grossman, R. G. (1979). Impaired recognition memory after head injury. *Cortex, 15,* 269–283.

Hecaen, H. (1976). Acquired aphasia in children and the otogenesis of hemispheric specialization. *Brain Lang., 3,* 114–134.

Jennett, B., & Bond, M. (1975). Assessment of outcome after severe brain damage. *Lancet, 1,* 480–487.

Kaufmann, P. M., Fletcher, J. M., Levin, H. S., Miner, M. E., & Ewing-Cobbs, L. (1993). Attentional disturbance after pediatric closed head injury. *J. Child Neurol., 8,* 348–353.

Levin, H. S., Aldrich, E. F., Saydjari, C., Eisenberg, H. M., Foulkes, M. A., Bellefleur, M., Jane, J. A., Marmarou, A., Marshall, L. F., & Young, H. (1992). Severe head injury in children: Experience of the Traumatic Coma Data Bank. *Neurosurgery, 31,* 435–444.

Levin, H. S., Amparo, E. G., Eisenberg, H. M., Miner, M. E., High, W. M. Jr., Ewing-Cobbs, L., Fletcher, J. M., & Guinto, F. C. Jr. (1989). Magnetic resonance imaging after closed head injury in children. *Neurosurgery, 24,* 223–227.

Levin, H. S., Culhane, K. A., Mendelsohn, D., Lilly, M. A., Bruce, D., Fletcher, J. M., Chapman, S. B., Harward, H., & Eisenberg, H. M. (1993). Cognition in relation to magnetic resonance imaging in head-injured children and adolescents. *Arch. Neurol., 50,* 897–905.

Levin, H. S., & Eisenberg, H. M. (1979a). Neuropsychological impairment after closed head injury in children and adolescents. *J. Pediatr. Psychol., 4,* 389–402.

Levin, H. S., & Eisenberg, H. M. (1979b). Neuropsychological outcome of closed head injury in children and adolescents. *Childs Brain, 5,* 1–10.

Levin, H. S., Eisenberg, H. M., Wigg, N. R., & Kobayashi, K. (1982). Memory and intellectual ability after head injury in children and adolescents. *Neurosurgery, 11,* 668–673.

Levin, H. S., High, W. M. Jr., Ewing-Cobbs, L., Fletcher, J. M., Eisenberg, H. M., Miner, M. E., & Goldstein, F. C. (1988). Memory functioning during the first year after closed head injury in children and adolescents. *Neurosurgery, 22,* 1043–1052.

Levin, H. S., O'Donnell, V. M., & Grossman, R. G. (1979). The Galveston Orientation and Amnesia Test. A practical scale to assess cognition after head injury. *J. Nerv. Ment. Dis., 167,* 675–684.

Russell, W. R., & Smith, A. (1961). Post-traumatic amnesia and closed head injury. *Arch. Neurol., 5,* 4–17.

Rutter, M., Chadwick, O., Shaffer, D., & Brown, G. (1980). A prospective study of children with head injuries: I. Design and methods. *Psychol. Med., 10,* 633–645.

Spreen, O., & Benton, A. L. (1969). *Neurosensory center comprehensive examination for aphasia: Manual of directions.* Victoria, BC: Neuropsychology Laboratory, University of Victoria.

Teasdale, G., & Jennett, B. (1974). Assessment of coma and impaired consciousness: A practical scale. *Lancet, 2,* 81–84.

Appendix: Children's Orientation and Amnesia Test (COAT)

General Orientation:

1. What is your name? first (2) _____   (5) _____
   last (3) _____
2. How old are you? (3) _____ When is your birthday?
   month (1) _____ day (1) _____   (5) _____
3. Where you you live? city (3) _____
   state (2) _____   (5) _____
4. What is your father's name? (5) _____
   What is your mother's name? (5) _____   (10) _____
5. What school do you go to? (3) _____   (5) _____
   What grade are you in? (2) _____
6. Where are you now? (5) _____   (5) _____
   (May rephrase question: Are you at home now? Are you in the
   hospital? If rephrased, child must correctly answer both questions
   to receive credit.)
7. Is it daytime or nighttime? (5) _____   (5) _____

General Orientation Total

Temporal Orientation: (administer if age 8–15)

8. What time is it now? (5) ————————————————   (5) ————
    (correct = 5; <hr. off = 4; 1 hr. off = 3; >1 hr. off = 2; 2 hrs.
    off = 1)
9. What day of the week is it? (5) ————————————   (5) ————
    (correct = 5; 1 off = 4; 2 off = 3; 3 off = 2; 4 off = 1)
10. What day of the month is it? (5) ———————————   (5) ————
    (correct = 5; 1 off = 4; 2 off = 3; 3 off = 2; 4 off = 1)
11. What is the month? (10) ————————————————   (10) ————
    (correct = 10; 1 off = 7; 2 off = 4; 3 off = 1)
12. What is the year? (15) ————————————————   (15) ————
    (correct = 15; 1 off = 10; 2 off = 5; 3 off = 1)

                         Temporal Orientation Total   ————

Memory:

13. Say these numbers after me in the same order. (Discontinue
    when the child fails both series of digits at any length. Score 2
    points if both digit series are correctly repeated; score 1 point if
    only 1 is correct.)

3	5 ————	35296	81493 ————	
58	42 ————	539418	724856 ————	
643	926 ————	8129365	4739128 ————	(14) ————
7216	3279 ————			

14. How many fingers am I holding up? Two fingers (2)————
    three fingers (3) ———————— 10 fingers (5) ————————   (10) ————
15. Who is on Sesame Street? (10) ————————————   (10) ————
    (can substitute other major television show)
16. What is my name? (10)————————————————   (10) ————

                                     Memory Total   ————
                                    OVERALL TOTAL   ————

From Ewing-Cobbs et al. 1990, with permission.

6

Discourse as an Outcome Measure in Pediatric Head-Injured Populations

SANDRA BOND CHAPMAN

Until recently, the prognosis for language recovery after a closed head injury (CHI) was viewed as highly favorable. This optimistic view was based on evidence of considerable improvement in language comprehension and production during the first 6 months after injury (Groher, 1977; Thomsen, 1975). Despite the evidence of relatively intact language systems within 6 months of the injury, however, a residual impairment in discourse was often noted (Groher, 1977; Levin et al., 1981; Sarno, 1980, 1984).

The subjective observation that discourse was often impaired after CHI despite adequate vocabulary and syntax underscored the fact that producing connected language (discourse) was not merely a "bottoms up" process. Indeed, discourse production is a complex process that cannot be explained by looking solely at the individual linguistic components. Prior to the 1970s, however, methodological approaches for characterizing suprasentential language were essentially nonexistent. Abstract constructs of discourse have only recently been identified and applied to the investigation of discourse ability in normal and brain-damaged populations.

Nature of Discourse

Definition

Discourse can be defined as a series of ideas typically expressed in sentences that serve the communicative function of conveying a message (Ulatowska et al., 1990). Discourse genres such as the narrative, procedural, or conversational have unique properties that define acceptability or coherence of their structure and content. The most extensively studied discourse type is narrative, which is the genre of interest in this chapter. Narrative discourse tells a story or relates an event oriented around

95

characters. Our group has investigated narrative discourse in pediatric CHI populations because it is developed early in life, is the most common discourse type, and
involves a complex interaction between language and cognition.

When the original models of discourse were being developed, they were characterized according to the language structures comprised by the discourse text,
such as individual words, clauses, and sentences. However, these models failed
to explain how individuals processed discourse. They processed discourse into
more global units of meaning (information structures) than were reflected in the
specific vocabulary and sentences (Kintsch & van Dijk, 1978).

Discourse Processing Model

Other discourse models were developed to include both information structures
and linguistic structures (Frederiksen & Stemmer, 1993). A conceptual schema
representing the components of discourse is illustrated in Figure 6-1. As depicted,
discourse representation can be described at multiple levels, some relating to language structures and some to information structures.

Information Structures. Whereas the linguistic structures are widely understood
and represent the building blocks of discourse, the information structures have
only recently been defined and reflect the more global organization of chunks of
language. The information structures used in this chapter include propositions,
superstructure, and macrostructure. A *proposition* represents a unit of meaning
that is conveyed through language structures but is not tied to specific vocabulary
or sentential form (Kintsch & van Dijk, 1978). A discourse *superstructure* represents a conventional organizing schema for discourse that varies across genre types
such as narratives, procedures, jokes, and letters, to mention a few. The most
canonical organization schema for a narrative is defined by episodic structure and
includes the components of setting, complicating action, and resolution (Labov,
1972). The superstructure defines the organization of information but not the spe-

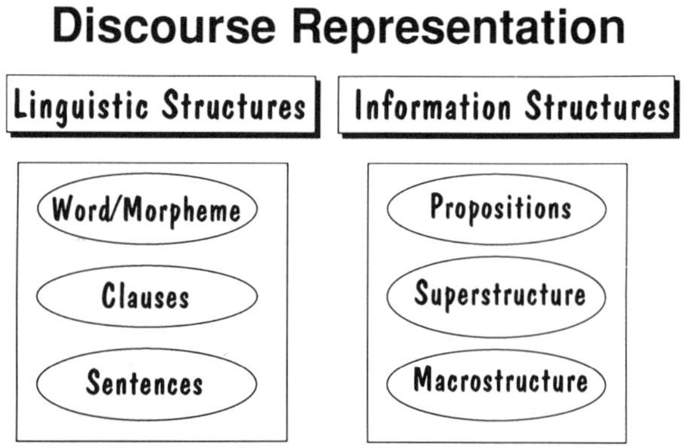

Discourse Representation

| Linguistic Structures | Information Structures |

Word/Morpheme	Propositions
Clauses	Superstructure
Sentences	Macrostructure

Figure 6-1. Multilevel discourse representation for language and information structures.

cific content. Discourse *macrostructures* organize all the propositions of a text into a higher level of semantic meaning and are expressed at different levels of generalization. Macrostructures are understood by notions such as theme, topic, main ideas or gist, and summaries, each of which involves selectively reducing the information while maintaining the central meaning (van Dijk, 1985). Examples of propositions, superstructure, and macrostructure appear in Appendix I.

Application. The recent development of methodologies for measuring discourse ability has made possible the study of differential breakdown and preservation of language and information structures. Multilevel discourse analysis, while tedious, has proven useful in analyzing individual and group differences in discourse processing in a variety of brain-damaged patient populations (Frederiksen & Stemmer, 1993; Glosser, 1993; Myers, 1993; Ska & Guenard, 1993).

Significance of Discourse Studies

During the last decade, researchers in psychology and language have applied discourse models to elucidate brain-language relations because of the explanatory power of discourse structures in documenting differential impairment of linguistic or conceptual factors (Joanette & Brownell, 1990). Studies of adult patients with left hemisphere lesions resulting in aphasia have revealed relative preservation of information structures despite marked impairment in linguistic abilities (Huber, 1990; Ulatowska et al., 1990; Ulatowska et al., 1983). In patient populations with less obvious language problems, such as dementia and stroke to the right hemisphere, information structures were found to be impaired relative to intact linguistic structures in discourse (Myers, 1993; Ska & Guenard, 1993; Ulatowska & Chapman, 1991).

Discourse Studies in Closed Head Injury

Recent discourse studies in head-injured populations suggest that discourse measures provide a way of examining the impact of cognitive and linguistic deficits on communication (Chapman et al., 1992; Chapman et al., in press; Dennis & Barnes, 1990; Dennis et al., 1994). Discourse studies in CHI populations revealed impairment in information structures manifesting itself by reduction of propositions, impairment of superstructure, and impairment of macrostructure (Glosser & Deser, 1990; Hartley & Jensen, 1991; Mentis & Prutting, 1991). For the most part, the linguistic structures of CHI patients were relatively preserved.

Compared to discourse studies in head-injured adults, there has been limited research on discourse in pediatric CHI populations. Dennis and Barnes (1990) identified discourse problems in most of their pediatric CHI patients. The problems were identified on separate tasks involving interpreting ambiguous sentences and metaphors, drawing inferences from a stereotypic event sequence, and generating sentences from key words.

The findings regarding discourse abilities in CHI children are equivocal. Jordan and coworkers (1991) found no significant differences among mild or severe CHI patients and normal individuals on narrative discourse measures of linguistic structures and information structures. Moreover, Campbell and Dollaghan (1990) failed to find significant deficits in a severely impaired CHI pediatric sample. These researchers suggested that the group data may have obscured individual differences, since over half the subjects (5 of 9) showed marked deficits 1 year after injury. Also, the measures used in this study involved linguistic structures at lexical and sentential levels. No measures of information organization were used.

Relevant Variables in Discourse Studies

While the prevailing view is that discourse is impaired following CHI in children, few studies have examined this claim. Discourse abilities in pediatric populations have not been studied systematically according to a number of variables including severity of injury, age of injury, stage of recovery (acute versus chronic) and pathophysiological profile (Dennis & Lovett, 1990).

Injury Variables

Severity and Pathophysiological Profile. Overall severity of injury as reflected by coma duration has been shown to be a reliable predictor of neurobehavioral outcome (Levin et al., 1981; Rutter et al., 1983).

An association between the presence, site, and size of mass lesions and outcome has been documented (Becker et al., 1982). With regard to language, the long-term outcome of posttraumatic language disruption is related to residual focal lesions (e.g., gliosis) superimposed on diffuse insult (Chapman et al., 1995). Damage to the frontal lobe is of particular interest, since it is the most common site of focal lesions in CHI (Adams et al., 1980). Discourse formulation deficits have been associated with frontal lobe damage in adults (Alexander et al., 1989; Kaczmarek, 1984; Stuss et al., 1978). The contribution of frontal injuries to discourse disability warrants investigation in pediatric CHI populations.

Age at Injury and Development of Discourse. Age at the time of injury is also relevant to understanding the recovery of discourse abilities in pediatric populations. Neurobehavioral recovery in children is influenced by how growth and development proceed in an injured brain (Fletcher et al., 1987). Of particular interest is the stage of discourse development at the time of injury, since language abilities in a rapid stage of development may be more vulnerable to brain injury than well-established abilities (Ewing-Cobbs et al., 1987).

Several critical stages in discourse development have been identified. Children are able to refer to past events by age 2 and to combine two events by age 3½. By age 4 to 5, normal children appear to have the cognitive and linguistic structures that enable them to produce well-structured stories (Applebee, 1978;

Westby, 1984). Elaborated narratives developed around a central theme with clear expression of causal relation are established by ages 9 to 10. Discourse recovery in pediatric populations must be examined using a developmental approach that focuses on rate, sequence, and transition effects. Children may have to recover from brain injury again and again at each subsequent stage of neurolinguistic development (Bates et al., 1992).

Summary of Discourse Studies

From a theoretical perspective, narrative discourse models are developed with enough specificity to establish measures to objectively characterize discourse ability in pediatric CHI populations. This chapter summarizes the particular discourse methodology used in our studies, followed by the findings from group and individual analyses of discourse. The issues considered include the following:

Research Questions

1. *Is narrative discourse impaired in CHI pediatric populations at 1 year postinjury according to severity of impaired consciousness and age at evaluation?*

   This question is relevant to determining whether deficits exist at a discourse level at chronic stages of recovery—a stage of recovery at which performance on traditional language measures is often normal. Additionally, this question addresses whether discourse measures are sensitive to deficits at different age levels in children and adolescents.
2. *Is narrative discourse more vulnerable in early versus late pediatric CHI?*

   This question asks whether children injured prior to the stage that basic story structure is well established (≤4 years) are more vulnerable than children injured after that stage.
3. *Is narrative discourse differentially impaired in CHI patients with frontal lobe injury superimposed on diffuse injury as opposed to those without frontal injury?*

   This question asks whether grouping patients according to pathophysiological profile helps define more homogeneous subgroups.
4. *Is there a relation between ability to organize discourse and ability to perform cognitive measures of organization?*

   This question asks whether deficits in organization can be seen across various tasks, reflecting possible association between global organizing strategies.

Discourse Method

Stimuli. The discourse tasks used in our studies, described below, varied across experiments. In the early studies, we used two comparable complex adventure stories—"Buried Alive" and "Shipwrecked" (Appendix II)—taken from the Xerox Education Publication and modified by Merritt and Liles (1987). These two stories were comparable in length and complexity of language (number of clauses, 45; number of sentences, 28) and in the amount of information (number of informational units or propositions, approximately 66; number of episodes, 4). In later studies, the discourse stories were altered to include less complex stories because pilot testing revealed that the original narratives were too difficult for normal children younger than age 8. Our goal was to include experimental stories that would show developmental changes through adolescence. In later studies, five stories were elicited, two presented auditorally and three visually. Performance on two stories has recently been analyzed and is reported in this chapter. These two stories were similar in length and complexity (16 propositions; 1 episode). The stories were comparable in the global semantic meaning (macrostructure) in that both stories portrayed a role-reversal situation of the main characters. One story involved retelling a verbally presented story ("The Rooster Story") and the other was elicited using five picture sequence cards ("The Cat Story").

Measures. The same methodology was used to assess all stories, using an approach developed by Ulatowska and colleagues and modified for our purposes (Ulatowska et al., 1981). The stories were analyzed according to the components-of-discourse representation for language and information structure domains (Figure 6-1). *Language structure* was assessed on four measures, including number of words, number of sentences, mean length of sentences, and complexity of sentences as reflected in the number of dependent clauses relative to the number of sentences.

The *information structure* measures included number of propositions or units of information, story structure or episodic structure, and global story content or gist/macrostructure. The measure of propositions involved comparing the propositions in the original story against the propositions produced by the individual subjects. That is, the children's story productions were matched against the a priori template of propositions. Story structure was measured by inclusion of the essential components of setting, action, and resolution. Just as the sentential grammar defines the necessary components for a well-formed sentence, the superstructure or story structure defines the necessary components for a well-formed story without specifying the content. The gist measure consisted of a smaller set of propositions established a priori as the essential information for conveying the central meaning of the story. For the cat and rooster stories, the gist measure represented the necessary information for conveying the role reversal of the main characters.

Subjects. All children were selected for study from the consecutive admissions to the neurosurgery service at Parkland Hospital, Dallas, and John Sealy Hospital, Galveston, Texas. All subjects were part of a larger study investigating long-term recovery of cognition-related to frontal lobe function. Criteria for admission in the larger study were (1) current age between 6 and 18 years; (2) a postinjury interval of 1 to 5 years; (3) no prior diagnosis of learning disability or other neuropsychiatric disorder; and (4) no evidence of child abuse. All CHI children underwent magnetic resonance imaging (MRI) within 1 month of the discourse assessment. Injury severity was assessed using the lowest postresuscitation Glasgow Coma Scale (GCS) score of Teasdale and Jennett (1974). If the GCS score was greater than 8, CHI was classified as mild/moderate. A GCS score of 8 or less was indicative of a severe head injury producing coma.

Discourse Outcome in Older and Younger Children with Closed Head Injury

Older Children. In a recent study of discourse processing in CHI, the effects of injury severity on narrative discourse were examined in children 9 years of age and older (Chapman et al., 1992). The patient population included three groups: a group of severely head-injured children and adolescents ($n = 9$; GCS $\leqslant 8$), a mild/moderate head-injured group ($n = 11$; GCS > 8), and a normal control group selected from the same local community comparable in age, gender, and socioeconomic levels ($n = 20$). At the time of testing, the subjects were within 1 to 5 years postinjury. The discourse task involved retelling one of the complex narratives described previously (Appendix II).

The results revealed persistent problems in discourse on measures of both language and information structures for children who had sustained a severe CHI at least 1 year earlier. On the language structures, the subjects with severe CHI produced fewer words and sentences than the mild/moderate CHI group and the normal control group (Figures 6-2 and 6-3). However, no significant differences were found for the measure of sentential complexity across groups. Thus, despite a reduction of language in the severe-CHI population, the brain injury did not have a long-term effect on the complexity of the sentences used.

On the measures of information organization, discourse performance for the children with severe CHI showed a significant reduction in the amount of information and significant deficits in organizational structure (superstructure) as well as in global semantic content (macrostructure) compared with both the mild/moderate CHI and normal control groups. Figure 6-4 shows the reduction of story information (propositions) and the impairment in producing complete episodes.

In seeking explanations for these findings, the roles of vocabulary and memory deficits were considered. It seems highly plausible that vocabulary deficits would be directly related to ability to manipulate language at a discourse level. Additionally, memory is an important variable because the experimental task involved retelling a relatively long story. The group effect on the vocabulary subtest from the Wechsler Intelligence Scale for Children—Revised (WISC-R) (Wechsler, 1974) approached significance ($p = 0.083$), but the differences on a measure of working memory, the first trial of the California Verbal Learning Test (CVLT)—Children's Version (Delis et al., 1987) were less impressive ($p = 0.2703$). Furthermore, the effects of injury severity on story recall remained significant ($p = 0.006$) even after controlling for memory scores. We concluded that the discourse deficits identified in the severe-CHI group could not be accounted for entirely by a disturbance in either vocabulary or working memory.

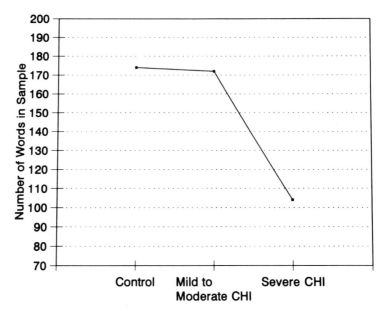

Figure 6-2. Amount of language in story retell as measured by number of words across three populations (9–18 years).

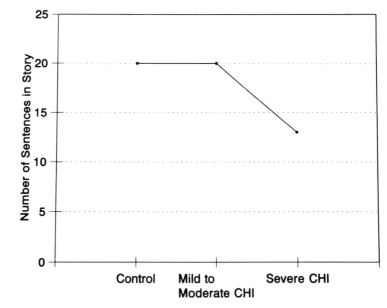

Figure 6-3. Amount of language in story retell as measured by number of sentences.

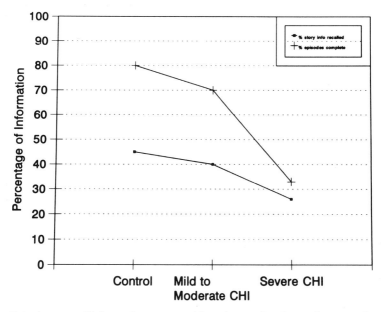

Figure 6-4. Amount of information or propositions (squares) and completeness of episodes as measured by the story components (crosses): setting, action, resolution in story retell.

Younger Children with CHI. In a more recent study (Chapman et al., in press), the long-term effects of severe head injury on discourse were examined in a younger group of children, between ages 6 and 8. The CHI group consisted of 23 children who sustained a severe head injury (GCS ≤ 8) at least 1 year prior to assessment of discourse. The control group (*n* = 26) did not differ from the head-injured group in age, gender, or socioeconomic level. Both subject groups were selected from the larger study of long-term cognitive recovery. The experimental discourse tasks for this study involved the two less complex narratives, i.e., "The Rooster Story" (Appendix I) and "The Cat Story."

In contrast to our findings in older severely injured children, group differences on all the language measures failed to reach significance for this younger sample. It is important to note that the complexity of the sentences did not differ between head-injured and control subjects for the older or younger samples. As in the older group, significant differences were found in information structure. The younger CHI group showed significant deficits on all the measures of information structure for both the visual (cat story) and auditory (rooster story) narratives. The differences between the CHI and control groups were highly significant for amount of information, ability to organize information within the story structure, and the ability to retain the most important information as reflected in the macrostructure/global story content.

The pattern-of-discourse deficits could not be accounted for solely on the basis of vocabulary or memory deficits. Although the CHI and control groups differed on the vocabulary and verbal memory measures, the effects of head injury on discourse remained significant in the analysis of variance even after controlling for these measures [$F(3,41) = 14.12; p = 30.0005$].

In summary, the findings from these two studies indicate that both younger children and older children and adolescents with severe head injuries show discourse problems at 1 year or more after injury. Perhaps the most important implication of our studies is the value of applying theoretical models of discourse processing for the analysis of communicative breakdown in pediatric CHI populations. Despite the frequent observation that CHI patients have problems in producing coherent discourse, it has been difficult to characterize these deficits empirically.

Relationship of Age to Discourse Outcome

Age at the time of injury is relevant to understanding the recovery processes in pediatric head-injured populations. The core question is whether children with early versus late injuries differ in long-term recovery. To investigate this issue, the sample of severely head-injured (GCS ≤ 8) young children, between 6 and 8 years of age, in the previously cited study (Chapman et al., in press) was divided into those who were injured before age 4 ($n = 9$) and those who were older at the

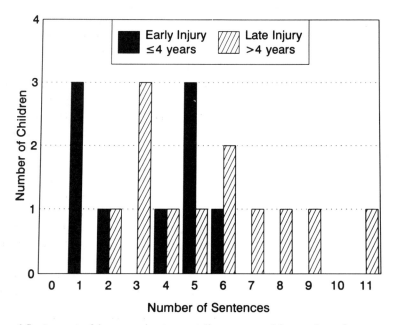

Figure 6-5. Amount of language in story retell as measured by number of sentences for early- and late-injured children. For example, three of the early-injured children produced only one sentence in their story retell.

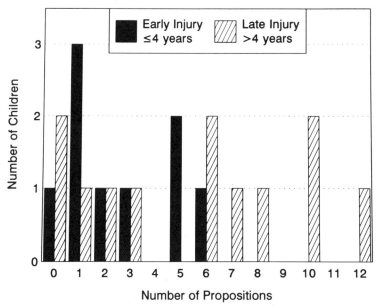

Figure 6-6. Amount of information (propositions) in story retell for individual children according to early versus late injury. For example, seven of the late-injured children produced six or more propositions and only one early-injured child produced six or more.

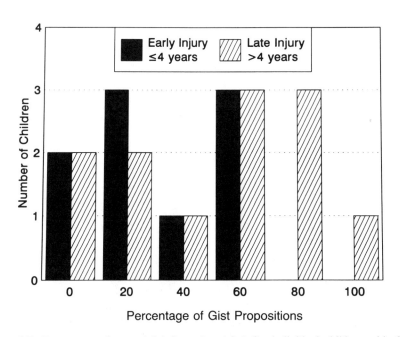

Figure 6-7. Percentage of essential information (gist) for individual children with CHI according to early versus late injury. For example, seven of the late-injured children produced 60% or more of the gist information and three of the early injured produced 60%.

time of injury ($n = 12$). No significant differences were found between groups in age at time of testing, gender, or socioeconomic level.

The preliminary pattern of scores for individual children reflected greater deficits in the early-injury group than the late-injury group. The early-injury group tended to perform worse on both language and information structures. As illustrated in Figures 6-5, 6-6, and 6-7, the early-injured children clustered at the lower end, indicating a tendency to produce less language, less propositional information, and less of the essential information (gist). No significant group differences were found on more structured measures of vocabulary (i.e., WISC-R, vocabularly subtest) and working memory (CVLT, children's Version, trial 1).

These results must to be interpreted cautiously due to the small sample size. Nonetheless, the consistent pattern of lower performance in the early-injured children suggests that injuries in young children may have a more deleterious effect on discourse recovery than injuries in older children.

Frontal Lobe Lesions and Discourse Ability

The case-study approach may help to elucidate certain effects of frontal lobe damage on discourse. Data averaging in groups with heterogeneous injuries can obscure distinct patterns of impairment evident in individual patients (Martin, 1990). To examine whether a relationship exists between frontal lobe injury and discourse, individual CHI cases were selected based on their MRI findings. The discourse samples were analyzed without knowledge of the MRI interpretations.

In the study of Chapman and colleagues (1992) of discourse in older children, 9 of the 13 CHI children with moderate to severe injuries manifested focal abnormalities on MRI, with 7 exhibiting frontal lobe lesions or atrophy. Of the 7 with frontal lobe involvement, 3 were chosen for study because of the relatively large size of their frontal lesions. Patients 1 and 2 had left frontal lesions. The lesion of patient 1 involved primarily the left gyrus rectus and that of patient 2 was located in the left middle and superior frontal gyri. Patient 3 exhibited involvement of the right superior and orbital frontal gyri. All three children had severe injuries (GCS 3, 6, and 4, respectively) and were in special education or resource classes at school. Stories produced by one normal control and by these three patients appear in Appendices III and IV.

Figure 6-8 depicts the relationship among scores on discourse components for the three CHI patients with MRI findings that included large frontal lobe injuries and the mean scores for the severely injured CHI group as a whole. The three children with large frontal injuries exhibited defects greater than those of the severely injured group in ability to organize information, as indicated by greater omission of essential story components (setting, complicating action, resolution, and evaluation) in ability to retain the central meaning as reflected in the macrostructure (gist), and in the number of complete episodes produced.

The children with large left and right frontal lobe injuries differed considerably in the language domain. The child with right frontal damage did not show a reduction in the amount and complexity of language relative to controls, as did the two children with left frontal damage. All three patients, however, showed a similar disruption in information structure, despite a relative preservation of the amount of language in the patient with right frontal damage.

Relation between Discourse and Cognitive Variables

To broaden our understanding of the discourse impairment in pediatric CHI populations, we investigated the relationship between the ability to organize discourse for stories and performance on more traditional cognitive tasks that rely on application of organizational schemas (Culhane et al., submitted). The subjects consisted of a group of 35 children and adolescents with CHI and a group of 58 uninjured controls taken from the larger study of cognitive recovery in pediatric CHI populations. Ages ranged from 9 to 18 years. The two groups did not differ significantly in gender, age, or indices of parental socioeconomic status.

The discourse stimuli involved the complex auditory retell narratives used in the study of Chapman and coworkers (1992). A composite discourse organization variable was constructed from two measures of information organization, i.e., episodic structure and macrostructure. These two measures represent the organization of the narrative information, with episodic structure defining the form of the story and macrostructure defining the global semantic meaning or gist of the story.

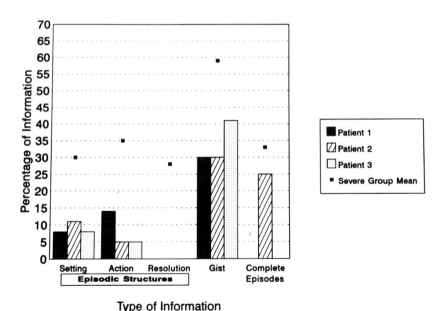

Type of Information

Figure 6-8. Comparison of three CHI subjects with frontal lobe damage to mean scores for the severely injured CHI group (*n* = 9) on the percentage of information for the story components of setting, action, and resolution, for gist, and the percentage of complete episodes.

A composite cognitive variable was made up of four neuropsychological tasks that were related to a semantic organization factor in a principal components analysis (Levin et al., 1991). The tasks were the Twenty Questions task (Denny & Denny, 1973), California Verbal Learning Test (CVLT)—Children's Version (Delis et al., 1987), semantic naming (i.e., naming animals in 90 seconds), and word fluency (i.e., generating words beginning with the letters F, A, and S).

All tasks involved verbal responses from which the subject's ability to use semantic organizing principles was assessed. For the Twenty Questions task, a stimulus card is used with 42 color pictures depicting items that can be grouped in various ways such as category, color, or function. The child is asked to determine which item the examiner has in mind by asking as few yes-no questions as possible. The measure of interest is the proportion of questions that refer to more than a single picture (e.g., "Is it an animal?" versus "Is it a dog?"). For the CVLT, the measure used was the percentage of responses that were clustered according to semantic category (i.e., fruit, clothing, and toys).

Nonverbal cognitive measures were also administered to determine whether discourse deficits simply reflect a generalized cognitive impairment or whether cognitive measures involving verbal semantic organizing principles are the better predictors of discourse ability. The nonverbal cognitive measures were the Tower of London task (Shallice, 1982), the Wisconsin Card Sorting test (Grant & Berg, 1948), and the Block Design subtest from the WISC-R (Wechsler, 1974).

The results showed that the composite cognitive variable significantly improved prediction on the composite discourse variable for both head-injured and control children (R^2 change = 0.055, $p < 0.01$). This improvement was over and above what could be explained by the nonverbal cognitive measures.

Discussion

The findings reviewed here support the use of narrative discourse structures as measures of neurobehavioral outcome after head injury in pediatric populations. The sensitivity of narrative discourse measures is apparent in the empirical documentation of reduced narrative abilities in populations with severe CHI at 1 year postinjury and beyond. The narrative disruptions were apparent at long-term follow-up in younger children and in older adolescents who had sustained a severe head injury (GCS ≤ 8). Discourse measures showed promise in documenting age-at-injury effects in young, severely head-injured children. The possibility of differences in discourse abilities in individual CHI patients with frontal lobe pathology warrants further investigation. The more severe discourse impairments were identified in individuals with focal frontal lesions superimposed on diffuse injury. Also, discourse patterns found in individual CHI patients suggest that the frontal lobes may contribute to the nature of the discourse impairment. This relationship may reflect frontal system dysfunction associated with areas of abnormal signal identified in various sites of the prefrontal region. Finally, preliminary evidence suggests that a relationship may exist between organized discourse and verbal cognitive tasks involving organizing principles. If the underlying processing deficits are the same, this information would be valuable in developing more integrated diagnostic and treatment paradigms.

There has been little research on discourse processing in head-injured pediatric populations. The models of narrative organization and its analysis were developed by linguists and psycholinguists relatively recently. These constructs have been applied to special populations such as CHI, hydrocephalic, and language-impaired children even more recently. Our studies extend the findings of Dennis and Barnes (1990), who identified problems on structured tasks relevant to discourse processing in nearly 80% of their head-injured population between 6 and 22 years of age. In contrast to our findings, Jordan and associates (1991) did not find significant differences among three groups of mild-CHI, severe-CHI, and matched control children on measures of story grammar and use of intersentential cohesive devices. This disparity may be due to task differences or to differences in how severity was specified. The task used by Jordan and colleagues (1991) involved generating a spontaneous narrative about a toy soldier, the G.I. Joe figure. The tasks for our studies required the subject to retell a verbal story and to generate a story given a sequence of pictures.

Creating a story would appear to be a more difficult task than retelling a story. One would expect to find greater deficits in the severely head-injured groups than in the mild-CHI or normal control children, so it is difficult to explain why no differences were found by Jordan. One possibility is that head-injured children may experience more problems in story productions when the semantic content is constrained, as in a retell task elicited by verbal or pictorial stimuli. In the more semantically constrained task, the child must comprehend the story, hold the information in short-term working memory, and then transform the story information into his or her own words, since individuals rarely retell a story verbatim. The examination of discrepancies among discourse studies can provide important insight into differences attributable to task demands.

Narrative discourse measures may provide a useful methodology for examining whether children injured early in development are at greater risk for discourse disabilities. If this pattern is substantiated in an empirical study, it would support the view that an injury to the brain before or during skill acquisition may have greater consequences than one occurring after skill acquisition (Dennis & Lovett, 1990; Ewing-Cobbs et al., 1989).

Clarifying whether a frontal lobe injury produces a selective discourse impairment has important implications from diagnostic and treatment perspectives. From a diagnostic perspective, the documentation of a relationship between localized areas of abnormal signal in the frontal lobes and selective discourse impairment would provide valuable information concerning the functional brain system subserving the ability to organize discourse information. From a treatment perspective, more effective rehabilitative interventions could be developed based on the relationship between the breakdown of organizing schemas and damage to the frontal lobes. Evidence from case studies suggests that discourse is more impaired when the frontal lobes are involved than when they are spared. Also, case studies suggest different impairments in discourse when the left frontal versus right frontal regions are involved. This possibility warrants investigation.

Future Directions for Research and Application to Rehabilitation

A number of issues remain to be resolved regarding discourse abilities in pediatric populations with CHI. One important issue that needs further study is whether mild to moderate head injuries affect discourse. Although no significant differences in discourse abilities were found between the mild/moderate CHI and normal control groups in our study, deficits may appear on more complex narratives or discourse genres other than narratives, such as expository discourse. We are in the process of analyzing performance in CHI populations using longer, more complex narratives that require inferences to create a story.

Another important issue is how discourse performance in children with other brain lesions (such as tumor, gunshot wound, or aneurysm) compares to discourse patterns of CHI children with similar foci of abnormal signal on MRI. This line of research would attempt to sort out the behavioral consequences associated with other brain pathologies versus those due to CHI.

With regard to recovery issues, it is not clear whether early-injured children eventually catch up to children with a later injury of similar severity. Moreover, the rate and degree of discourse recovery in children beyond 1 year after CHI is relatively unknown. The roles of injury severity, neuropathological profile, age at injury, and environmental factors will need careful investigation in tracking long-term recovery curves.

Perhaps the most important contribution of discourse studies to rehabilitation could develop from establishing relationships between discourse and certain academic abilities. Research findings in the area of learning disabilities indicate that narrative discourse is an indicator of academic ability and a precursor to reading (Roth & Spekman, 1989; Westby, 1989). Assessing narrative discourse in CHI and an association with academic performance may provide insight into why a child is failing in the classroom. The process of storytelling is similar to what goes on in a classroom setting. Story organization and manipulation of verbal text for classroom purposes may rely heavily on the ability to apply organizational schemas in order to comprehend text material (Roth & Spekman, 1989).

Discourse studies appear to have important implications for improving the quality of patient care. These measures evaluate communication abilities which are more likely to reflect language problems than the traditional structured measures such as naming. Understanding the nature of communication breakdown is an essential first step to improving the interventions of speech-language pathologists. At present, discourse as an outcome measure of functional language appears promising.

Acknowledgments

This investigation was supported by NIH Grant NS-21889. I am grateful to Lori Kusnerik and Joe Kufera for assistance in data analyses and to Cathy Smiley for assistance in manuscript preparation. I sincerely appreciate the contributions of Kathy Culhane, my research assistants (Alicia Wanek, Julie Weyrauch, Sarah Harrison), and the children and families whose commitments made these projects possible.

References

Adams, J. H., Graham, D. I., Scott, G., Parker, L. S., & Doyle, D. (1980). Brain damage in non-missile head injury. *J. Clin. Pathol., 33,* 1132–1145.

Alexander, M. P., Benson, D. F., & Stuss, D. T. (1989). Frontal lobes and language. *Brain Lang., 37,* 656–691.

Applebee, A. N. (1978). *The child's concept of story.* Chicago: University of Chicago Press.

Bates, E., Reilly, J., & Marchman, E. (1992). Discourse and grammar after early focal brain injury. Abstract from Academy of Aphasia Meeting, Toronto, October 25–27.

Becker, D. P., Miller, J. D., & Greenberg, R. P. (1982). Prognosis after head injury. In J. R. Youmans (Ed.), *Neurological surgery* (p. 2124). Philadelphia: Saunders.

Campbell, T. F., & Dollaghan, C. A. (1990). Expressive language recovery in severely brain-injured children and adolescents. *J. Speech Hearing Dis., 55,* 567–581.

Chapman, S. B., Culhane, K. A., Levin, H. S., Harward, H., Mendelsohn, D., Ewing-Cobbs, L., Fletcher, J. M., & Bruce, D. (1992). Narrative discourse after closed head injury in children and adolescents. *Brain Lang., 43,* 42–65.

Chapman, S. B., Levin, H., & Culhane, K. (1995). Language impairment in closed head injury. In H. Kirschner (Ed.), *Handbook of neurological speech and language disorders.* (pp. 387–414). New York: Marcel Dekker.

Chapman, S., Levin, H., Wanek, A., Weyrauch, J., & Kufera, J. (In press). Discourse after closed head injury in young children. *Brain Lang.*

Culhane, K., Chapman, S. B., & Levin, H. S. (submitted). The relationship of discourse and cognitive task performance following closed head injury. *Brain Cogn.*

Delis, D. C., Kramer, J. H., Kaplan, E., & Ober, B. A. (1987). *The California Verbal Learning Test—Children's Version—Research Edition.* New York: Psychological Corporation.

Dennis, M., & Barnes, M. A. (1990). Knowing the meaning, getting the point, bridging the gap, and carrying the message: Aspects of discourse following closed head injury in childhood and adolescence. *Brain Lang., 39,* 428–446.

Dennis, M., Jacennik, B., & Barnes, M. A. (1994). The content of narrative discourse in children and adolescents after early-onset hydrocephalus and in normally developing age peers. *Brain Lang., 46,* 129–165.

Dennis, M., & Lovett, M. W. (1990). Discourse ability in children after brain damage. In Y. Joanette & H. H. Brownell (Eds.), *Discourse ability and brain damage: Theoretical and empirical perspectives* (pp. 199–223). New York: Springer-Verlag.

Denny, D. R., & Denny, N. W. (1973). The use of classification for problem-solving: A comparison of middle and old age. *Dev. Psychol., 9,* 275–278.

Ewing-Cobbs, L., Levin, H. S., Eisenberg, H. M., & Fletcher, J. M. (1987). Language functions following closed-head injury in children and adolescents. *J. Clin. Exp. Neuropsychol. 9,* 575–592.

Ewing-Cobbs, L., Miner, M. E., Fletcher, J. M., & Levin, H. S. (1989). Intellectual, motor, and language sequelae following closed head injury in infants and preschoolers. *J. Pediatr. Psychol., 14,* 531–547.

Fletcher, J. M., Miner, M., & Ewing-Cobbs, L. (1987). Age and recovery from head injury in children: Developmental issues. In H. S. Levin, J. Graufman, & H. M. Eisenberg (Eds.), *Neurobehavioral recovery from head injury* (pp. 279–292). New York: Oxford University Press.

Frederiksen, C. H., & Stemmer, B. (1993). Conceptual processing of discourse by a right hemisphere brain-damaged patient. In H. H. Brownell & Y. Joanette (Eds.), *Narrative discourse in neurologically impaired and normal aging adults* (pp. 239–273). San Diego, CA: Singular Publishing Group.

Glosser, G. (1993). Discourse production patterns in neurologically impaired and aged populations. In H. H. Brownell & Y. Joanette (Eds.), *Narrative discourse in neurologically impaired and normal aging adults* (pp. 191–211). San Diego, CA: Singular Publishing Group.

Glosser, G., & Deser, T. (1990). A comparison of changes in macrolinguistic aspects of discourse production in normal aging. *J. Gerontol., 47,* 266–272.

Grant, D. A., & Berg, E. A. (1948). A behavioral analysis of degree of reinforcement and ease of shifting to new response in a Weigl-type card sorting problem. *J. Exp. Psychol., 38,* 404–411.

Groher, M. (1977). Language and memory disorders following closed head trauma. *J. Speech Hearing Res., 20,* 212–223.

Hagen, C. (1984). Language disorders in head trauma. In A. Holland (Ed.), *Language Disorders in Adults* (pp. 245–282). San Diego, CA: College Hill Press.

Hartley, L. L., & Jensen, P. J. (1991). Narrative and procedural discourse after closed head injury. *Brain Inj., 5,* 3:267–285.

Huber, W. (1990). Text comprehension and production in aphasia: Analysis in terms of micro- and macrostructure. In Y. Joanette & H. Brownell (Eds.), *Discourse ability and brain-damaged: Theoretical and empirical perspectives* (pp. 154–179). New York: Springer-Verlag.

Joanette, Y., & Brownell, H. (Eds.) (1990). *Discourse ability and brain damage.* New York: Springer-Verlag.

Jordan, F. M., Murdoch, B. E., & Buttsworth, D. L. (1991). Closed head-injured children's performance on narrative tasks. *J. Speech Hearing Res., 34,* 572–582.

Kaczmarek, B. L. J. (1984). Neurolinguistic analysis of verb utterances in patients with focal lesions of frontal lobes. *Brain Lang., 21,* 52–58.

Kintsch, W., & van Dijk, T. (1978). Toward a model of text comprehension and production. *Psycholog. Rev., 85,* 363–394.

Labov, W. (1972). *Language in the inner-city: Studies in the black vernacular.* Philadelphia: University of Pennsylvania Press.

Levin, H. S., Culhane, K. A., Hartmann, J., Evankovich, K., Mattson, A. J., Harward, H., Ringholz, G., Ewing-Cobbs, L., & Fletcher, J. (1991). Developmental changes in performance on tests of purported frontal lobe functioning. *Dev. Neuropsychol.,* *7,* 377–395.

Levin, H. S., Grossman, R. G., Sarwar, M., & Meyers, C. T. (1981). Linguistic recovery after closed head injury. *Brain Lang., 12,* 360–374.

Martin, A. (1990). Neuropsychology of Alzheimer's disease: The case for subgroups. In M. F. Schwartz (Ed.), *Modular deficits in Alzheimer-type dementia* (pp. 143–176). Cambridge, MA: MIT Press.

Mentis, M., & Prutting, C. A. (1991). Analysis of topics as illustrated in a head-injured and normal adult. *J. Speech Hearing Res., 34,* 583–595.

Merritt, D. D., & Liles, B. Z. (1987). Story grammar ability in children with and without language disorder: Story generation, story retelling, and story comprehension. *J. Speech Hearing Res., 30,* 539–552.

Myers, P. S. (1993). Narrative expressive deficits associated with right hemisphere damage. In H. H. Brownell & Y. Joanette (Eds.), *Narrative discourse in neurologically impaired and normal aging adults* (pp. 279–296). San Diego, CA: Singular Publishing Group.

Roth, F. P., & Spekman, N. J. (1989). Higher-order language processes and reading disabilities. In A. G. Kamhi & H. W. Catts (Eds.), *Reading disabilities: A developmental language perspective* (pp. 159–197). Boston/Toronto: Little, Brown.

Rutter, M., Chadwick, O., & Shaffer, D. (1983). Head injury. In M. Rutter (Ed.), *Developmental neuropsychiatry.* New York: Guilford Press.

Sarno, M. T. (1980). The nature of verbal impairment after closed head injury. *J. Nerv. Ment. Dis., 168,* 685–692.

Sarno, M. T. (1984). Verbal impairment after closed head injury: Report of a replication study. *J. Nerv. Ment. Dis., 172,* 475–479.

Shallice, T. (1982). Specific impairments of planning. *Philos. Trans. R. Soc. Lond. [Biol.]., 298,* 199–209.

Ska, B., & Guenard, D. (1993). Narrative schema in dementia of the Alzheimer's type. In H. H. Brownell & Y. Joanette (Eds.), *Narrative discourse in neurologically impaired and normal aging adults* (pp. 299–314). San Diego, CA: Singular Publishing Group.

Stuss, D. T., Alexander, M. P., Lieberman, A., & Levine, H. (1978). An extraordinary form of confabulation. *Neurology, 28,* 1166–1172.

Teasdale, G., & Jennett, B. (1974). Assessment of coma and impaired consciousness: A practical scale. *Lancet, 2,* 81–84.

Thomsen, I. V. (1975). Evaluation and outcome of aphasia in patients with severe closed head trauma. *J. Neurol. Neurosurg. Psychiatry, 3,* 713–718.

Ulatowska, H. K., Allard, L., & Chapman, S. B. (1990). Narrative and procedural discourse in aphasia. In Y. Joanette & H. H. Brownell (Eds.), *Discourse ability and brain damage.* New York: Springer-Verlag.

Ulatowska, H. K., & Chapman, S. B. (1991). Discourse studies. In R. Lubinski (Ed.), *Dementia and communication: Research and clinical implications.* Philadelphia: Decker.

Ulatowska, H. K., Freedman-Stern, R., Doyel, A. W., & Macaluso-Haynes, S. (1983). Production of narrative discourse in aphasia. *Brain Lang., 19,* 317–334.

Ulatowska, H. K., North, A. J., & Macaluso-Haynes, S. (1981). Production of narratives and procedural discourse in aphasia. *Brain Lang., 13,* 345–371.

van Kijk, van Dijk, T. T. (1985). Introduction: Discourse analysis as a new cross-discipline. In T. van Dijk (Ed.), *Handbook of discourse analysis*. New York: Academic Press.

Wechsler, D. (1974). *Wechsler Intelligence Scale for Children—Revised*. New York: Psychological Corporation.

Westby, C. E. (1984). Development of narrative language abilities. In G. Wallach & K. G. Butler (Eds.), *Language learning disabilities in school-age children* (pp. 103–177). Baltimore, MD: Williams & Wilkins.

Westby, C. (1989). Assessing and remediating test comprehension problems. In S. Kamhi & H. Catts (Eds.), *Reading disabilities: A developmental language perspective* (pp. 199–259). Boston: College-Hill Press.

Appendix I: Exemplification of Propositions, Superstructure, and Macrostructure for the Rooster Story

Superstructure (story structure)	A Priori Propositions
Episode 1	
Setting	1. There were two roosters.
	2. They were in the chicken yard.
Action	3. The roosters were fighting.
Resolution	4. One rooster was defeated.
Episode 2	
Setting	5. He hid himself in the corner.
	6. The other rooster flew to the top of the roost.
Action	7. He began crowing/singing.
	8. He began flapping his wings.
	9. He boasted of his victory.
	10. An eagle/hawk/crow swooped down/came by.
	11. The eagle grabbed the rooster.
	12. The eagle carried him away.
Resolution	13. This was good for the defeated rooster.
	14. He could rule over the chickens.
	15. He could have all the hens.
	16. He desired to have the hens.

Macrostructure (gist propositions)

1. The two roosters are fighting/there is a fight.
2. Someone won/lost the fight.
3. The winner bragged/showed off.
4. The eagle carried the winner away.
5. The defeated rooster/the one that remained won/ruled over the chickens.

The five gist propositions reflect the role reversal of the winning rooster being the loser in the end.

Appendix II: Sample of Complex Narrative Used in the Chapman et al. (1992) Study

"Shipwrecked"

Once there were three brothers who fished together in the ocean. They were good sailors and usually were gone from home for only a short time. One day, they all fell asleep on their boat. While they slept, the anchor broke loose and the boat drifted away in the dark night. It finally crashed against some rocks. The boys woke up frightened but then saw an island about a mile from the wrecked boat. They swam for their lives and finally all reached the island. The boys were grateful to be alive but they knew they were lost.

In the beginning, life on the island was very hard. The boys could not find fresh water or food. But they knew they could survive if they worked together. First, they looked for coconuts. Then they caught birds with their bare hands and cooked them over an open fire. They always had enough to eat and drink and never felt hungry again.

The blazing sun was always hot on the island. But one day the rainy season began. The brothers knew they had to build a shelter. They searched the island and found parts of their wrecked boat. They tied the wood together and built a simple cabin and kept dry when the rain came.

The boys still dreamed every night of returning home to their family. One day, they spotted a ship. They became excited and set fire to some large bushes. The black smoke rose high in the sky and the ship's captain spotted it. He ordered his men to go ashore, where the sailors were welcomed by the three brothers. They shouted their thanks. After 15 long months on the island, they were finally going home.

Appendix III: Example Story from Control Subject

"Shipwrecked" Discourse Sample: 9-year-old male control subject. The following story shows a general reduction in story information; however, structure of all four episodes is intact:

Once there was three brothers who fished in the ocean. Once they fell asleep and the boat, and the anchor broke loose. The boat floated far away, finally hit a rock. And the brothers woke up. They were very scared. They saw an island and swam to it. They were very glad to be on the island but they knew it would be hard. First they looked for coconuts then birds and caught them with their hands. They built a little place with grass and leaves which kept them warm. In the morning they saw a boat go by and they started a fire in the bushes. They dreamed of being home every night. Then they saw a boat and the boat saw the fire. The captain sent some of his men out to find them. The boys were going to be off the island.

Appendix IV: Frontal Lobe Case Examples (See text for Details of Patients)

Patient 1

"Shipwrecked" Story Sample: Severe CHI patient with primarily left frontal damage. The following story shows disruption of story structure and loss of the most important content ("gist"). Only information from the first episode is produced and even this information is sparsely elaborated. The resolution is inaccurate:

Three little boys were sailing in their boat. They fell asleep in the water. The boat crashed. The little boys were killed.

Patient 2

"Shipwrecked" Story Sample: Severe CHI patient with primarily left frontal damage. The following story shows a disruption of story structure. Setting is unclear in that identification of the story characters is ambiguous. The resolution is omitted for the only episode attempted. It is unclear what "hit the rocks," but it appears to be the anchor. Repetition of information interferes with the sequence of events. Story content is extremely sparse and the most important information is omitted:

First they were sailing and they fell asleep. And after that they got up they were frightened because the anchor broke and hit a bunch of rocks. And they woke up and got frightened.

Patient 3

"Shipwrecked" Story Sample: Severe CHI patient with primarily right frontal damage. The following story shows a disruption of story structure as manifested by omission of setting, action, and resolution for episodes attempted. Also evident is confabulation of story content. Sequence of events is difficult to follow:

There were three boys camping in the woods . . . there were three boys camping in the woods. They got into a boat sail and sailed so they catch some fish. The boat started to flood, flooded the water. People started to fuss each other and say bad words and stuff. Also, they was trying to swim out the water they were trying to swim out the water and swim to shore. After that they fished on the shore and on the grass. They got ropes and stuff. They brought all their supplies off the boat and jumped out and got a little boat. And they split . . . a pet canary that talks.

7

The UCLA Study of Mild Closed Head Injury in Children and Adolescents

ROBERT F. ASARNOW, PAUL SATZ, ROGER LIGHT,
KENNETH ZAUCHA, RICHARD LEWIS,
and CAROL McCLEARY

This chapter is the first presentation of the results of the UCLA Study of Closed Head Injuries in Children and Adolescents. The first section presents the background of this study, which was designed to correct methodological problems of earlier studies. The next section briefly describes the experimental design and methods of the UCLA study, emphasizing those aspects that were designed to correct some key methodological problems. Last, the major findings of the UCLA study are summarized. The statistical analyses reported here are preliminary. More sophisticated analyses will be conducted to address some of the more complex questions and to provide more rigorous tests of certain hypotheses.

Background

Head trauma is a major cause of morbidity, disability, and mortality in children. Among children aged 5 to 14, *mild* head injuries are the most prevalent, while fatal and severe head trauma makes up only about 10% of the total (Annegers, 1986). There is general agreement that in children and adolescents as in adults, there is significant functional morbidity associated with *severe* CHI. In contrast, there are conflicting views about whether there is significant functional morbidity associated with *mild* CHI.

Some investigators question whether mild CHI produces any significant morbidity (Ewing-Cobbs et al., 1985; Levin et al., 1987; Rutter, 1981). Other investigators contend that the functional morbidity caused by mild CHI is underestimated:

> Mild head injury is a quiet disorder. It is common, typically bloodless and without call for significant medical intervention. It seems even more quiet because

the noise it does make (its symptoms) is often attributed to other causes. Nevertheless, the disruption in coping capacity and attendant breakdown in usual behavioral patterns causes more psychological and academic-economic hardship than has begun to be appreciated. (Boll, 1983)

In part, this disagreement reflects a relative paucity of data. While mild CHI accounts for the vast majority of head injuries, there have been relatively few studies of the sequelae of mild CHI as opposed to severe CHI in children and adolescents.

Table 7-1 summarizes 14 peer-reviewed articles, found through a Medline computer search and published from 1970 through 1994, that examined the neurobehavioral sequelae of mild head injury in children. In addition, abstracts published in the *Journal of Clinical and Experimental Neuropsychology* during the same period are included. The studies differ dramatically in both methodology and results. Table 7-1 shows that some studies reported adverse effects of a mild CHI while others reported no adverse neurobehavioral effects. Because of the numerous differences among studies, it is difficult to isolate the key methodological factors that might account for the discrepant results. Studies differed in (1) definition of mild head injury; (2) inclusion and exclusion criteria; (3) presence/absence of control groups (other injury and/or noninjury); (4) breadth of outcome domains assessed and types of outcome measures; (5) intervals between injury and follow-up assessments; (6) retrospective vs prospective design; (7) assessment or control for preinjury level of functioning; (8) assessment or control for preinjury history of central nervous system (CNS) insults and learning problems; and (9) age differences among study groups. Interpretation of some studies is complicated by their small sample size, which limits their power to detect any subtle neurobehavioral effects of mild CHI.

How can these discrepant results be resolved? Our review of this literature suggests that many of the conflicting findings are accounted for by differences between studies in (1) how subjects are ascertained, (2) how mild head injury is operationally defined, and (3) whether and how key preinjury factors are controlled for.

Subject Ascertainment

Inspection of Table 7-1 shows that subjects in studies of mild CHI were drawn from such diverse sources as neurosurgery units, consecutive admissions to emergency rooms, outpatient referrals for assessment, chart reviews from hospital records, or combinations of these methods. The source of the subjects may be an implicit descriptor of injury severity. Some of the studies reporting adverse effects of mild CHI have recruited subjects from referrals for postacute follow-up evaluation (e.g., Horowitz et al., 1983; Light et al., 1987; Prigatano & Papero, 1991; Winogron et al., 1984). There may be more patients with residual problems in a sample ascertained in this manner. Conversely, studies of patients ascertained from emergency rooms (e.g., Snoek et al., 1984) are less likely to find adverse effects of a mild CHI. Recruiting subjects from clinics that provide follow-up evaluations also increases the possibility of inaccurate assessment of acute injury severity due to the retrospective nature of the screening.

Definition of Mild Head Injury

A major cause of conflicting results is differences between studies in how mild CHI is operationally defined. Table 7-1 summarizes the operational definitions of mild CHI used in studies of children with mild and moderate CHI published since 1971. Inspection of Table 7-1 reveals that there is currently no consensus on how to define the severity of head injury in the mild/moderate range. The majority of studies to date have relied on either length of alteration of consciousness (e.g., length of coma, LOC) or depth of altered consciousness (e.g., lowest Glasgow Coma Scale Score). The criteria for a mild head injury have ranged from a CHI with no loss of consciousness and no signs of concussion (Casey et al., 1986) to any head injury that results in a period of posttraumatic amnesia (PTA) less than 24 hours (Mahalick et al., 1990; Lundar et al., 1985; Gronwall and Wrightson, 1974). Studies utilizing the duration of PTA as a criterion for severity of mild CHI are problematic, since it is difficult to obtain a reliable measure of PTA in children. Part of the difficulty in measuring PTA in children arises from the lack of normative developmental data on temporal orientation in children. Most studies reporting cognitive and/or behavioral impairments in children with mild head injuries seem to include children with apparently more severe injuries, such as those with complications and/or extended loss of consciousness (e.g., Ewing-Cobbs et al., 1989; Gronwall & Wrightson, 1974; Gulbrandsen, 1984; Horowitz et al., 1983; Klonoff et al., 1977; Light et al., 1987; Mahalick et al., 1990; Winogron et al., 1984).

The absence of an operational definition of mild and moderate CHI that is well agreed upon reflects a fundamental problem. Severity of head injury is really a dimension. Assigning labels such as "mild" and "minor" to arbitrary cut points along that dimension so as to establish categories of severity only ends up reifying the arbitrary cut points. The critical need is not to establish a consensus about the definition of the terms "mild" and "moderate CHI." Rather, what is needed is an operational definition of CHI severity along multiple dimensions (e.g, LOC and PTA). A related issue is the need to employ measures of severity of acute head injury that have satisfactory interrater reliabilities. In all likelihood, multiple functional dimensions of severity may need to be measured.

A recent intriguing report (Williams et al., 1990) may help to account for some of the conflicting reports of the effects of mild CHI on neurobehavioral outcome. The morbidity produced in adults by an otherwise mild CHI (i.e., GCS score of 13 to 15) complicated by an intracranial lesion on computed tomography (CT) was comparable to that of a moderate CHI (i.e., GCS score of 9 to 12) without an intracranial lesion on CT. Extrapolating from this study of adults, the presence of an intracranial lesion on CT may adversely affect the outcome of children and adolescents with mild/moderate CHI.

TABLE 7-1. Range of Operational Definitions Used for Mild and Moderate Head Injury in Children

Reference	Subject Source[a]	Operational Definition
	Adverse Effect	
Asarnow et al., 1991	3	*Mild* = PTA < 4 hours, no coma or only transient LOC *Severe* = LOC > 9 hours
Butterbaugh et al., 1993	4	*Mild/Mod* – GCS > 8 *Severe* = GCS 3–8
Casey et al., 1986	4	*Minor* = HI with no signs of concussion, LOC, skull fx, no hosp. admission, memory loss or neurological impairment.
Chadwick et al., 1981	1	*Minor* = PTA > 1 hour and < 1 week *Severe* = PTA > 1 week
Gulbrandsen, 1984	1	*Light HI* = dx of concussion (LOC < 15 min or two symptoms: amnesia, nausea, drowsiness, or somnolence)
Horowitz et al., 1983	7	*Mild* = Local pediatric hospitalization with head injury *Severe* = District neurosurgical referral
Levin et al., 1994	1	*Less severe* = GCS > 8 *Severe* = GCS < or equal to 8
Levin & Eisenberg, 1979	1	*Grade 1* = conscious on admission, only momentary LOC, no neurological deficits *Grade II* = LOC < 24 hours or neurological deficits *Grade III* = LOC > 24 hours
Mattson, et al., 1990 (P)	1	*Mild* = GCS 13–15 those with abnormal CT or upper extremity injuries excluded
Snoek et al., 1984	7	*Delayed Deterioration Mild* = No LOC or less than 5 min LOC and later decrease in consciousness or focal neurological signs.
	No Effect	
Bawden et al., 1985	6	*Mild* = LOC < 20 min (incl. linear skull fx) *Moderate* = LOC > 20 min or neurological signs; EEG or CT abnormality *Severe* = GCS 3–7 and required ICP monitoring
Bijur et al., 1990	2	*Mild* = ICD-9 code of concussion or LOC and no more than 1 night of hospitalization
Black et al., 1971	4	Only children suffering LOC, skull fx or neurological effects were included. Severity was not subdivided.
Chapman et al., 1992	1	*Mild/Mod* = GCS > 8 *Severe* = GCS < or equal to 8
Ewing-Cobbs et al., 1987	1	*Mild* = Normal CT; LOC < 15 min; no neurological deficits *Moderate/Severe* = Positive CT; LOC > 15 min
Ewing-Cobbs et al., 1989	4	*Mild/Moderate* = impaired consciousness > 24 hours: GCS on admit 9–15 *Severe* = impaired consciousness > 1 day

TABLE 7-1. (*continued*)

Reference	Subject Source[a]	Operational Definition
		No Effect
Ewing-Cobbs et al., 1990	1	*Group 1* = PTA < 7 days (Using COAT) *Group 2* PTA 8–14 *Group 3* PTA > 14 days
Fletcher et al., 1990	1	*Mild* = Admission GCS 13–15; LOC < 20 min, no skull fx/mass lesion/swelling, no deterioration after admission *Moderate* = Admission GCS 9–12; or 13–15 with skull fx/mass lesion *Severe* = Initial GCS 3–8
Gronwall et al., 1974	4	*Minor* = PTA < 24 hours, no skull fx, hematoma, contusion, or other complications
Hannay & Levin, 1988	1	Two methods (1) *Mild* GCS, 13–15 (no mass lesion/skull fx) *Moderate* = GCS 9–12 or 13–15 with abnormal CT *Severe* = GCS 3–8 (2) *Group 1* = no coma, conscious on admission *Group 2* = if impaired consciousness < 24 hours *Group 3* = impaired consciousness > 24 hours
Kewman et al., 1992 (P)	6	*Mild* = GCS 13–15 *Moderate* = GCS 9–12 *Severe* = GCS < 9
Klonoff et al., 1977	4	*Minor* = suspected but unproven LOC, no concussion *Mild* = suspected but unproven LOC, concussion *Moderate* = LOC < 5 min, concussion *Severe* = LOC 5–30 min, concussion or skull fx *Serious* = LOC > 30 min, skull fx or other sequelae
Knights et al., 1991	4	*Mild* = GCS 13–15, LOC < 20 min, admitted overnight, linear fx, no LOC *Moderate* = GCS 8–12, LOC > 20 min, abnormal CT, neurological deficit *Severe* = GCS 7 or less, signs of neurological deficits on CT
Leahy et al., 1987	1	Z score derived from GCS and length of hospital stay (if Z = 0 or below = mild)
Levin et al., 1982	1	*Group 1* = initial GCS < 8 *Group 2* = initial GCS > 8
Light et al., 1987	3	*Mild* = PTA < 4 hours, no coma or only transient LOC *Moderate* = PTA > 24 hours and < 7 days *Severe* = PTA > 7 days

TABLE 7-1. (*continued*)

Reference	Subject Source[a]	Operational Definition
	No Effect	
Lundar et al., 1985	4	*Mild* = PTA < 24 hours
		Severe = PTA > 24 hours
Tompkins et al., 1990	4	Several measures of severity treated as continuous variables
Thompson et al., 1990 (P)	1	*Mild* = GCS 13–15 normal CT, no neurological deficit
		Moderate = GCS 9–12, LOC < 1 day or GCS > 13 with abnormal CT or neurological deficit
		Severe = GCS 8 or less, LOC > 1 day
Winogron et al., 1984	6	*Mild* = LOC < 20 min (includes linear skull fx)
		Moderate = LOC > 20 min or neurological signs; EEG or CT abnormality
		Severe = GCS 3–7 and required ICP monitoring

Abbreviations: PTA = posttraumatic amnesia; HI = head injury; LOC = loss of consciousness; GCS = Glasgow Coma Scale; COAT = Children's Orientation and Amnesia Test; dx = diagnosis; fx = fracture; EEG = electroencephalogram, CT = computed tomography; ICP = intracranial pressure; ICD = International Classification of Diseases.

[a] Subject source codes:
  1 = Recruited through pediatric neurosurgery department of hospital/medical center.
  2 = All children born in 1 week on follow-up who were ages 5–10 in England.
  3 = Recruited through an outpatient pediatric treatment center.
  4 = Consecutive admissions to hospital(s).
  5 = Recruited for longitudinal research project.
  6 = Both inpatient and outpatient cases to pediatric hospital.
  7 = Chart review. All referred for hospitalization with head injury for a certain period of time.

Another factor that may moderate the effects of a particular level of severity of acute CHI is the presence of multiple organ traumas. Unintentional injuries that produce mild CHI in adults often produce multiple organ traumas (e.g., fractures, abrasions, etc.). Dikmen and colleagues (1986) found that the presence of multiple traumas (e.g., long bone fracture) increases the rate of functional morbidity in adults who have incurred mild CHI as compared to adults with mild CHI without multiple traumas.

Control of Key Preinjury Factors

Even when significant functional morbidity is found in children and adolescents who have incurred a mild CHI, there is still the question of whether that morbidity is a *direct* result of the head injury. For example, Brown and colleagues (1981) found that children with mild CHI had an unusually high rate of behavioral disturbance *prior* to the accident and concluded that the behavior problems detected postinjury antedated the accident. It is now widely recognized that prior to the index injury, children who incur mild CHI have elevated rates of behavioral and school problems as well as prior histories of head injuries and other CNS insults (Brooks, 1984). Establishing a direct link between mild CHI and adverse outcomes clearly requires a rigorous evaluation of preinjury status. Few studies have adequately evaluated and controlled for preinjury status other than by *excluding* subjects with problems prior to the index injury. Unfortunately, this type of study design may limit generalization to the population of children with mild CHI, many of whom have already sustained other injuries (including head injuries). Equally important, it precludes a determination of the effects of preinjury risk factors on outcome. The importance of adequately measuring key preinjury factors is underscored by the results of the UCLA study indicating that for certain outcome measures, the effects of certain preinjury factors (e.g., history of learning and school problems) are larger than the effects of a very mild CHI. In addition, it is possible that certain preinjury risk factors (e.g., prior head injury) may interact with the current injury to lower the minimal threshold of acute CHI severity necessary to produce significant functional morbidity.

Specificity of Outcomes and Sample Size

Prior studies have rarely evaluated the specificity of the outcomes of mild CHI. It is possible that some of the adverse psychosocial outcomes associated with a mild CHI are not caused by a head injury per se but rather reflect the generalized emotional distress caused by having an injury that requires emergency medical care. Both the child and caretakers might experience this distress. For example, Casey and colleagues (1986) studied a large sample of 2- to 14-year-old patients with minor head injuries 1 month postaccident; they attributed the excessive rate of behavioral problems (27%) and functional morbidity in these youngsters to "parental overreaction and possibly family dysfunction" possibly exacerbating the child's emotional response to the accident. This underscores the need for an "other injury" control group. A group of patients with injuries not involving the head and drawn from the same hospitals as the CHI group helps control for the effects of factors that convey a general risk for injuries, thereby providing a test of the specificity of the effects of a mild CHI (see Chapters by Bijur and by Taylor, this volume).

Another source of conflicting results among studies is the relatively small sample size used in almost all studies to date. The effect size of mild CHI is not large, and large sample sizes are needed to obtain stable estimates of this effect. In addition, estimating the effects of mild CHI requires having reliable estimates of what is normal for that population. Most prior studies have used small, nonrepresentative samples of normal controls.

Methods

The UCLA study was designed to avoid some of the major methodological problems discussed above. To avoid the ascertainment biases of prior studies, the

UCLA study obtained a large representative sample of children with mild closed head injury by identifying them through a primary portal of care-emergency rooms. By studying injury patients *prospectively* at the point of first contact with the health care system, we were able to avoid the biases that arise when patients are retrospectively ascertained through follow-ups at clinics. We obtained multiple measures of acute head-injury severity from emergency room records and parental interviews, including number of concussive symptoms, length of PTA, and duration of unconsciousness.

A major focus of the UCLA study was to control adequately for preinjury level of functioning by carefully assessing relevant preinjury factors and utilizing two comparison groups. The specific methods used to accomplish this are described in some detail below.

An important aspect of obtaining a representative sample in a multicultural city like Los Angeles was to ensure that we included ethnic minorities (e.g., African Americans and Latinos) in the study sample. To accomplish this, ethnic minorities were well represented among the project staff. Many of the field testers were bilingual, so they were able to conduct the evaluations in Spanish for those subjects who did not speak English. In addition, test materials were translated into Spanish.

Major efforts were made in this study to minimize attrition. As demonstrated below, we were quite successful in this regard. This was accomplished, in large measure, by conducting the evaluations in the patients' homes rather than requiring them to come to a clinic. In addition, small monetary reinforcements were used to maintain the children's participation in the study.

Study Design

The UCLA study is a prospective cohort follow-up. The design for determining the outcomes following mild brain injury, the influence of preinjury functioning on outcome, and the identification of prognostic factors that predict adverse outcomes following injury are presented in Figure 7-1. The major study objectives were addressed as follows.

1. *The sequelae or outcomes specific to mild brain injury* were determined by prospective follow-up of three different groups of children and adolescents: a group with mild CHI, a group with mild injuries but not to the brain (the "other injury" group, matched on age and sex); and a group without injuries (the "noninjury" group, matched on age and sex). The prospective nature of this design, especially the collection of data shortly after the injury to characterize preinjury functioning, avoids one of the important methodological problems of previous studies—the inability to determine preinjury levels of parameters that may have changed following injury. For example, if school failure is thought to be caused by a mild brain injury, then it is important to evaluate scholastic functioning before the injury. One method we used to determine the sequelae of mild brain injury was to compare the outcomes of the CHI and noninjury groups. A related problem is whether changes in important factors noted postinjury were, in fact,

STUDY DESIGN

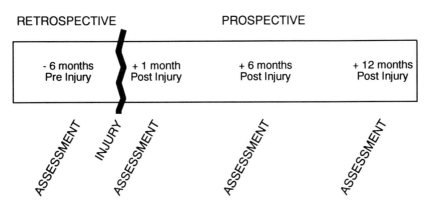

Figure 7-1. Study design.

due to the brain injury itself or to the general effect of any injury irrespective of anatomic location. The specificity of outcome is evaluated by comparing the outcomes of the CHI and the other-injury groups.

2. *The influence of preinjury functioning on outcome* was addressed in the UCLA study by determining whether preinjury factors predict adverse neuropsychological and behavioral outcomes *within* the CHI group and by statistically controlling for the effects of preinjury functioning on outcome variables. The preinjury factors of major interest include history of learning, school, and behavior problems (particularly attention deficit and conduct disorders), use of alcohol, and prior injury history.

Subjects

Three groups of children, age 8 to 16, were studied: (1) CHI, (2) other injured, and (3) noninjured. The CHI and other-injured children were recruited from 14 emergency rooms located throughout Los Angeles, Riverside, and Orange counties. The geographical placement of the participating emergency rooms resulted in the inclusion of frequently understudied African American and Latino populations. Emergency room (ER) treatment logs were reviewed on a weekly basis. All children whose parents or guardians could be contacted by letter or phone within 4 weeks of their child's accident were invited to participate.

Definition of Mild Closed Head Injury

We defined mild CHI as an uncomplicated closed brain injury from blunt forces characterized as concussion resulting in an Abbreviated Injury Scale (AIS) score of 1, 2, or 3. Children with a CHI and other injuries of the same or lesser severity (i.e., AIS 1 to 3) were "cases." The AIS criteria are as follows:

AIS 1: History of or observed presence of any two of the following: nausea, vomiting, headache, dizziness. Or a diagnosis of "concussion" with any of the above or following symptoms: diplopia, ringing in the ears, or seeing stars as long as these symptoms are not treated as neurological deficits and the symptoms usually disappear in the ER.

AIS 2: History of or observed length of coma in ER for less than 1 hour; some symptoms with or without skull fracture; level of consciousness and sensorium improving; no neurological deficits, ER Glasgow Coma Scale rating between 13 and 14.

AIS 3: Observed length of coma 1 to 6 hours; symptoms of amnesia, lethargy, stupor with or without skull fracture; no neurological deficits, surgery, or other brain injury; *transient* neurological deficits; Glasgow Coma Scale rating of 12.

Inclusion and Exclusion Criteria for the Mild-CHI Group (Cases)

Children were included in the CHI group if they had experienced nonintentional injury to the head possibly resulting in mild CHI. These head injuries fell within AIS injury severity levels 1 to 3, assuring that all head-injured children had a minimum of two concussive symptoms documented in the ER records. Injuries to the head area resulting in fewer than two concussive symptoms or injuries that had unclear documentation of symptoms were not included.

The CHI group included children or adolescents with the following characteristics:

1. An acute brain injury equivalent to AIS 1, 2, or 3 either admitted to a hospital or discharged from an ER
2. No injuries above AIS level 3 at any anatomic location
3. Injured from unintentional external causes
4. No litigation related to the index accident pending at time of first contact
5. No serious injuries or deaths involving others due to the same accident
6. A resident of Los Angeles, Riverside, or Orange County who sought ER treatment at one of the participating hospitals
7. Aged 8 through 16 years at time of injury
8. No significant preexisting CNS damage or serious chronic diseases (i.e., cancer, congenital malformation)
9. Parental willingness and ability to give informed consent to be contacted for follow-up
10. Child residing with parent(s) or legal guardian

Comparison Groups

Two comparison groups were included in the study design, "other injured" and "noninjured."

Other-Injured Group. Injured children admitted to the same hospital ER as the cases but not having a brain/head injury were members of this comparison group. Children seen in the ER with injuries at AIS levels 1 to 3 were part of an eligibility pool. Because the experimental tasks required the use of hands, children with injuries resulting in discomfort or restricted movement of the hands and arms were excluded. Members of this comparison group met characteristics 2 to 10 listed above.

Noninjured Group. This comparison group provided "normative" data on neuropsychological and school functioning and was an important contrast group for causal modeling. For each CHI case, an age- and sex-matched noninjured control was identified. Each control met characteristics 7 to 10 above.

Children in this group were enrolled in schools in a district centrally located within our catchment area and, as shown in Table 7-2, were similar demographically to the children in the CHI and other-injury groups. Children in the noninjury group were drawn from a larger pool of children who were recruited to provide normative data on the experimental measures used in the study. Children were asked when tested at their school if they had ever had a head injury and if they had an injury to another part of the body *within the past year* that resulted in a clinic or ER visit. The parents of children who reported no injuries of *either* type were contacted by phone. The "no injury" status of the child was confirmed by the parent's report according to the same criteria. An in-home appointment with willing parents was made to obtain initial interview and questionnaire data for the child. Children were excluded from this group if the family did not speak either English or Spanish, if siblings were already participating in the study, or if the child had a history of significant CNS disease or insult.

TABLE 7-2.   Demographic Information for Study and Comparison Groups

	Head Injury ($n = 137$)	Other Injury ($n = 132$)	No Injury ($n = 114$)
Gender			
Percentage male	64%	61%	42%
Percentage right-handed	89%	86%	93%
AIS scores[a]			
Percentage AIS 1	36%	54%	0%
Percentage AIS 2	60%	39%	0%
Percentage AIS 3	4%	7%	0%
Mean age at injury	12.0 (2.5)	12.9 (2.5)	12.2 (2.4)
Mean SES	39.26 (16.8)	43.46 (18.7)	37.12 (14.6)
Race			
Percentage white	49%	45%	55%
Percentage Latino	34%	42%	36%
Percentage African/Asian American	17%	13%	9%

[a]AIS = Abbreviated Injury Scale.

Normative Data

For certain secondary analyses, it is important to have estimates of what is "normal" for the age group being studied. It was particularly important to collect age-appropriate normative data for the neuropsychological tasks developed for this study because many of the cognitive measures have age effects. Data were collected in elementary, junior high, and high schools, resulting in at least 40 subjects in each 1-year age group for each sex for our test battery and interview and questionnaires. This procedure yielded approximately 500 subjects. We will use this extensive set of normative data to determine (for secondary analyses) whether certain scores are outliers.

Subject Characteristics

A total of 137 children in the head-injury group, 132 children in the other-injury group, and 114 children in the noninjury group were entered into the study. We had originally planned to include 120 subjects in each group. The two injury groups were oversampled to protect against attrition. The attrition rate from the 1- to 12-month assessments was 11.7% for the head-injury group, 15.2% for the other-injury group, and 7.0% for the noninjury group. Inspection of Table 7-2 shows that the 3 groups are in general comparable across major demographic variables. The groups were comparable in socioeconomic status (SES) as measured by the education and employment scales of the Hollingshead index. There was a nonsignificantly higher proportion of females in the noninjury than in the head- and other-injury groups. The head-injury group tended to be slightly younger than the other-injury group.

Injury Severity

Table 7-3 describes the severity of injury for the CHI group. As noted earlier, subjects in the CHI and other-injury groups had injuries of AIS levels 1 to 3. This meant that all children in the head-injured group had at least two concussive symptoms noted in the parental reports. Thirty percent of the head-injury group had three concussive symptoms and 31% had four or more concussive symptoms.

The overwhelming majority of the CHI group were either never unconscious (53%) or were unconscious less than 10 minutes (43%). The data on length of PTA are similar. Forty-four percent of the CHI group reported no PTA while 24% reported a PTA of less than 10 minutes. Sixty-six percent of the CHI group were disoriented for less than 10 minutes.

When compared with the studies summarized in Table 7-1, the UCLA cohort was clearly in the most minimal range of mild CHIs.

Three general factors were examined: preinjury status, the injury itself, and outcome.

TABLE 7-3. Description of Injury Severity
for the Head-Injury Group

Number of postconcussive symptoms	
0 or 1 postconcussive symptoms	—
2 Postconcussive symptoms	39%
3 Postconcussive symptoms	30%
4 Postconcussive symptoms	23%
5 Postconcussive symptoms	8%
Loss of Consciousness	
Never unconscious	53%
Unconscious < 10 minutes	43%
Unconscious > 10 minutes	4%
Disorientation	
No disorientation	36%
Disoriented < 10 minutes	30%
Disoriented > 10 minutes	34%
Posttraumatic Amnesia	
No PTA	44%
PTA < 10 minutes	24%
PTA > 10 minutes	32%

Preinjury Factors

Indices of preinjury status were derived from parental interviews and question-naires and a medical/developmental questionnaire that provided, among other data, a history of previous injuries. These measures were completed during the initial visit 1 month postinjury. Additional information about preinjury status was provided by the Child Behavior Checklist (CBCL), which was completed by the parent 1 month postinjury, and by school records. For the CBCLs collected 1 month postinjury, informants were instructed to describe the child's behavior for the 6-month period prior to the injury. This was only a minor modification of the standard instructions for the CBCL that require informants to describe the child's behavior over the previous 6-month period.

Injury-Related Factors

The injury-related factors of primary interest were (1) acute injury severity and (2) a number of measures abstracted from the medical records, including the characteristics of the injury, specific immediate postinjury sequelae, the type of treatment, and sociodemographic factors.

Outcome Factors

Three major domains of outcome were examined: (1) 1-month postinjury measures of neuropsychological functioning; (2) 12-month postinjury rates of behavior problems as measured by the CBCL; and (3) 12-month postinjury measures of school functioning derived from school records and parent CBCL ratings of school problems.

Measures

Data were collected from school and medical records, parental questionnaires and interviews, and neuropsychological testing.

School Records

Local school districts routinely collect several types of information on all of their students, including school grades and the California Test of Basic Skills. This annual test measures math and reading proficiency. We received parental consent to obtain the school records for the year prior to and the year after the injury.

Medical Records

Hospital records for the head-injury and other-injury subjects were reviewed and the following information was abstracted by our staff:

1. Emergency room diagnosis
2. Hospital admission diagnosis and complaint(s)
3. AIS level(s)
4. Descriptions of injuries
5. External cause of injury
6. Name, age, gender
7. Parents' names, current address and telephone number
8. Hospital name
9. Usual care provider (if name was available)
10. Results of standard neurological examinations

Parent Questionnaire and Interview

Parents completed the CBCL (Achenbach & Edelbrock, 1983), a 113-item behavioral checklist. The CBCL surveys a broad range of child behavior problems including anxiousness, social withdrawal, depression, immaturity, self-destruction, inattention, delinquency, and aggressive behavior typically seen in children referred to child guidance clinics. Second-order principal components analysis has consistently identified two broad groupings of behavior problems—internalizing and externalizing (Achenbach & Edelbrock, 1983). The internalizing factor includes "fearful, inhibited, overcontrolled behavior," whereas the externalizing factor includes "aggressive, antisocial, and undercontrolled behavior." The total behavior problem scale of the CBCL provides a measure of global psychopathology.

We developed a brief medical/developmental questionnaire that was completed by the parent. This questionnaire reviewed the child's medical and developmental history with a focus on factors suggesting the presence of CNS disturbances. The questionnaire also reviewed health care utilization since the index injury, the parents' reaction to the child's injury, and their expectations of how the injury might affect the child over the next year. A parental interview asked detailed questions about the index injury and any prior injuries.

Neuropsychological Measures

The neuropsychological tests were selected to tap various aspects of executive functions (i.e., insight, self-awareness), attention, and memory. Assessment of these domains have been shown to detect deficits in children who have incurred a mild to moderate brain injury. To circumscribe the nature of the cognitive deficits in children with mild brain injuries, additional tasks (Peabody Picture Vocabulary Test-Revised [PPVT-R] and the PIN Test) were included to assess the general level of intellectual functioning and fine motor speed. The number of tests was constrained by the necessity of conducting the testing in one 2-hour session in the child's home. For a test to be included in the study, it had to be suitable for administration to children and adolescents between 8 and 16 years of age. The tasks are briefly described in Table 7-4. A key reference describing each task is provided for the reader desiring further details about a task.

Initial statistical analyses of key variables are summarized in the following section. We are currently conducting more sophisticated analyses to address some of the more complex issues in this study. After a brief summary of analyses of preinjury functioning, analyses of four major outcome domains are summarized.

Results

Preinjury Functioning

Preinjury functioning and medical/developmental history were obtained from the best-informed parent via interview and questionnaire during the assessment conducted 1 month postinjury. Individual questions were aggregated into four a priori global indices: (1) history of pregnancy and birth complications; (2) history of early developmental delays; (3) history of learning and later developmental problems; and (4) history of medical problems. Analyses of variance showed significant group differences for pregnancy and birth complications only [$F(2,312) = 3.15$, $p < 0.05$]. Both injury groups had higher scores on this index than the noninjury group. Both injury groups also tended to have higher scores on the remaining three indices than the noninjury group.

Outcome Domains

Behavior Problems. Initial analyses of the CBCL data focused on the Total Behavior Problem scale, since scores on this broad-band scale can be computed for both boys and girls between 4 and 16 years of age, and it is the CBCL scale that best predicts clinic referral. Table 7-5 shows the CBCL Total Behavior Problem

TABLE 7-4. Description of Neuropsychological Tasks

Instrument	Tasks Required	Function Measured	Key Reference
Prospective Memory Test	Subjects are required to respond to 5 tasks that approximate everyday memory situations embedded in the standard protocol (e.g., remembering to tell or give something, remembering to do something at an appointed time, etc.).	Prospective memory	Experimental
Word List Memory Test/Release from Proactive Interference	Four lists of words consisting of 10 animals are presented one at a time for free recall. Correct recall, recall intrusions from previous lists, and non-list intrusions are recorded. A fifth list of 10 weather terms is presented for free recall as a release from proactive interference.	Verbal recall of auditorially presented material	Wickens, 1970
Picture Memory Test	Three groups of 20 target pictures are presented to the subject at the rate of 2 seconds per picture. After each group, subjects pick out target pictures for each group from a larger "recognition" group of pictures. In recognition groups 2 and 3, previous target pictures are presented again, increasing the likelihood of false alarms. Finally, temporal coding of targets is assessed when 5 pictures from each target group are randomly presented and the subject is asked to indicate in which group the picture was first seen.	Visual recognition memory, temporal coding of visual material	Experimental
Span of Apprehension	Subjects are instructed to search for two predesignated target letters, T or F, which appear in 3-, 5-, and 10-letter arrays on a computer monitor. Either T or F occurs on half the trials, and these targets are varied to appear equally in each of the 16 possible array positions of the 4×4 array template used to arrange the letters. Arrays appear on the screen for 50 milliseconds to prevent subjects from initiating multiple eye scans. Subjects indicate if a T or F was present by pressing one of two response buttons. Dependent variables are the detection rates by array size. Response latencies for both correct and incorrect trials are recorded to permit analysis	Selective attention, assessment of early aspects of visual information processing	Asarnow et al, 1977

Test	Description	Measures	Source
Degraded Stimulus Continuous Performance Test	Subjects view a computer monitor on which numbers 0 through 9 are presented one per second for a duration of 50 milliseconds. Subjects are instructed to press a response button whenever they see a 0. This target stimulus appears randomly on one-third of the trials. Number of correct detections (hits) and errors of commission (false alarms) are measured, along with response latencies for both. A total of 480 trials is presented and the sensitivity of the task is increased by randomly removing 40% of the pixels from the images.	Sustained attention, Vigilance	Nuechterlein, 1983
Color Trails Test (Child Version)	In Part A, the subject is to connect numbered circles in order as quickly as possible without lifting the pencil from the page. Time to completion and number of errors are recorded for Parts A and B. Part B varies from the traditional Halstead version by introducing a second set of numbers that appear in contrasting colored circles. The subject is to connect the numbers in order; however, each subsequent number must be in the alternating colored circle (e.g., pink 1 to yellow 2, etc.).	Speed of visual search, mental flexibility, motor function and attention	Modified from Reitan & Wolfson, 1985
Stroop Test	Dependent variables in each of 3 trials are time to complete the task and number of errors made. During Trial 1, subjects are to point to and say the colors of groups of X's that are printed in red, blue, yellow, and green ink. In Trial 2, the identical response pattern as Trial 1 is duplicated with the colors printed as words using black ink. The subject is to point to and read the words in order as quickly as possible. In Trial 3, color names are printed but using an interfering ink (e.g., the word red is printed using blue ink, etc.), and the subject is to ignore the meaning of the word and to say the ink color that was used to print the word.	Ability to shift perceptual set or to suppress an automatized process in favor of a nonautomatized process	Modified from Golden, 1976

(continued)

TABLE 7-4. *(continued)*

Instrument	Tasks Required	Function Measured	Key Reference
Symbol Digit Substitution Test	Adapted from the Digit-Symbol subtest of the Wechsler scales, the subject is presented with rows of blanks printed underneath nonsense symbols. The subject's task is to fill in the blanks with the number that is matched to the symbol in the key at the top of the page. The number of correct responses and errors made in 90 seconds is recorded.	Cognitive flexibility and speeded performance, incidental learning, fine motor function	Smith, 1968
Peabody Picture Vocabulary Test (Revised)	Subjects are required to point to a picture corresponding to a target word that is read.	Receptive vocabulary, estimate of general intellectual functioning	Dunn and Dunn, 1981
PIN Test	Subjects are required to push a pin through the holes of a metal template, puncturing a piece of paper underneath. The subject uses only one hand at a time, and two 45-minute trials are performed for each hand. The combined total punctures (total hits) for each hand are recorded and an Advantage Index is obtained by dividing the total hits for the dominant hand by the total hits for the nondominant hand.	Fine motor speed, lateral dominance	Satz and D'Elia, 1989
UCLA Attention, Impulsivity and Memory Questionnaire	Subjects respond to 24 questions about everyday situations involving memory, attention, and impulsivity. Possible responses are contained on a 4-point Likert scale ranging from "Not At All True" to "Very True."	Subjective report to cognitive difficulties experienced during everyday activities	Experimental, based on Connors Check List, Goyette, et al., 1978

TABLE 7-5.   Total Behavior Problem Scale Scores for Three Groups of Children

Total Behavior Problems	6 Months Preinjury		12 Months Postinjury	
	Mean	Standard Deviation	Mean	Standard Deviation
Head injury	57.2	11.2	54.5	11.6
Other injury	56.8	11.5	51.8	11.1
No injury	53.3	10.0	48.1	10.5

scores for the three groups during the 6 months prior to the index injury as assessed at 1 and 12 months postinjury. For the 6-month period prior to the index injury, an analysis of variance indicated a significant main effect of group $[F(2,299) = 5.65; p < 0.01]$. Posthoc tests using Bonferroni-corrected t-tests revealed that the CHI group had an increased number of behavior problems compared to the noninjury group. The other-injury group did not differ significantly from the head-injury or the noninjury groups during the 6-month period prior to the index injury. These analyses show that a number of the children in the head-injury group and to a lesser extent in the other-injury group had behavior problems antedating their injuries. This is consistent with previous reports indicating that elevated rates of behavior problems may contribute to the risk of incurring an accident (Brown et al., 1981).

Analyses of the assessment at 12-months postinjury revealed similar results. There was a significant effect of group $[F(2,299) = 7.23, p < 0.001]$. Bonferroni-corrected t-tests revealed that the head-injury group had a significantly higher score on the Behavior Problem Scale than the noninjury group. The other-injury group did not differ significantly from the head-injury or noninjury groups. Of critical importance, *all* groups showed some decline in the rate of behavior problems reported by the parent at 12 months postinjury relative to the 6 months prior to the injury. There was *no* evidence that the index head injury produced an increased rate of reported behavior problems. The other-injury and noninjury groups tended to show a somewhat greater decline in the rates of behavior problems than the head-injury group. The absence of an increased rate of behavior problems 12 months postinjury compared to the preinjury baseline is *not* consistent with the hypothesis that the index injury caused behavior problems.

Analysis of the internalizing and externalizing scales of the CBCL produced, not surprisingly, parallel results. There was no evidence of an increased rate of internalizing or externalizing behavior problems in either the head-injury or other-injury groups at the 12-month follow-up relative to the 6-month period prior to the injury.

The finding that the head-injury and other-injury groups did not differ significantly on any behavior problem scale at any test occasion suggests that the range of severity of head injury sampled thus far falls below the minimal threshold of acute severity necessary to produce significant functional morbidity.

Finally, it is important to note that the mean scores obtained by the three groups on the CBCL fell well within the normal range. Contrary to our prior study (Asarnow et al., 1991), which examined children with somewhat more serious injuries in the mild range, there was no indication in these data that a disproportionate number of the children in the head-injury group show elevated rates of behavior problems.

Data from the CBCL on the rate of placement in special classes prior to injury paralleled the behavioral problem data. Prior to the index injury, a greater proportion of the children in the head-injury and other-injury groups were placed in special education classes compared to the children in the noninjury group. Again, this finding is consistent with prior research (e.g., Brown et al., 1981) indicating that children with school problems have an elevated risk of incurring a subsequent accident. These findings underscore the importance of properly evaluating preinjury factors and the usefulness of the other-injury comparison group.

School Records Data. At this writing only portions of the school record data have been analyzed. Releases for school records have been obtained for nearly 90% of the head-injury and other-injury groups thus far, and the records have been obtained for 75% of these subjects. Data collection for the noninjury group has recently been completed in the schools where they were initially recruited. A collection rate approaching 100% is anticipated.

The two major measures derived from the school records data were the mean school grades and mean achievement-test scores prior to and at one year postinjury. These measures were computed by excluding the quarter or semester (depending on the school) during which the children were injured or, for the noninjury group, the quarter/semester in which they were first tested. Grades from the quarter/semester immediately prior to the injury (or first testing) were converted to a 5-point scale, with A equal to 1 and F equal to 5, and were then averaged over all academic classes to produce a single mean score for this grading period. The same procedure was used for the available grading period closest to 1 year postinjury or initial testing. The preliminary data are presented in Table 7-6. Comparisons were made via mixed-design ANOVA with group as the between factor and occasion the within factor. The results were not significant for group, test-occasion, or group-by-occasion interaction.

The pre- and postinjury achievement scores were derived by obtaining the standardized testing records for the test occasion immediately prior to injury (or first testing) and averaging the national percentile scores for all available academic subtests. This procedure provided a mean achievement test score (in percentile) for subjects pre- and postinjury. Analyses were performed via ANOVA. With only partial data analyzed, the mean scores of the head-injury and other-injury groups were very similar both pre- and postinjury. There were no significant group or test occasion effects or group-by-occasion interactions.

Neuropsychological Functioning. Neuropsychological impairments in the head-injury group should be most apparent at the assessment conducted 1 month postin-

TABLE 7-6.   Mean School Grades and Mean School Test Scores Preinjury
and Postinjury

	Most Recent Preinjury			1 Year Postinjury		
	N	Mean	Standard Deviation	*N*	Mean	Standard Deviation
Mean School Grades (one 1-to-5 scale)						
Head injury	71	2.3	0.8	74	2.3	0.7
Other injury	67	2.4	0.8	73	2.4	0.7
Mean School Test Scores (percentile)						
Head injury	59	59.5	23.4	41	64.1	24.6
Other injury	58	56.1	23.6	46	54.3	22.9

Note: Student grades are coded as 1 for A and 5 for F. Mean values, averaged over all academic classes, correspond to a C. Percentiles for achievement test scores are averaged over all available academic subjects.

jury, because the normal course of CHI (in the absence of medical complications such as seizures or stroke) is toward restitution of function. Table 7-7 summarizes the results on key variables 1 month postinjury for the head-injury and two comparison groups.

For each task we designated on an a priori basis either one or two key dependent variables. This reduced to 22 the number of dependent variables from an original set of more than 70. Confirmatory factor analyses have been initiated to test our working hypotheses concerning the domains under which each task falls. That work is not yet far enough along to be reported. The frequency distributions of all the neuropsychological tasks within each group were examined to determine if there were significant deviations from normality. In those instances, scores were transformed using a logarithmic transformation.

Because there were small differences between the groups in age at entry into the study, we used, for initial analyses, multivariate analysis of covariance with age and SES as covariates to test for the effects of group. The neuropsychological variables were grouped on an a priori basis into five domains: (1) memory, (2) attention, (3) language, (4) executive and motor functions, and (5) handedness. The individual tasks are grouped by these domains in Table 7-7.

Four separate analyses of covariance were used to test for group differences on the variables contained in domains 1 to 4. A univariate analysis of covariance was used to test for group differences for domain 5 because only one variable was included in this domain. The results of the multivariate analysis of covariance showed a significant effect of group at 1 month postinjury on the memory domain $[F(14,718) = 2.51, P < 0.002]$ and an almost significant effect of group $[F(12,710)$ $p < 0.06]$ on the attention domain. As predicted from the results of prior studies, the groups did not differ in language functioning as indexed by PPVT-R or handedness. The groups also did not differ on the measures included in the executive and motor domains. The same analyses were conducted on the neuropsychological

TABLE 7-7. Neuropsychological Variables by Domain and Test 1 Month Postinjury

	Head Injury (N = 137)	Other Injury (N = 132)	No Injury (N = 114)	Effect of Group (F)				
				Adjusted for Age/SES	Adjusted for Age, SES and Pregnancy + Birth	Adjusted for Age, SES, and Developmental Delay	Adjusted for Age, SES, and History of Learning	Adjusted for Age, SES, and History of Medical Problems
Memory Domain								
Prospective Memory: total score	3.72 (1.1)	3.70 (1.1)	3.98 (1.1)	1.29	2.01	2.02	2.17	2.61
Picture Memory Interference: total correct	50.28 (6.6)	51.85 (5.3)	50.66 (6.0)	2.09	1.98	2.42	1.90	1.92
Picture Memory Interference: temporal coding	10.24 (2.5)	10.72 (2.1)	10.73 (2.2)	1.77	1.70	1.90	1.85	1.80
Word List Memory: total correct	18.89 (4.4)	19.25 (3.9)	20.16 (4.0)	3.01	2.94	3.02[a]	2.42	4.08[a]
Word List Memory: total extr + intru errors	2.54 (2.0)	2.91 (2.5)	1.96 (1.9)	8.58[c]	10.32[d]	10.32[d]	9.51[d]	10.48[d]
Word List Memory: release—total correct	6.03 (1.7)	6.03 (1.5)	6.26 (1.5)	0.87	0.63	0.83	0.42	0.97
Word List Memory: release—extr + intru errors	1.01 (1.0)	0.98 (1.1)	0.88 (1.0)	1.15	0.71	1.01	0.91	0.85
Attention Domain								
CPT: Summary hit rate	0.907 (0.11)	0.907 (0.13)	0.911 (0.09)	0.30	0.49	0.36	0.37	0.48
CPT: Summary false alarm rate	0.042 (0.08)	0.046 (0.10)	0.032 (0.04)	1.78	1.50	1.34	1.11	1.26
CPT: Summary sensitivity P(A)	0.969 (0.03)	0.964 (0.05)	0.966 (0.04)	2.12	2.41	2.24	2.21	2.62
SOA-3: letters-number correct out of 32	30.44 (1.8)	30.54 (1.7)	30.20 (2.4)	2.05	1.98	1.92	2.54	2.03
SOA-5: letters-number correct out of 64	60.10 (3.3)	59.48 (4.6)	59.77 (5.0)	1.31	1.36	1.45	1.46	1.32
SOA-10: letters-number correct out of 64	52.46 (7.5)	52.64 (6.6)	52.50 (6.1)	0.31	0.31	0.26	0.29	0.23

Language Domain

PPVT-R: standard score	100.22 (20.1)	96.00 (16.5)	103.25 (16.6)	2.06	2.44	2.46	1.91	2.84

Executive and Motor Functions Domain

Pin Test: advantage index	1.34 (0.2)	1.29 (0.2)	1.36 (0.2)	2.63	0.19	0.21	0.15	0.25
Symbol Digit: total correct	42.04 (13.2)	46.08 (13.0)	46.4 (13.2)	3.10[a]	3.48[a]	3.59[a]	3.03[a]	3.75[a]
Stroop Test: color naming time	50.27 (14.7)	46.86 (12.5)	46.49 (15.0)	1.84	2.86	3.15[a]	2.41	2.96
Stroop Test: reading time	38.09 (10.8)	36.92 (10.8)	35.11 (8.0)	3.40[a]	3.90[a]	4.31[a]	3.06[a]	4.33[a]
Stroop Test: interference time	82.79 (29.2)	76.44 (24.0)	77.56 (24.5)	0.72	1.27	1.23	0.85	1.29
Color Trails: trials 1 time	21.49 (12.9)	21.06 (19.3)	17.94 (8.8)	2.04	4.65[b]	5.23[b]	4.61[a]	4.94[b]
Color Trails: trials 2 time	45.44 (29.0)	39.56 (13.7)	37.76 (17.9)	1.89	1.67	1.95	1.42	1.94

Handedness

Handedness Check: total right hand	6.11 (2.1)	6.09 (2.1)	6.49 (1.6)	1.71	1.87	1.60	1.58	1.48

Abbreviations: extr + intru = extra- and intralist intrusions; CPT = continuous performance test; SOA = span of apprehension.

[a] $p < 0.05$.
[b] $p < 0.01$.
[c] $p < 0.001$.
[d] $p < 0.0001$.

data collected at 6 and 12 months postinjury. Those analyses revealed no significant effects of group in any domain.

Inspection of Table 7-7 reveals that on the tasks within the memory domain, the head-injury group tended to perform more poorly, with lower scores on measures of accuracy and higher scores on measures of errors than the noninjury group. Further inspection reveals that the head-injury and other-injury groups obtained similar scores on the tasks included within the memory and attention domains. The main effect of group reflects the differences between both injury groups and the noninjury group. This is seen most clearly on the total number of extra- and intralist intrusions on the Word List Memory Test, the single task that best differentiated between the groups.

Both injury groups had higher rates of errors than the noninjury group. In fact, the other-injury group had a somewhat higher rate of extra- and intralist intrusion errors than the head-injury group. If the other-injury group had not been included in this study and we had used the contrast between the head-injury and noninjury groups as the only test of the effect of a brain injury, we would have concluded erroneously that the head injury had produced subtle impairments in memory. The other-injury group controls for the nonspecific effects of incurring a head injury as well as for differences in preinjury functioning that were not captured by our measures of preinjury status. This is one of the more important methodological implications of the UCLA study.

To control for the effects of the four preinjury factors on neuropsychological functioning, each of these factors was entered in a separate analysis of covariance as a covariate after age and SES were first entered. The results of these analyses are summarized in the last four columns of Table 7-7. Correcting for these key preinjury factors had a relatively small effect.

Effect of Acute Head-Injury Severity. Within this study design there are two ways of determining the effects of CHI severity. The first (as just described) is to compare the neuropsychological performance of head-injured children with that of two groups of children who have not incurred a recent head injury. This analysis collapses across levels of severity within the head-injury group. It is possible that even within the attenuated range of acute head-injury severity sampled in this project, there may be an effect of degree of acute head-injury severity. This question is particularly important because only a relatively small proportion of children within the CHI group had injuries of AIS level 3. Similarly, relatively few of the children in the current sample had any significant periods of unconsciousness or posttraumatic amnesia (see Table 7-2). Perhaps children in the head-injury group with the more serious acute head injuries showed significant neuropsychological impairments relative to those with less severe injuries (AIS level 1). Could some of the children in the CHI group have incurred injuries that reached the minimal threshold for producing neuropsychological impairments? To evaluate this possibility, the children in the head-injury group were stratified using multiple measures of acute head-injury severity, including length of posttraumatic amnesia (PTA), length of unconsciousness, and the AIS level recorded in the hospital emergency room logs. We compared children with PTAs of zero with children with PTAs > 10 minutes; children with PTAs < 10 minutes with children of PTAs > 10 minutes; children who had never been unconscious to children who had been unconscious for > 10 minutes; and children with AIS scores of 1 versus AIS scores of 3. Multivariate analyses of covariance were used with age and SES forced in first as covariates; the four key preinjury factors also entered as covariates. We found no significant effects of acute head-injury severity. Only 7 of the 176 contrasts reached a 0.05 level of significance, well within the level of chance findings.

To conclude, the head-injury group did not show impaired neuropsychological functioning relative to the other-injury group. In the few instances where there were statistically significant differences between the two injury groups and the noninjury group, those differences were not judged to be clinically significant. Our previous experience with these tests both in clinical practice and in research suggests that the magnitude of the difference in scores between the head-injury and noninjury groups is very unlikely to have any adaptive significance in the children's everyday life.

Attention, Impulsivity, and Memory Scale (AIMS). During the course of conducting this study, it became clear that there was a need to add a measure of the child's subjective appraisal of his or her cognitive functioning. We modified a widely used self-report questionnaire—the Conners's Check List (Goyette et al., 1978)—by adding items to tap both prospective and retrospective memory. The wording of the items was changed so that they could be more readily understood by the children in the study sample who were not being referred to a clinic for psychological evaluations but were rather drawn from the community. After extensive pilot testing, we began collecting AIMS data. The AIMS had a satisfactory reliability coefficient, as measured by the Cronbach Coefficient Alpha, of 0.82. The AIMS was administered at each follow-up interval to assess the child's subjective appraisal of problems in attentiveness, memory, and impulsivity. Results of analysis of variance showed that the three groups did not differ on this instrument at any follow-up assessment. There was no indication that children in the head-injury group reported more cognitive complaints than children in the comparison groups.

Comments and Conclusions

The initial results of the UCLA study indicate that children admitted to ERs with mild CHI (AIS levels 1 to 3, with two or more concussive symptoms) do not show clinically significant neuropsychological impairments at either 1, 6, or 12 months postinjury. The mild-CHI group also did not show an increased rate of behavior problems at 12 months postinjury compared to the 6-month period before the index injury. There were no changes in the academic performance of the children in the mild-CHI group 1 year postinjury relative to their academic performance during the year prior to the injury. Finally, the children in the head-injury group did not report more cognitive complaints than the children in the other two groups.

These findings clearly indicate that the level of acute head-injury severity sampled in this phase of the UCLA study does not produce significant functional morbidity. As noted earlier, approximately 84% of the children in the CHI group had periods of unconsciousness < 30 minutes, with 62% having PTA < 30 minutes. Apparently this level of severity of acute injury is below the minimal threshold of head-injury severity necessary to produce significant functional morbidity. This study has helped to define an anchor point for injury severity which does *not* produce significant functional morbidity. What is left unanswered is how much more severe an injury has to be before it causes significant functional morbidity in a child.

Fundamentally different conclusions would have been reached had we not controlled for preinjury level of functioning. The head-injury group had elevated scores on the total behavior problem scale of the CBCL 12 months postinjury as compared to the noninjury group. Virtually all of the studies summarized in Table 7-1 did not use other-injury control groups, and very few assessed preinjury level of functioning. We would have concluded that the index head injury resulted in elevated rates of behavior problems had we not measured preinjury level of functioning. We found, however, that the children in the head-injury group (consistent with prior studies) had elevated rates of behavior problems *prior* to the index injury. Their rates of behavior problems actually *declined* at 12 months relative to their preinjury level, providing compelling evidence that the index head injury did not produce an increased frequency of *new* behavior problems. In addition, at both preinjury and 12 months postinjury, the head-injury and other-injury groups had similar rates of behavior problems, providing additional evidence that the index head injury did not produce a brain insult that directly caused elevated rates of behavior problems.

A similar situation pertains to neuropsychological functioning. There was a tendency at 1 month postinjury, particularly on certain measures tapping memory and executive functions, for the head-injury group to perform below the level of the noninjury group. These differences, even when statistically significant, were quite small and of little or no clinical significance. One could have argued, however, that there were subtle impairments in memory and certain executive functions. These small differences were not appreciably affected by controlling for the four indices of preinjury functioning. But when preinjury functioning was controlled by examining the contrast between the CHI and other-injury group, a different picture emerged. There were no significant differences between the CHI and other-injury groups on any of the neuropsychological variables. Given the relatively large sample size, the lack of group differences is not due to the absence of statistical power. Rather, it indicates that when aspects of preinjury functioning not adequately measured by our questionnaires and interviews are controlled by a comparison group that had incurred an accidental injury not involving the brain, there is no effect of the index head injury. This constellation of findings underscores the importance for subsequent studies of including an other-injury control group to determine the neurobehavioral sequelae of mild head injuries.

The results of the present study are largely consistent with the results of studies summarized in Table 7-1. Studies that rigorously screened for preexisting CNS impairments, developmental delays, and behavior problems tended to find less functional morbidity postinjury than studies that did less extensive screening of the child's preinjury status.

The results of the present study clearly demonstrate the level of acute head-injury severity that *does not* produce significant functional morbidity in children and adolescents. We intend to build upon these results by extending the present study to examine children with more serious head injuries in order to identify the minimal threshold of severity necessary to produce significant functional morbidity in children and adolescents.

Acknowledgments

This work was supported by a grant from the National Institute of Neurological Disorders and Stroke (RO1 NS26801). The authors gratefully acknowledge the assistance of the patients, parents, and hospitals that participated in this study. We are also grateful for the assistance of the Downey School District and Mrs. Wendy Marino, who provided invaluable help in word processing.

References

Asarnow, R. F., Satz, P., Light, R., Lewis, R., & Neumann, E. (1991). Behavior problems and adaptive functioning in children with mild and severe closed head injury. *J. Pediatr. Psychol., 16,* 543–555.

Achenbach, T., & Edelbrook, C. (1983). *Manual for the Child Behavior Checklist and the Revised Behavior Profile.* Burlington, VT: Department of Psychiatry, University of Vermont.

Annegers, J. F. (1986). The epidemiology of head trauma in children. In K. Shapiro (Ed.), *Pediatric head trauma.* Mt. Kisco, NY: Futura.

Bawden, H. N., Knights, R. M., & Winogron, H. W. (1985). Speeded performance following head injury in children, *J. Clin. Exp. Neuropsychol., 7,* 39–54.

Bijur, P., Haslum, M., & Golding, J. (1990). Cognitive and behavioral sequelae of mild head injury in children. *Pediatrics, 86,* 337–344.

Black, P., Blumer, D., Wellner, A. M., & Walker, A. E. (1971). The head-injured child: Time-course of recovery, with implications for rehabilitation. In *Head Injuries, Proceedings of an International Symposium.* Edinburgh and London: Churchill Livingstone.

Boll, T. J. (1983). Minor head injury in children—Out of sight but not out of mind. *J. Clin. Child Psychol., 12,* 74–80.

Brooks, D., Deelman, A., Zomeren, H., Dongen, H., Harskamp, F., & Aughton, M. (1984). Problems in measuring cognitive recovery after acute brain injury. *J. Clin. Neuropsychol., 6,* 71–85.

Brown, G., Chadwick, O., Shaffer, D., Rutter, M., & Traub, M. (1981). A prospective study of children with head injuries: III. Psychiatric sequelae. *Psychol. Med., 11,* 1227–1232.

Butterbaugh, G., Roochvarg, L., Slater-Rusonis, E., Miranda, D., & Heald, F. (1993). Academic abilities in adolescents with traumatic brain injuries: An 18-month follow-up study. *J. Clin. Exp. Psychol., 15,* 84 (abstract).

Casey, R., Ludwig, S., & McCormick, M. C. (1986). Morbidity following minor head trauma in children. *Pediatrics, 78,* 497–502.

Chadwick, O., Rutter, M., Brown, G., Shaffer, D., & Traub, M. (1981). A prospective study of children with head injuries: II. Cognitive sequelae. *Psychol. Med., 11,* 49–61.

Chapman, S. B., Culhane, K. A., Levin, H. S., Harward, H., Mendelsohn, D., Ewing-Cobbs, L., Fletcher, J. M., & Bruce, D. (1992). Narrative discourse after closed head injury in children and adolescents. *Brain Lang., 43,* 42–65.

Dikmen, S., McLean, A., & Temkin, N. (1986). Neuropsychological and psychosocial consequences of minor head injury. *J. Neurol. Neurosurg. Psychiatry, 49,* 1227–1232.

Dunn, L. M., & Dunn, L. M. (1981). *Peabody Picture Vocabulary Test—Revised Manual.* Circle Pines, MN: American Guidance Service.

Ewing-Cobbs, L., Fletcher, J. M., & Levin, H. S. (1985). Neuropsychological sequelae following pediatric head injury. In M. Ylvisaker (Ed.), *Head injury rehabilitation: Children and adolescents* (pp. 71–90). San Diego, CA: College-Hill.

Ewing-Cobbs, L., Levin, H. S., Eisenberg, H. M., & Fletcher, J. M. (1987). Language functions following closed head-injury in children and adolescents. *J. Clin. Exp. Neuropsychol., 9,* 575–592.

Ewing-Cobbs, L., Levin, H. S., Fletcher, J. M., Miner, M. E., & Eisenberg, H. M. (1990). The Children's Orientation and Amnesia Test: Relationship to severity of acute head injury and to recovery of memory. *Neurosurgery, 27,* 683–691.

Ewing-Cobbs, L., Miner, M. E., Fletcher, J. M., & Levin, H. S. (1989). Intellectual, motor, and language sequelae following closed head injury in infants and preschoolers. *J. Pediatr. Psychol., 14,* 531–547.

Fletcher, J. M., Ewing-Cobbs, L., Miner, M. E., Levin, H. S., & Eisenberg, H. M. (1990). Behavioral changes after closed head injury in children. *J. Consult. Clin. Psychol., 58,* 93–98.

Golden, J. C. (1976). Identification of brain disorders by the Stroop Color and Word Test. *J. Clin. Psychol., 32,* 654–658.

Goyette, C. H., Conners, C. K., and Ulrich, R. F. (1978). Normative data for Revised Conners Parent and Teacher Rating Scales. *J. Abnorm. Child Psychol., 6,* 221–236.

Gronwall, D., & Wrightson, P. (1974). Delayed recovery of intellectual function after minor head injury. *Lancet, 2,* 605–609.

Gulbrandsen, G. B. (1984). Neuropsychological sequelae of light head injuries in older children 6 months after trauma. *J. Clin. Neuropsychol., 6,* 257–268.

Hannay, H. J., & Levin, H. S. (1988). Visual continuous recognition memory in normal and closed-head-injured adolescents. *J. Clin. Exp. Neuropsychol., 11,* 444–460.

Horowitz, I., Costeff, H., Sadan, N., Abraham, E., Geyer, S., & Najenson, T. (1983). Childhood head injuries in Israel: Epidemiology and outcome. *Int. Rehab. Med., 5,* 32–36.

Kewman, D. G., Warschausky, S., & Jordan, C. (1992). Canonical relationships between achievement and intelligence of children with traumatic brain insult. *J. Clin. Exp. Neuropsychol., 14,* 114 (abstract).

Klonoff, H., Low, M. D., & Clark, C. (1977). Head injuries in children: A prospective five year follow-up. *J. Neurol. Neurosurg. Psychiatry, 40,* 1211–1219.

Knights, R. M., Ivan, L. P., Ventureyra, E., Bentivoglio, C., Stoddart, C., Winogron, W., & Bawden, H. N. (1991). The effects of head injury in children on neuropsychological and behavioral functioning. *Brain Injury, 5,* 339–351.

Leahy, L. F., Holland, A. L. & Frattalli, C. M. (1987). Persistent deficits following closed-head injury. *J. Clin. Exp. Neuropsychol., 9,* 55 (abstract).

Levin, H. S., & Eisenberg, H. M. (1979). Neuropsychological impairments after closed head injury in children and adolescents. *J. Pediatr. Psychol., 4,* 389–402.

Levin, H. S., Mattis, S., Ruff, R. M., Eisenberg, H. M., Marshall, L. F., Tabaddor, K., High, W. M., & Frankowski, R. F. (1987). Neurobehavioral outcome following minor head injury: A three center study. *J. Neurosurg., 66,* 234–243.

Levin, H. S., Mendelsohn, D., Lilly, M. A., Fletcher, J. M., Culhane, K. A., Chapman, S. B., Harward, H., Kusnerik, L., Bruce, D., & Eisenberg, H. M. (1994). Tower of London performance in relation to magnetic resonance imaging following closed head injury in children. *Neuropsychology, 8,* 171–179.

Light, R., Neumann, E., Lewis, R., Morecki-Oberg, C., Asarnow, R., & Satz, P. (1987). An evaluation of a neuropsychologically based re-education project for the head-injured child. *J. Head Trauma Rehabil., 2,* 11–25.

Lundar, T., & Nestvold, K. (1985). Pediatric head injuries caused by traffic accidents: A prospective study with 5-year follow-up. *Childs Nerv. Syst., 1,* 24–28.

Mahalick, D. M., Yalamanchi, K., & Bowen, M. (1990). Spontaneous recovery in pediatric head injury. *Proceedings of the National Head-injury Foundation 9th Annual National Symposium.* New Orleans, LA.

Mattson, A. J., Levin, H. S., Evankovich, K. E., Ewing-Cobbs, L., & Fletcher, J. M. (1990). Longitudinal assessment of memory and motor skills after mild closed head injury in children and adolescents. *J. Clin. Exp. Neuropsychol. 12,* 104 (abstract).

Nuechterlein, K. H., (1983). Signal detection in vigilance tasks and behavioral attributes among offspring of schizophrenic mothers and among hyperactive children. *J. Abnorm. Psychol., 92,* 4.

Prigatano, G. P., & Papero, P. H. (1991). The effects of age, severity, and chronicity of head injury on neuropsychological test performance of children, *J. Clin. Exp. Neuropsychol., 13,* 437 (abstract).

Reitan, R. M., & Wolfson, D. (1985). *The Halstead-Reitan Neuropsychological Test Battery.* Tucson, AZ: Neuropsychology Press.

Rutter, M. (1981). Psychological sequelae of brain damage in children. *Am. J. Psychiatry, 138,* 1533–1544.

Satz, P., & D'Elia, L. (1989). *The Pin Test Professional Manual.* Odessa, FL: Psychological Assessment Resources.

Smith, A. (1968). The Symbol Digit Modalities test: A neuropsychologic test for learning and other cerebral disorders. *J. Learning Dis., 3,* 83–91.

Snoek, J. W., Minderhoud, J. M., & Wilmink, J. T. (1984) Delayed deterioration following mild head injury in children. *Brain, 107,* 15–36.

Tompkins, C. A., Holland, A. L., Ratcliff, G., Costello, A., Leahy, L. F., & Cowell, V. (1990). Predicting cognitive recovery from closed head-injury in children and adolescents. *Brain Cogn., 13,* 86–97.

Thompson, N. M., Francis, D., Fletcher, J. M., Ewing-Cobbs, L., Levin, H. S., & Miner, M. (1990). Recovery of spatial, motor, and perceptual skills following closed head injury in children. *J. Clin. Exp. Neuropsychol., 12,* 104 (abstract).

Wickens, D. (1970). Encoding categorized words: An empirical approach to memory. *Psychol. Rev., 77,* 1–15.

Williams, D. H., Levin, H. S., & Eisenberg, H. M. (1990). Mild head injury classification. *Neurosurgery, 27,* 422–428.

Winogron, H. W., Knights, R. M., & Bawden, H. N. (1984). Neuropsychological deficits following head injury in children, *J. Clin. Neuropsychol., 6,* 269–286.

8

Cognitive, Behavioral, and Motoric Sequelae of Mild Head Injury in a National Birth Cohort

POLLY E. BIJUR and MARY HASLUM

It is evident from the studies comparing sequelae across varying degrees of severity of injury that if there are persistent deficits due to mild head injury, they are more subtle and are expressed with greater variability than the deficits associated with more extensive damage to the brain. The lack of clarity about the outcome of mild head injury may be due in large part to the increased importance methodology assumes in the study of weak associations (see Asarnow et al., this volume). Differences in definition of mild head injury, choice of outcomes, measurement of outcomes, length of follow-up, choice of comparison groups, and characteristics to be controlled analytically may all lead to different conclusions about the sequelae of mild head injury.

Goldstein and Levin (1985) have nicely summarized the literature on cognitive outcomes of head injury in the pediatric age range with a focus on the various methodologies used to study this issue. Investigations of behavioral and psychiatric sequelae have been reported by numerous authors (Brown et al., 1981; Casey et al., 1986; Coonley-Hoganson et al., 1984; Light et al., 1993; Rutter, 1981; see also Shaffer, this volume).

An issue that has not been addressed in the pediatric literature is the possibility that repeated mild injuries to the head result in cumulative damage that may lead to adverse cognitive, behavioral, or motoric outcomes. Two studies of multiple head injury in adults have suggested that the effects are cumulative (see also, Klonoff et al., this volume). Gronwall and colleagues, (1974, 1975) have shown that information processing abilities are affected by concussion, and that recovery of these abilities takes substantially longer in subjects with a previous concussion than in those with only one mild head injury. Roberts (1969) described a syndrome in boxers who suffer multiple head trauma which includes dysarthria, ataxia, pyramidal and extrapyramidal signs, and dementia.

The observed association between mild head injuries (measured in a variety of ways) and adverse behavioral and cognitive sequelae can be explained by several models. The most straightforward is a model that posits a direct causal relationship between damage to the brain and specific behaviors and cognitive functions. An elaboration of this model is one in which the brain injury causes cognitive disturbances that lead to behavioral problems. The relationship between cognitive deficits and brain injury is direct, but the relationship with behavior is indirect. Alternatively, the primary relationship could be between behavior and brain injury with a secondary impact on cognition and academic achievement. A second model posits that children with and without injuries of any kind differ on a variety of personal, familial, and social characteristics, and that these differences are associated with differential injury risk. One specific form of this model is that the observed behavioral problems of children with head injuries precede the injuries temporally and increase the risk of injury. The observed association is therefore an epiphenomenon with no causal implications. There is a discrepant literature on the preinjury behaviors of children with head injury. Brown and colleagues (1981) found a higher rate of premorbid behavioral problems in children with mild head injuries than in the controls, and Bijur and coworkers (1990) similarly found higher scores on measures of aggression and activity before the injury than in children without any injuries. In contrast, Pelco and associates (1992) and Donders (1991) found the prevalence of preexisting behavioral difficulties to be the same in head-injured children as in children in the communities studied.

Two other models address the association between behavioral/emotional problems and head injury but apply less directly to cognitive sequelae except insofar as cognitive problems are associated with emotional or behavioral disorders. In a model suggested by Casey and coworkers (1986), the parental response to a child with head injury, (e.g., indulgence, overprotection, excess concern) leads to behavioral problems. Another model described by Basson and colleagues (1991) proposes that all injuries, not just those involving the head, have the potential to lead to behavioral and emotional problems, the most extreme of which could be classified as posttraumatic stress disorder.

The study described in this chapter was undertaken to specifically test the model in which premorbid differences in behavior, cognition, and familial and social factors are causally related to subsequent injury of all kinds and the observed association between head injury and adverse outcomes is a spurious one (Bijur et al., 1990). This study also addresses the impact of multiple mild injuries to the head on cognitive, behavioral, and motoric outcomes. As the head is the body part most frequently injured in children (Manheimer et al., 1966) and given the high rate of head injuries (Kraus et al., 1986), it is likely that a substantial number of children have sustained multiple head injuries during their childhoods (see Kraus, this volume).

The British Birth Cohort

The existence of the 1970 British Birth Cohort, which included measures of behavior and intellectual functioning on approximately 12,000 children around the time of their fifth birthday, provided an unusual opportunity to examine the outcome of mild injury in children for whom there were independent premorbid measures of behavior and cognition. This is a rich data set with multiple measures of the familial, social, and physical environment that allow comparisons between single and multiple head injuries while appropriately taking into account the role of non-injury-related factors that distinguish children with varying numbers of injuries.

Data Collection and Analysis

The subjects were sampled from the 1970 British Birth Cohort, which consists of approximately 12,000 children born during 1 week in 1970 and assessed at ages 5 and 10 under the auspices of the Child Health and Education Study (Butler et al., 1986; Child Health and Education Study, 1982). The children's parents were extensively interviewed by visiting nurses from the National Health Service at the time of the children's fifth and tenth birthdays. At the time of the children's 10-year interview, the parents were asked the following question:

> Since the fifth birthday, has the child had an accident requiring medical advice or treatment? Please include accidents at home, in school, on the road and elsewhere, accidental ingestion of medicines/poisons, burns/scalds, eye injuries, near-drowning, bad cuts, and other injuries with and without unconsciousness. If yes, please state total number of accidents.

At the time of the 5-year interview, the parents were asked the same question, although the question then focused on the period between birth and age 5. Parents' descriptions of the children's injuries in both time periods were coded using the International Classification of Diseases, 9th revision (World Health Organization, 1978).

In the first set of analyses, the cognitive, academic, behavioral, and motoric outcomes of children with one or more mild head injuries experienced after the fifth birthday were compared to the outcomes of children without injury from age 5 to age 10 and to those with limb fractures, lacerations or burns. The definition of mild head injury for this set of analyses was a parental report of a head injury that resulted in concussion (ICD-9 code 850), or loss of consciousness (ICD-9 code 780) and a head-injury code: 800, 801, 803, 804, 851 to 854. The injured child had to have been treated as an outpatient or admitted to hospital for one night. There were 114 children who had head injuries between ages 5 and 10 who met these criteria. Nine of the head-injured children had two head injuries that met the criteria and two children had three head injuries between their fifth and tenth birthdays. Forty-three percent of the children in the sample were hospitalized following the head injury.

The head-injured children were compared with four other groups of children: (1) a random sample of 1726 children who had no injuries between the ages of 5 and 10; (2) 601 children who had limb fractures (ICD-9 code 810-829); (3) 605 children with lacerations of the limbs (ICD-9 code 880-884, 890-894); and (4) 136 children with burns (ICD-9 codes 940-949). Children with multiple injuries from a single accident or multiple accidents were assigned to an injury group using the following hierarchy: head injury, burn, fracture, laceration.

Other inclusion criteria included no head injury between birth and age 5, mother present at interview, family primarily English-speaking, child never in residential care, more than half the behavioral data available, singleton birth, and hospitalized for no more than one night for injury.

In the analyses of multiple head injuries, a less stringent definition of head injury was used than in the first set of analyses, so that there would be a sufficient number of subjects. In these analyses, a head injury was defined as a parental report of a head injury (ICD-9 codes 800, 801, 803, 804, 851 to 854) regardless of whether there was any evidence of concussion or loss of consciousness. Head injuries that occurred in the entire 10-year age period, from birth to age 10, were counted in these analyses. There were 1698 children with one head injury that met these criteria, 296 with two head injuries, and 53 with three or more. These children were matched to children who did not experience any injuries to the head between birth and age 10 on the total number of injuries in the 10-year period and on sex. Thus the children matched to the children with one head injury had a minimum of one injury, those matched to children with two head injuries had a minimum of two injuries, and the controls for those with three or more head injuries had a minimum of three injuries not to the head. Children with head injuries who had a large total number of injuries (i.e., five or more) could not all be matched with children without head injuries. A hierarchy was therefore established, so that the children with three or more head injuries were first matched to children without head injuries on the basis of their total number of injuries and sex; then the children with two head injuries were matched to the remaining children without head injuries; and finally those with one head injury were matched. Matches could not be found for 4% of the children with three or more head injuries, 6% of children with two head injuries, and 7% of children with one head injury. The inclusion criteria were the same for this set of analyses as the prior set except that children with head injuries before age 5 were also included in the analyses, again to increase the number of subjects.

The cognitive outcomes came from group testing of the children at school during the 10-year interview. They include four subscales of the British Abilities Scale (word definitions, recall of digits, similarities and matrices), the Child Health and Education Study Language Pictorial Comprehension Test (based on the English Picture Vocabulary Test), and a shortened version of the Edinburgh Reading Test. A mathematics test, the Friendly Maths Test, was devised for the study. The cognitive scales and achievement tests were all standardized to a mean of 100 and a standard deviation of 15.

The behavioral outcome measures come from parents' and teacher's reports of child behaviors on the Rutter and Conner's questionnaires (Conners, 1969; Rutter et al., 1970). Subscales were derived through factor analysis of these scales to measure aggressive behavior such as bullying other children, destroying belongings, and hyperactive behavior (e.g., hardly ever sits still, is restless and overactive). Preinjury intelligence was measured by the English Picture Vocabulary Test (Brimer and Dunn, 1963), a British modification of the Peabody Picture Vocabulary Test, and preinjury behavior was assessed by parent's report of aggressive and hyperactive behavior on the Rutter Child Behavior Questionnaire (Rutter et al., 1970). The behavioral scales were all standardized to a mean of zero and a standard deviation of one.

During the 10-year survey, the children were given a series of motoric tests by National Health Service physicians in the school, and teachers and parents were administered questionnaires concerning the fine and gross motor coordination of their children. The motoric outcomes included the maximum number of times the child clapped after throwing a ball in the air and before catching it; the average time a child could balance on one leg without moving hands or feet; the number of steps a child could walk backward without error; and the number of seconds it took a child to sort matches.

Many social, familial, and personal factors are known to differ between children with and without injury. Therefore, even after statistical control for preexisting measures of behavior and cognition, differences between head-injured children and noninjured controls could result from differences in these other characteristics. The following factors were controlled analytically: socioeconomic status, housing quality, mother's depression, mother's employment, number of household moves from birth to age 5, number of siblings, child's sex, number of non-accident-related hospitalizations, and number of injuries between birth and age 5.

Analysis of covariance was used to compare the mean outcome measures among groups. The Scheffé criterion was used to test the difference between pairs of groups while adjusting the significance level for the effect of multiple significance tests.

Sample Characteristics

Many of the social and demographic characteristics measured at age 5 varied among the five groups of children, as shown in Table 8-1. Compared to the uninjured children, the children with burns and lacerations had substantially lower mean scores on the index of socioeconomic status (SES), while the head-injured had somewhat higher SES and those with fractures were quite similar to the uninjured. The quality of the injured children's housing was lower than that of the uninjured, their mothers were younger, the children were more likely to be male, and they had substantially higher rates of injuries not to the head prior to their fifth birthdays than the children who were uninjured between ages 5 and 10. There were also differences among the injured children; those with burns and lacerations

TABLE 8-1.   Social and Personal Characteristics of the Sample[a]

	No Injuries (N = 1726)[b]	Head Injury (N = 114)	Burns (N = 136)	Fractures (N = 601)	Lacerations (N = 605)	p
Socioeconomic status	0.00 ± 0.99	0.13 ± 0.98	−0.34 ± 74[c]	−0.02 ± 0.98	−0.14 ± 0.96[c]	<0.00
Quality of housing	0.03 ± 1.00	−0.04 ± 1.08	−0.16 ± 0.96	0.01 ± 0.95	−0.10 ± 1.00	<0.05
Mother's age	26.21 ± 5.36	25.06 ± 5.04	25.64 ± 5.99	25.79 ± 5.14	25.27 ± 5.44[c]	<0.01
Mother's depression	4.12 ± 3.46	4.29 ± 3.53	4.64 ± 3.49	4.40 ± 3.59	4.64 ± 3.59[c]	<0.05
Number of siblings	1.44 ± 0.98	1.43 ± 0.89	1.62 ± 1.11	1.44 ± 0.94	1.64 ± 1.12[c]	<0.00
Mother's full-time work (% full time)	11.6	17.5	10.9	11.4	15.1	<0.05
Sex of child (% male)	43.6	64.9[c]	50.7	51.9[c]	64.8[c]	<0.00
Number of hospitalizations not related to injury	0.26 ± 0.64	0.50 ± 0.85[c]	0.26 ± 0.62	0.30 ± 0.69	0.27 ± 0.63	<0.01
Number of injuries, birth to 5 years	0.35 ± 0.61	0.52 ± 0.79	0.55 ± 0.77[c]	0.52 ± 0.77[c]	0.57 ± 0.86[c]	<0.00
Aggression score at age 5	−0.12 ± 0.91	0.28 ± 1.24[c]	0.03 ± 0.86	0.10 ± 1.05[c]	0.26 ± 1.12[c]	<0.00
Hyperactivity score at age 5	−0.04 ± 0.97	0.00 ± 1.06	0.09 ± 1.02	0.06 ± 1.03	0.17 ± 1.05[c]	<0.00
Verbal intelligence (EPVT) at age 5	0.10 ± 0.94	0.11 ± 0.94	−0.14 ± 0.88	0.03 ± 0.95	−0.07 ± 0.94[c]	<0.00

[a] Mean ± standard deviation unless otherwise noted.

[b] Number of subject varies for different measures due to missing data.

[c] Significantly different from No Injuries group, Scheffé criterion.

came from the most disadvantaged families. The head-injured children differed significantly from the uninjured only on the proportion of males. Their rate of other injuries prior to the fifth birthday and average maternal age were similar to those of the other injured children and quite different from those of the uninjured children, although not statistically significant because of the smaller sample size.

As a group, the injured children had higher scores on aggression and hyperactivity at age 5, before the occurrence of the injuries, than the uninjured children. The children with head injuries after age 5 and those with lacerations had the highest means scores on aggression at age 5, and those with lacerations had the highest mean scores on hyperactivity as well. The measure of verbal intelligence at age 5 presents a somewhat more complex picture. There were no differences between the verbal intelligence of the head-injured children, those with fractures, and the uninjured children, while the children with burns and lacerations had lower mean scores than the uninjured children on the English Picture Vocabulary Test at age 5.

Cognitive and Achievement Outcomes

The mean scores on the British Ability Scale at age 10 of the head-injured children were indistinguishable from those of the noninjured children both before and after

TABLE 8-2.   Cognitive Outcomes by Injury Group: Unadjusted and Adjusted Means

		British Ability Scale			Ches Language Comprehension Test	
Injury Group	N	Unadjusted Mean	Adjusted Mean[a]	N	Unadjusted Mean	Adjusted Mean[a]
No injury	1374	101.4	100.9	1395	101.6	101.2
Head injury	91	102.2	101.0	92	102.2	101.1
Burns	107	95.3[b]	97.8	96	98.4	100.3
Fractures	466	100.4	100.4	479	101.8	101.6
Lacerations	504	96.9[b]	98.1[b]	512	99.2	100.2
F		11.17	5.44		3.54	0.80
p		<0.001	<0.001		<0.01	0.53

Source: From Bijur et al., 1990, with permission.

[a] Adjusted for sex of child, socioeconomic status, housing quality, age of mother, maternal malaise inventory, mother's employment, number of siblings in household at age 5, number of non-accident-related hospitalizations of the child from birth to age 5, number of other injuries between birth and age 5, and English Picture Vocabulary Test at age 5.

[b] Significantly different from no-injury group, Scheffé criterion.

adjustment for the social factors and the measure of intelligence at age 5, as shown in Table 8-2. The mean scores of children with burns and lacerations were significantly lower than the means of the uninjured children, and this remained significant for the children with lacerations after statistical adjustment for all the covariates. The language comprehension test had almost identical results.

The head-injured children had slightly lower math scores than the uninjured children, but the only significant differences were again between the children with burns and lacerations versus the uninjured children before control of the estimate of their preinjury intelligence (Table 8-3). The results of the reading test were

TABLE 8-3.   Academic Achievement by Injury Group: Unadjusted and Adjusted Means

		Friendly Maths Test			Edinburgh Reading Test	
Injury Group	N	Unadjusted Mean	Adjusted Mean[a]	N	Unadjusted Mean	Adjusted Mean[a]
No injury	1392	101.3	100.7	1398	102.1	101.2
Head injury	92	99.6	98.7	92	99.1	98.6
Burns	108	95.7[b]	97.9	109	97.0[b]	99.5
Fractures	475	100.2	100.1	479	100.5	100.5
Lacerations	512	97.8[b]	99.0	513	96.7[b]	98.5[b]
F		7.64	2.63		14.14	4.85
p		<0.001	0.03		<0.001	0.001

Source: From Bijur et al., 1990, with permission.

[a] Adjusted for sex of child, socioeconomic status, housing quality, age of mother, maternal malaise inventory, mother's employment, number of siblings in household at age 5, number of non-accident-related hospitalizations of the child from birth to age 5, number of other injuries between birth and age 5, and English Picture Vocabulary Test at age 5.

[b] Significantly different from no-injury group, Scheffé criterion.

similar, in that the head-injured children had slightly lower scores than the uninjured group, but these mean scores were statistically indistinguishable. The magnitude of both the math and reading scores was similar for the children with head injuries and those with burns and lacerations. Because of the larger number of children with lacerations, however, only their mean math and reading scores were statistically distinguishable from those of the uninjured children.

Behavioral Outcomes

All the injured children had higher mean aggression scores than the uninjured children before adjustment for the covariates (Table 8-4). The mean score based on the mother's report of the head-injured children's aggressiveness was about one-fifth of a standard deviation higher than the mean aggression scores of the noninjured controls. These differences were attenuated after control for mother's report of aggression and the other covariates at age 5. The teacher's report of aggression was less affected by control of the preinjury reports of aggression but follows the same pattern in that all the injured children had higher mean aggression scores as rated by the teacher, and the head-injured children's scores are no worse and, in fact, better than those of some of the other injured children.

All the injured children had higher mean hyperactivity scores than the uninjured controls (Table 8-5). Mother's report of child's hyperactivity at age 10 was about three-tenths of a standard deviation higher than the mean of the uninjured children. This was reduced to about two-tenths of a standard deviation after the covariates were introduced, and the association was not statistically significant. The teacher's report of child's hyperactivity, in contrast, was the only outcome that distinguished the head-injured children from the noninjured, even after full statistical control. The head-injured children had hyperactivity scores that were half a standard deviation higher than those of the uninjured children and remained

TABLE 8-4.   Measures of Aggression by Injury Group: Unadjusted and Adjusted Means

| | | Mother's Report | | | Teacher's Report | |
Injury Group	N	Unadjusted Mean	Adjusted Mean[a]	N	Unadjusted Mean	Adjusted Mean[a]
No injury	1678	−0.07	0.01	1469	−0.11	−0.07
Head injury	113	0.13	0.01	95	0.14	0.06
Burns	134	0.18	0.11	113	0.27[b]	0.25[b]
Fractures	596	0.07	0.03	515	0.04	0.03
Lacerations	595	0.23[b]	0.08	532	0.24[b]	0.16[b]
F		10.76	0.86		15.74	7.17
p		<0.001	0.49		<0.001	<0.001

[a] Adjusted for sex of child, socioeconomic status, housing quality, age of mother, maternal malaise inventory, mother's employment, number of siblings in household at age 5, number of non-accident-related hospitalizations of the child from birth to age 5, number of other injuries between birth and age 5, and mother's report of child's aggression at age 5.

[b] Significantly different from no-injury group, Scheffé criterion.

TABLE 8-5.   Measures of Hyperactivity by Injury Group: Unadjusted and
Adjusted Means

		Mother's Report			Teacher's Report	
Injury Group	N	Unadjusted Mean	Adjusted Mean[a]	N	Unadjusted Mean	Adjusted Mean[a]
No injury	1680	−0.07	−0.02	1469	−0.10	−0.05
Head injury	113	0.20	0.17	95	0.43[b]	0.36[b]
Burns	134	0.17	0.10	113	0.24[b]	0.19
Fractures	595	0.06	0.03	515	0.03	0.01
Lacerations	597	0.23[b]	0.11	532	0.23[b]	0.13[b]
F		12.38	3.31		17.65	7.59
p		<0.001	<0.01		<0.001	<0.001

[a]Adjusted for sex of child, socioeconomic status, housing quality, age of mother, maternal malaise inventory, mother's employment, number of siblings in household at age 5, number of non-accident-related hospitalizations of the child from birth to age 5, number of other injuries between birth and age 5, and mother's report of child's hyperactivity at age 5.
[b]Significantly different from no-injury group, Scheffé criterion.

about four-tenths of a standard deviation higher after control for preinjury behavior.

Due to the significant association between hyperactivity and head injury, further analyses of this relationship were performed in order to assess whether the association was likely to be causal. It was hypothesized that if the overall association observed was causal, it would be stronger for those injured more recently than those injured earlier, as the children injured earlier would have had more time to recover. There is a statistically significant relationship between the age at injury and mother's rating of hyperactivity ($p = 0.02$). It is opposite, however, to the hypothesized direction, with children injured between their fifth and sixth birthdays having the highest scores on hyperactivity while those injured when they were older had lower scores. In contrast, there was no linear relationship between the teacher's rating of hyperactivity and age of injury. Children injured at ages 6 to 7 and those injured between 9 and 10 years had the highest mean scores on hyperactivity.

Motoric Outcomes

The mean scores of all five groups of children on the four observed motoric measures were indistinguishable both before and after adjustment for the covariates, as shown in Table 8-6. Unlike the cognitive and behavioral outcomes, the motoric outcomes were not associated with the social and demographic variables, which differ among the five groups of children. While the observed motoric measures were virtually identical across the five groups, the mothers' rating of clumsiness was significantly associated with injury status (Table 8-7). The mothers rated the head-injured children and those with lacerations as clumsier than those without injuries. Again, because of the larger number of children with lacerations and the slightly higher mean clumsiness score, it was only the children with lacerations

TABLE 8-6. Observed Motoric Outcomes at Age 10 by Injury Group: Unadjusted and Adjusted Means

Injury Group	Number of Claps			Balance Time			Steps Backwards			Sort Matches		
	N	Unadjusted Mean	Adjusted Mean[a]	*N*	Unadjusted Mean	Adjusted Mean[a]	*N*	Unadjusted Mean	Adjusted Mean[a]	*N*	Unadjusted Mean	Adjusted Mean[a]
No injury	1520	2.97	2.94	1503	25.7	25.6	1489	15.5	15.5	1499	46.5	46.6
Head injury	104	3.12	3.16	100	25.4	25.8	102	15.3	15.4	104	45.0	44.8
Burns	123	2.88	2.91	119	26.0	26.2	118	15.8	15.8	121	46.1	46.0
Fracture	528	2.96	2.96	518	25.1	25.2	526	15.6	15.6	527	45.3	45.5
Lacerations	538	2.98	3.03	526	25.0	25.3	523	15.8	15.9	533	46.6	46.2
F		0.61	1.32		2.31	1.09		0.41	0.50		0.69	0.73
p		0.65	0.26		0.06	0.36		0.80	0.74		0.60	0.57

[a]Adjusted for sex of child, socioeconomic status, housing quality, age of mother, maternal malaise inventory, mother's employment, number of siblings in household at age 5, number of non-accident-related hospitalizations of child from birth to age 5, number of other injuries between birth and age 5.

who were statistically distinguishable from the uninjured children. While the injury status was not significantly associated with teachers' rating of clumsiness, the teachers rated all the children who had sustained injuries between ages 5 and 10 years as clumsier than the uninjured children. The magnitude of the differences was only about one- to two-tenths of a standard deviation. The teachers' scale was further broken down into fine and gross motor skills. Neither of these was significantly associated with injury status. The head-injured children, however, had the highest mean score on the fine motor deficits scale (0.21 standard deviation above the mean versus -0.01 for the uninjured controls).

TABLE 8-7. Teachers' and Mothers' Ratings of Children's Clumsiness: Unadjusted and Adjusted Means

Injury Group	Teacher's Rating of Clumsiness			Mother's Rating of Clumsiness		
	N	Unadjusted Mean	Adjusted Mean[a]	*N*	Unadjusted Mean	Adjusted Mean[a]
No injury	1353	-0.04	-0.01	1555	0.01	0.02
Head injury	90	0.18	0.14	107	0.10	0.09
Burns	106	0.20	0.17	125	-0.07	-0.10
Fracture	481	0.04	0.04	559	.01	0.01
Lacerations	501	0.13[b]	0.09	559	0.18[b]	0.16[b]
F		4.28	1.91		3.57	2.84
p		<0.002	<0.11		0.007	0.02

[a]Adjusted for sex of child, socioeconomic status, housing quality, age of mother, maternal malaise inventory, mother's employment, number of siblings in household at age 5, number of non-accident-related hospitalizations of the child from birth to age 5, number of other injuries between birth and age 5.

[b]Significantly different from no-injury group, Scheffé criterion.

Multiple Head Injuries

A second set of analyses focused on the relationship between multiple mild head injuries from birth to age 10 and behavioral outcomes, as the only outcomes associated with mild head injury in the first set of analyses were behavioral. In these analyses, children with head injuries were matched to children with other types of injury on the total number of injuries from birth to age 10 and sex.

The children with one head injury had an average of 1.86 total injuries, those with two head injuries had an average of 3.14 injuries, and those with three head injuries had an average of 4.8 total injuries in the 10-year period. Because the controls were matched to the head-injured children on the total number of injuries, the controls also had this same average number of injuries. The proportion of males in the groups increased with the number of head injuries. Fifty-seven percent of those with one head injury and their matched controls were male, 68.7% of those with two head injuries and their controls were male, and 80.4% of those with three or more head injuries and their controls were male.

The number of head injuries in the 10-year period was strongly related to many of the social, demographic, and behavioral characteristics of the children, as shown in Table 8-8. As the number of head injuries increased, there was also a decrease in socioeconomic status, quality of housing, and mother's age. The total number of injuries occurring before age 5 and after age 5 increased with increasing numbers of head injuries, as did the number of hospitalizations not for injuries. Both the aggression and hyperactivity scores measured at age 5 were significantly higher in children with increasing numbers of head injuries. The direction of the relationships between the social characteristics and the total number of injuries experienced by the control children was similar to the relationship between these variables and the number of the cases' injuries, although only mother's age was significantly associated with the number of injuries. Their total number of injuries both before and after age 5 was significantly associated with the 10-year total of injuries, as was the aggression score measured at age 5.

Significance tests were performed comparing the social and demographic characteristics of the cases and the matched controls. The matching resulted in closely similar groups on all variables except the social class indicator, which was lower in the children matched to cases with one head injury ($t = 2.96$, $p = 0.003$), and the number of hospitalizations not for injuries, which was higher in head-injured children with two head injuries than in their matched controls ($t = 2.27$, $p = 0.02$) and in head-injured children with three injuries ($t = 2.17$, p = 0.03). The most striking difference between the groups was in the timing of their injuries. Although they were matched on the total number of injuries from birth to age 10, the head-injured children in all three groups had significantly more injuries before age 5 than their matched controls ($t = 10.4$, p < 0.001; $t = 6.19$, $p <$ 0.001; $t = 3.27$, $p = 0.001$); conversely, the matched controls had significantly more injuries after age 5 than the head-injured cases ($t = -9.30$, $p < 0.001$; $t = -5.5$, $p < 0.001$; $t = -3.49$, $p = 0.001$). Younger children injure their heads at a higher rate than older children, which is the likely explanation of this

TABLE 8-8. Social and Personal Characteristics of Head-Injured Cases and Non-Head-Injured Controls

	Head-Injured Cases				Controls			
	One Head Injury (N=1586)	Two Head Injuries (N=278)	Three Head Injuries (N=51)	p^a	One or More Injuries (N=1586)	Two or More Injuries (N=278)	Three or More Injuries (N=51)	p^a
Socioeconomic status (Z)[b]	0.03	−0.04	−0.25	0.04	−0.07	−0.05	−0.18	ns
Quality of Housing (Z)[b]	−0.02	−0.11	−0.52	0.001	−0.04	−0.13	−0.13	ns
Mother's age	25.6	25.3	23.9	0.02	25.6	25.2	23.3	0.006
Mother's employment (% full-time)	14.0	18.0	14.0	ns	12.0	14.0	13.0	ns
Number of injuries birth to age 5	1.12	1.92	2.90	<0.001	0.84	1.41	2.00	<0.001
Number of injuries ages 5 to 10	0.74	1.23	2.00	<0.001	1.02	1.74	2.84	<0.001
Number of hospitalizations not for injuries	0.32	0.42	0.53	0.005	0.28	0.27	0.21	ns
Aggression score at age 5 (Z)[b]	0.05	0.18	0.52	<0.001	0.12	0.28	0.45	0.001
Hyperactivity score at age 5 (Z)[b]	0.01	0.20	0.24	0.002	0.11	0.27	0.07	ns

[a] Analysis of variance, test of linear trend.
[b] Standardized score with mean = 0, SD = 1.

AGGRESSION

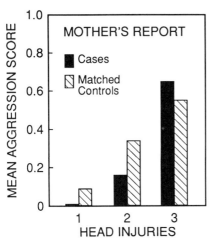
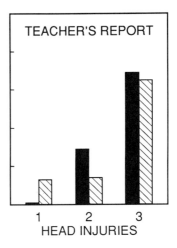

HYPERACTIVITY

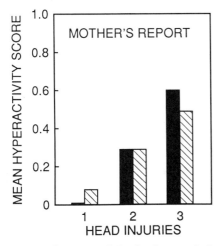
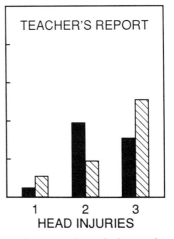

Figure 8-1. Mean behavioral scores in head-injured cases and matched controls.

difference. As a result of this finding, the number of injuries before and after age 5 was also controlled statistically to take into account the difference in timing of the injuries.

Three of the four measures of behavioral problems at age 10 were associated in a linear fashion with the number of head injuries, as shown by the black bars in Figure 8-1. It is clear, however, that the matched controls—those children with the same total number of injuries who had experienced no injuries to the head—also had increasing levels of behavioral problems as the number of injuries increased. Significance tests were performed between each of the three sets of cases and controls adjusted for social class, housing quality, employment of the mother, other hospitalizations not associated with injuries, and the number of injuries before and after age 5. In none of these tests was the mean score on the behavioral scale of the head-injured cases significantly higher than the mean score of the matched controls. In pairwise comparisons, however, the controls matched to the head-injured cases with one head injury did have significantly higher mean scores on mother's and teacher's rating of aggression (mother's report: $F = 6.56$, $p = 0.03$; teacher's report: $F = 10.10$, $p = 0.002$) and mother's report of child's hyperactivity ($F = 4.69$, $p = 0.03$). The children with three or more head injuries had mean scores on the aggression and hyperactivity scales as reported by their mothers which were one-tenth of a standard deviation higher than the mean scores of their matched controls. These differences, however, were not statistically significant. In contrast, the controls matched to those with three or more head injuries had a mean score on hyperactivity reported by the teachers that was two-tenths of a standard deviation higher than the that of cases, again, not a statistically significant difference.

Discussion

The results of this study are concordant with those of several other studies that have found little evidence for adverse long-term sequelae of mild head injury and have extended this finding to multiple mild head injuries. There is no indication that there are any adverse cognitive sequelae of head trauma in this series of mildly head-injured children 1 to 5 years after the head injury. In the absence of comparison groups with other types of injuries, one might have inferred that the consistent 2- to 3-point difference between the scores of the head-injured children and the controls on achievement tests, while not statistically significant, suggest a small but real decrement in cognitive functioning following head injury. Because the children with other injuries, most notably those with lacerations, also had decrements of the same or greater magnitude, it is more likely that any remaining difference between the injured and noninjured groups is due to other unmeasured or poorly controlled social or psychological differences but not to damage resulting from trauma to the head. It is possible that the overall measure of intelligence used in this study was too gross a measure and that head injury may have more subtle effects that could be detected with more specific measures. However, the UCLA studies of mild closed head injury (see Asarnow and colleagues, this volume) have used a variety of tests designed to be sensitive to the specific types of cognitive deficits associated with closed head injury and have similarly been unable to distinguish the mildly head-injured children from children with other injuries and a group of uninjured children.

The observed motoric outcome measures differentiated between the groups even less than did the cognitive outcomes. The head-injured group was indistinguishable from the uninjured group on the three measures of gross motor function and the one fine motor function. While the teachers rated the head-injured children as more clumsy than the uninjured children, the inclusion of the children with the other three types of injuries allows us to infer that clumsiness is not associated causally with head injuries, as all the injured children had higher clumsiness ratings than the uninjured children.

The findings were less clear for behavior. The mean hyperactivity score as rated by the mother was highest in the head-injured group, although it was not significantly higher than in the other groups. Furthermore, the head-injured children had a mean hyperactivity score reported by the teachers that was relatively high and significantly different from that of the uninjured controls. However, the fact that the children with other injuries also had higher mean scores than the noninjured controls, even after control for preinjury behavior and other social and personal factors, suggests that the observed differences between the head-injured and the controls may be largely due to factors that increase the risk of any injury rather than being due to adverse sequelae of damage associated with head trauma. The inverse association between age at head injury and hyperactivity at age 10 as reported by the mother, and the flat relationship using teachers' rating, suggests that the observed association was not causal, as it was expected that injuries closer to the time of behavioral assessment would be more strongly related than those that occurred earlier. An alternative hypothesis, however, is that younger children are more vulnerable than older children.

A number of studies have found an association between behavioral problems and a diverse set of injuries for which there is little or no basis for hypothesizing that the injuries lead to the observed problems (Bijur et al., 1986, 1988; Davidson et al., 1988, 1992). These studies have been based on a model in which behavioral problems of children with injuries precede the injuries and contribute to risk of injury rather than resulting from the injuries. There is also a growing body of literature suggesting that nonneurological trauma can lead to behavioral disturbances. Basson et al. (1991) found that 34% of children hospitalized for injuries not involving the head had substantial behavioral change following the injury, versus 28% in children hospitalized for mild head injuries. No children in a comparison group of children who underwent appendectomies met the criterion for "substantial psychobehavioral change." Wesson et al. (1992) similarly found a high rate of behavioral disturbance that lasted for at least 1 year following multisystem injuries in children with serious trauma (Injury Severity Score > 16), and this was found in children with and without head injury. This line of research suggests that children's responses to trauma per se are responsible for the observed behavioral disturbances. Some authors suggest that their findings may be consistent with posttraumatic stress disorder in response to physical trauma (Basson et al., 1991; Martini et al., 1990). There are a number of inferential problems with these studies, including the assessment of premorbid functioning and the measurement of posttraumatic stress disorder, which is poorly defined in children. Despite these limitations, however, the investigators do not provide evidence that head injury (substantially more severe than the head injuries in this study) conveys any more risk of behavioral or emotional disturbance than other trauma of similar severity.

As for the effect of repeated mild head injury, the findings do not support the inference that two or three mild head injuries result in increased behavioral problems. The inclusion of a control group with a similar number of injuries, not to the head, was essential for disentangling the effect of the head injury from the complex set of personal, social, and behavioral characteristics associated with the phenomenon of multiple injury. Given the frequency with which children injure their heads, this is an area that warrants further research.

There are a number of limitations to the current study. While it is in fact prospective and there are measures of some of the outcomes at age 5 the measures are imprecise and may not be sensitive to the specific types of intellectual, behavioral, and motoric problems that might be associated with mild head injury. Second, the data were gathered 1 to 5 years after the head injury. If adverse sequelae are relatively short-lived, then this design would miss morbidity that might warrant short term intervention. This long and variable time period is also, clearly, not optimal for assessing premorbid behavior, which should ideally be measured shortly before the head injury. Third, injuries were reported by the parent after a 5-year period. A well-known feature of reported health events is that there is substantial memory decay, and more severe events are more likely to be recalled and reported than less severe events (Harel et al., 1994). Therefore some of the children categorized as uninjured may have had head injuries, thus attenuating the findings if there is truly an association. It seems, however, that head injuries resulting in observed behavioral change would be more likely to be recalled than those that do not have any adverse sequelae. This bias would result in observed findings that overestimate the association between adverse sequelae and head injuries.

These analyses of the 1970 British Birth Cohort underscore the importance of considering head injury in the context of other injuries and the very real likelihood that children with head injuries are quite different from uninjured children prior to the occurrence of the head injuries. It also raises the question of the impact of multiple mild head injuries on children's functioning, a question that deserves further consideration.

References

Basson, M. D., Guinn J. E., McElligott, J., Vitale, R., Brown, W., & Fielding, L. P. (1991). Behavioral disturbance in children after trauma. *J. Trauma, 31,* 1363–1368.

Bijur, P., Golding, J., Haslum, M., & Kurzon, M. (1988). Behavioral predictors of injury in school-age children. *Am. J. Dis. Child., 42,* 1307–1312.

Bijur P. E., Haslum M., & Golding J. (1990). Cognitive and behavioral sequelae of mild head injury in children. *Pediatrics, 86,* 337–344.

Bijur, P. E., Stewart-Brown, S., & Butler, N. R. (1986). Child behavior and accidental injury in 11,966 preschool children. *Am. J. Dis. Child., 140,* 487–492.

Brimer, M. A., & Dunn, L. M. (1963). *Manual for the English Picture Vocabulary Test,* Bristol, England: Educational Evaluation Enterprises.

Brown, G., Chadwick, O., Shaffer, D., Rutter, M., & Traub, M. (1981). A prospective study of children with head injuries: III. Psychiatric sequelae. *Psychol. Med., 11,* 63–78.

Butler, N. R., Golding, J., & Howlett, B. (1986). *From birth to five: A study of the health and behaviour of Britain's five year olds.* Oxford, England: Pergamon Press.

Casey, R., Ludwig S., & McCormick M. C. (1986). Morbidity following minor head trauma in children. *Pediatrics, 78,* 497–502.

Chadwick, O., Rutter M., Shaffer D., & Shrout P. E. (1981). A prospective study of children with head injuries: IV. Specific cognitive deficits. *J. Clin. Neuropsychol., 3,* 101–120.

Child Health and Education Study. (1982). First report to the Department of Health and Social Security on the 10 year follow-up. Bristol, England: Department of Child Health, University of Bristol.

Conners, C. K. (1969). A teacher rating scale for use in drug studies with children. *Am. J. Psychiatry, 126,* 152–156.

Coonley-Hoganson R., Sachs N., Bindu D., & Whitman, S. (1984). Sequelae associated with head injuries in patients who were not hospitalized: A follow-up survey. *Neurosurgery, 14,* 315–317.

Davidson, L. L., Hughes, S. J., & O-Connor, P. A. (1988). Preschool behavior problems and subsequent risk of injury. *Pediatrics, 82,* 644–651.

Davidson, L. L., Taylor, E. A., Sandberg, S. T., & Thorley G. (1992). Hyperactivity in school-age boys and subsequent risk of injury. *Pediatrics, 90,* 697–702.

Donders J. (1992). Premorbid behavioral and psychosocial adjustment of children with traumatic brain injury. *J. Abnorm. Child Psychol., 20,* 233–246.

Filley, C. M., Cranberg, M. D., Alexander, M. P., & Hart E. J. (1987). Neurobehavioral outcome after closed head injury in childhood and adolescence. *Arch. Neurol., 44,* 194–198.

Goldstein, F. S., & Levin, H. S. (1985). Intellectual and academic outcome following closed head injury in children and adolescents: Research strategies and empirical findings. *Dev. Neuropsychol., 1,* 195–214.

Gronwall, D., & Wrightson, P. (1974). Delayed recovery of intellectual function after minor head injury. *Lancet, 2,* 605–609.

Gronwall, D., & Wrightson, P. (1975). Cumulative effect of concussion. *Lancet, 2,* 995–997.

Gulbrandsen, G. B. (1984). Neuropsychological sequelae of light head injuries in older children 6 months after trauma. *J. Clin. Neuropsychol., 6,* 257–268.

Harel, Y., Overpeck, M. D., Jones, D. H., Scheidt, P. C., Bijur, P. E., Trumble, A. C., & Anderson, J. (1994). The effects of recall on estimating annual nonfatal injury rates for children. *Am. J. Epidemiol., 84,* 599–605.

Klonoff, H., Low, M. D., & Clark C. (1977). Head injuries in children: A prospective five year follow-up. *J. Neurol. Neurosurg. Psychiatry, 40,* 1211–1219.

Kraus, J. F., Fife, D., Cox, P., Ramstein, K., & Conroy, C. (1986). Incidence, severity and external causes of pediatric brain injury. *Am. J. Dis. Child., 140,* 687–693.

Levin, H. S., High, W. M., Ewing-Cobbs, L., Fletcher, J. M., Eisenberg, H. M., Miner, M. E., & Goldstein, F. C. (1988). Memory functioning during the first year after closed head injury in children and adolescents. *Neurosurgery, 22,* 1043–1052.

Light, R., Asarnow, R., Satz, P., Zaucha, K., & Lewis, R. (1993). UCLA studies of mild closed head injury: III. Behavioral and academic outcomes. *J. Clin. Exp. Neuropsychol., 15,* 20–21.

Manheimer, D. I., Dewey, J., Mellinger, D., & Corsa, L. (1966). 50,000 child-years of accidental injuries. *Public Health Reports, 81,* 519–533.

Martini, D. R., Ryan, C., Nakayama, D., & Ramenofsy, M. (1990). Psychiatric sequelae after traumatic injury: The Pittsburgh regatta accidents. *J. Am. Acad. Child Adolesc. Psychiatry, 29,* 70–75.

Pelco, L., Sawyer, M., Duffield, G., Prior, M., & Kinsella, G. (1992). Premorbid emotional and behavioural adjustment in children with mild head injuries. *Brain Inj., 6,* 29–37.

Roberts, A. H. (1969). *Brain damage in boxers.* London: Pittman.

Rutter, M. (1981). Psychological sequelae of brain damage in children. *Am. J. Psychiatry, 138,* 1533–1544.

Rutter, M., Tizard, J., & Whitmore, K. (1970). *Education, health and behaviour.* London: Longman.

Wesson, D. E., Scorpio, R. J., Spence, L. J., Kenney, B. D., Cipman, M. L., Netley, C. T., & Hu, X. (1992). Physical, psychological and socioeconomic costs of pediatric trauma. *J. Trauma, 33,* 252–257.

Winogron H. W., Knights R. M., & Bawden, H. N. (1984). Neuropsychological deficits following head injury in children. *J. Clin. Neuropsychol. 6,* 269–286.

World Health Organization. (1978). *International classification of diseases: Manual of the international classification of diseases, injuries, and causes of death* (Vol. 1). Geneva: World Health Organization.

Zaucha, K., Asarnow, R., Satz, P., Light, R., & Lewis, R. (1993). The UCLA studies of mild closed head injury in children and adolescents: II. Neuropsychological outcomes. *J. Clin. Exp. Neuropsychol., 15,* 20.

9

Attention Deficits in the Long Term after Childhood Head Injury

MAUREEN DENNIS, MARGARET WILKINSON,
LISA KOSKI, and ROBIN P. HUMPHREYS

Cognitive outcome is highly variable after childhood head injury, both within and between groups of head injured children. An analysis of subject and intratask variables can provide useful information about some factors that contribute to the observed variability. The analysis of *subject variables* is pertinent to identifying some factors responsible for long-term variability in cognitive outcome in childhood head injury populations. The analysis of *intratask variables* is important for understanding the defective processing responsible for performance deficits. This chapter briefly reviews the neuropsychological effects of childhood head injury, focusing on the cognitive skills of memory and attention that are involved in both academic work and daily function; it then summarizes a recent study from our laboratory concerned with some putative processes of attention in children who had earlier sustained a closed head injury.

Neuropsychological Outcome and Age

For many years, the relation between age at time of brain insult and later cognitive function was viewed in terms of two interconnected hypotheses: the protective function of a young age and the functional plasticity of a young brain. Accordingly, it was believed that infants and preschoolers could sustain considerable brain damage with relative impunity (Lenneberg, 1967). But as neuronal plasticity proved to be a feature of mature as well as immature brains (e.g., Finger & Stein, 1982), and as a fuller range of behavioral observations on brain-damaged children were made, it became apparent not that children are deficit-free after brain injury but that different types and patterns of cognitive deficit are evident at different points in the life span.

Some of these insights about age and childhood brain damage came from research that referenced cognitive outcome, not against models of adult brain damage but against the normal course of cognitive development. More than half a century ago, Kennard's (1940, 1942) studies of infant monkeys showed that brain lesions normally producing motor deficits in adult animals had no immediate effect on motor function in infants, a finding superficially congruent with the idea of greater plasticity in the infant. As the infant monkeys matured, however, significant motor deficits emerged, a finding quite inconsistent with the infant plasticity viewpoint. Kennard concluded that (1) behavioral impairments occurring immediately after brain insult in the immature brain were different from those that appeared immediately after lesions in the mature brain; (2) the difference between the behavioral effects of immature and mature brain lesions varied with the type of behavior being considered; and (3) certain functional or behavioral impairments were not apparent immediately after early brain damage but emerged only later in development, at a time when the relevant behavior would normally appear. Later research (Goldman, 1972) confirmed and extended Kennard's important idea that many effects of brain damage or dysfunction in the immature organism have their greatest impact on cognitive function at a point in development far removed from the time of the brain insult.

Current clinical practice does not yet reflect awareness of the implications of Kennard's work of 50 years ago: that brain injury early in life may be associated with a wide range of outcomes later in development, and that a young age at brain insult will not protect the child from long-term cognitive deficits. Even today, the working principle of many clinicians who evaluate head-injured children is that younger children will sustain head injury with more cognitive impunity than will older children. Hart and Faust (1988) asked practicing clinicians with specialized neuropsychological training to predict cognitive outcome for two case histories, each of which described a bicycle accident in which the patient hit his head, experienced a brief loss of consciousness and posttraumatic confusion, and suffered chronic personality change and forgetfulness. Clinicians were significantly more likely to judge the adolescent case (as opposed to the child case) as having cognitive impairment, despite the fact that the fictional case histories differed only in the age of the child.

The assumption that young children are somehow protected from cognitive deficits following brain injury has had direct and continuing implications for the neuropsychological evaluation of children after head injury. If it is believed that younger head-injured children will have no cognitive deficits or only minor ones, then a thorough evaluation of their cognitive function may not be undertaken. The incidence of cognitive deficits after childhood head injury will certainly be underestimated when the domain of such deficits is not even assessed. It is important, therefore, to consider empirical research designed to evaluate directly the effects of age at brain damage on cognitive outcome.

Age is an independent variable that marks the time course of development, demarcates periods of developmental change, and delineates developmental phases (Siegel et al., 1983; Wohlwill, 1973). An early age at brain injury, however, is not an explanation of the presence or absence of cognitive morbidity, so it should not be invoked as a form of recovery mechanism (Fletcher, et al., 1984; Fletcher et al., 1987; Fletcher & Satz, 1983). Nevertheless, age is an important variable in deciding how cognitive deficits might best be identified and ameliorated after childhood brain injury (e.g., Johnson et al., 1989; Lehr, 1990). The behavioral effects of childhood brain lesions are developmentally time-lagged; that is to say, some are evident soon after the lesion, but others take some years to become manifest. The existence of a range of age-related outcomes after childhood brain damage means that cognitive morbidity must be specified, not only according to the pathology of brain damage but also to a set of age variables that include the age at which brain injury was sustained, the time elapsed since the brain injury, and the age of the child at cognitive evaluation.

Recent research has explored age as a factor in the variability of cognitive outcome after childhood brain damage and has compared outcomes in both children and adults and in younger and older children. After brain damage, cognitive function is not always spared more in younger than in older children, as was once believed under the older view of a negative linear relationship between age at brain injury and amount of functional plasticity (still termed the "Kennard principle," although, as noted earlier, it is neither a principle nor something Kennard actually proposed). Nevertheless, the relation between cognitive status and age at onset of brain disorder or treatment is proving to be a complex one.

The idea of greater sparing in young children arose from earlier studies in which age at brain injury was confounded with brain pathology. In comparing the incidence of aphasia in head-injured children and adults with cerebrovascular accidents, for example, it appeared that aphasia was more common in adults, a finding that was used to infer greater functional brain plasticity in children. But cerebrovascular accidents are more likely to produce persisting clinical aphasic conditions than are head injuries, regardless of age at brain injury, so differences in brain pathology and onset age cannot be ascribed solely to differences in age at brain insult.

Recent studies in which children with the same brain pathology are compared at different ages (of disease onset or of treatment) now provide a clearer perspective on age effects than did older studies comparing recovery in children and adults with different underlying brain pathologies (e.g., Lenneberg, 1967). Considerable evidence now suggests that cognitive function is not always spared more in younger than in older children who have incurred brain damage. Particularly in instances where brain damage is acquired during childhood (rather than being congenital) and is diffuse and/or multifocal in nature, a younger age at onset appears to be associated with a higher risk of long-term cognitive morbidity (Dennis & Barnes, 1994).

The young brain appears to be particularly vulnerable to diffuse or multifocal insult. Studies of leukemia and brain tumor show a younger age to be associated with greater vulnerability to cognitive deficit (reviewed in Ris & Noll, 1994). Intellectual impairment is more likely in younger-radiated than in older-radiated children (e.g., Danoff et al., 1982; Mulhern et al., 1992a; Spunberg et al., 1981). After treatment for acute lymphoblastic leukemia, younger-treated children are overall more vulnerable to neuropsychological dysfunction than are older-treated children (Halberg et al., 1991; Meadows et al., 1981; Mulhern et al., 1992b;

1992c). Age at treatment is also related to cognitive skill profiles (Waber et al., 1992); for example, younger-treated leukemic children are less phonologically accurate spellers than are older-treated children (Kleinman & Waber, 1992).

Time since onset of brain pathology, trauma, or treatment is an important issue, and it should be considered in its own right. Disruption of neurocognitive function early in life affects not only the skills that are already acquired or are shortly to be acquired but also the ability to acquire new skills and to develop an age-appropriate knowledge base. The latter, in particular, might be reflected in IQ test scores.

For children with acquired focal lesions, a relationship between time since lesion and IQ has been demonstrated. Many children with focal brain lesions have normal levels of intelligence (Aram & Ekelman, 1986). In children with early brain lesions from diverse etiologies, however, there is an association between increasing time since lesion and decreasing IQ scores (Banich et al. 1990). That is, when age of lesion onset is held constant, increasing time since lesion brings about lower, not higher, intelligence. This finding has been reported in groups of children with focal lesions tested at one point in time (Nass et al., 1989) and also in a more homogeneous group of children with left or right focal lesions, in whom it was found that injury sustained earlier in development, particularly prenatally or in the first years of life, was more debilitating of performance on intelligence tests than was later-onset brain injury (Aram & Eisele, 1994).

Such data have important implications for the understanding of long-term cognitive morbidity in children after brain injury, because they suggest that domains like general intelligence that depend on the continual acquisition and retention of a complex knowledge base may be vulnerable to brain injury early in life. To the extent that some forms of focal brain injury in children are associated with increasing cognitive morbidity as the child develops, it is important to monitor the long-term cognitive effects of childhood brain injury.

Neuropsychological Outcome and Childhood Head Injury

Having considered the effects of age and other temporal variables on cognitive outcome after childhood brain injury in general terms, it is now useful to review what empirical research shows about the effects of childhood head injury on specific cognitive functions. Broadly, the data suggest that childhood head injury disrupts the development of a range of cognitive functions that include discourse (Dennis & Barnes, 1990) and academic skills (Chadwick et al., 1981) but which are most obviously apparent in the domains of memory and attention (Ewing-Cobbs & Fletcher, 1987; Ewing-Cobbs et al., 1989a). Further, many cognitive deficits persist through the acute stage into the chronic stage of recovery, with the result that cognitive morbidity is evident several years posttrauma in a proportion of head-injured children.

Attention is an important regulator of cognitive activity that has to with what is selected for awareness. It involves selecting among competing data so as to bias a response to one set of contents rather than to another. Attention is engaged by almost all neuropsychological tasks except perhaps those like implicit memory that involve the unconscious processing of information. In consequence, a particular test (such as the WISC Digit Span; Wechsler, 1974) may be characterized by some investigators as a test of short-term memory and by others as a test of attention (Van Zomeron & Brouwer, 1992). Certainly, persisting difficulties with attention may contribute to observed memory impairments after childhood head injury (Kaufmann et al., 1993). While memory and attention are certainly not identical processes, any overview of the literature on cognitive morbidity and childhood head injury will consider them together.

Memory deficits have long been known to occur after head injury in adults (Levin et al., 1982a). Recent work suggests that this cognitive deficit is also common in head-injured children and adolescents (e.g., Ewing-Cobbs & Fletcher, 1987; Ewing-Cobbs et al., 1989a; Lehr, 1990; Levin et al., 1982a). Attention problems occur after closed head injury in adults, not only in the acute phase of the injury but also in the long term. Disorders of attention are also common after childhood head injury (Johnson & Roethig-Johnson, 1989; Murray et al., 1992). It was once proposed that attention deficits after childhood head injury were not evident beyond 4 months postinjury (Chadwick et al., 1981; Gulbrandsen, 1984), but more recent studies suggest that measurable attention deficits continue beyond this time period (Kaufmann et al., 1993). Thus, cognitive function is not spared in children as contrasted with adults after head injury, as was once believed, and memory and attention problems may persist.

With increasing evidence that cognitive deficits exist, research into cognitive morbidity after childhood head injury has now become concerned with explaining outcome variability—that is, with identifying some of the factors that increase or decrease particular forms of posttraumatic cognitive morbidity. Recent studies have attempted to identify which medical features might make one head-injured child more vulnerable than another to poor memory or attention (Ewing-Cobbs et al., 1989a). Two subject variables emerging as important are the severity of the head injury and the age of the child at the time of head injury. While there exists a relation between injury severity and outcome, some proportion of children having sustained mild head injuries experience persisting cognitive deficits in specific areas. Younger head-injured children may be even more vulnerable than older head-injured children to deficits in memory and attention. Increasingly, recent studies are addressing the issue of which intratask variables are sensitive to the effects of head injury, an important step in accounting for outcome variability.

Much of the emphasis in recent studies of cognitive morbidity has been focused on the child with severe head injury. But mild or moderate head injuries (the typical diagnostic criteria for which include temporary loss of consciousness for less than 15 to 20 minutes (Vogenthaler, 1987); high-end Glasgow Coma Scale (GCS) scores (Jane et al., 1985); normal neurological status (Binder, 1986); and a 72-hour or less hospitalization) are common: Of the 100,000 children under 15 who are admitted each year to U.S. hospitals, over 90% have sustained mild or moderate head injury (Kraus et al., 1987; see also Kraus, this volume).

While mild or moderate head injury to adults is associated with low mortality (Snoek, 1989), it is clear that it brings a risk of cognitive morbidity in both the acute phase and in the long term, especially in memory and attention (Papanicolau et al., 1985; Stuss et al., 1985; Trexler & Zappala, 1988; Van Zomeren & Deelman, 1978; Zappala & Trexler, 1992). Memory and attention deficits in the long term are not well predicted by indices of clinical severity like the GCS in adult populations (Lieh-Lai et al., 1992; Trexler & Zappala, 1988). In children, GCS score 72 hours posttrauma is one of a set of factors predicting survival (Michaud et al., 1992), and, further, emergency room GCS scores are related to memory and motor speed 3 weeks postinjury (Jaffe et al., 1992). It is not clear whether GCS scores predict longer-term cognitive function in childhood head injury.

Structural brain imaging provides an index of severity of head injury aside from the evidence about severity of disturbed consciousness derived from GCS scores. Computed tomography (CT) and magnetic resonance imaging (MRI) provide important information about traumatic brain injury. Computed tomography reveals the majority of surgically relevant lesions, features of structural brain injury independently prognostic of outcome such as subarachnoid hemorrhage, and morphological features associated with raised intracranial pressure such as compression of the cisterns, shift of the ventricles, and diffuse brain swelling. Magnetic resonance imaging is more sensitive than CT to small nonhemorrhagic lesions, diffuse axonal injury, and altered brain metabolism (Salcman & Pevsner, 1992). As structural neuroimaging techniques provide better resolution of certain forms of traumatic brain injury, it is becoming apparent that even head injuries traditionally considered mild or moderate may create measurable disturbances of the brain.

Focal brain lesions occur in more than two-thirds of children with moderate or severe head injury (Mendelsohn et al., 1992). Mild or moderate head injury, even in individuals who appear neurologically intact (Binder, 1986), produces diffuse lesions that include axonal compression and stretching (Povlishock & Coburn, 1989) and diffuse, microscopic neuronal loss (Rimel et al., 1981). Further, MRI has revealed more focal lesions in mild and moderate head injury than were earlier thought to exist (see Han et al., 1984; Luerssen et al., 1987). These lesions are evident in the frontal and temporal lobes as well as in the temporal poles and the limbic system, including the connections with the orbitofrontal surface of the frontal cortex (Levin et al., 1987; Sekino et al., 1981).

Neuropsychological function in mild or moderate head injury is correlated with size and localization of the lesions on MRI, and the postinjury reduction in lesion size is paralleled by improvements in neuropsychological function (Levin et al., 1987). Even in the chronic stage of recovery from head injury, children show many more focal areas of abnormal signal on MRI than on CT, particularly in terms of frontal parenchymal damage (Levin et al., 1993). In attempting to account for cognitive outcome in head-injured children, it is useful to take account of focal lesions as well as GCS scores (Levin et al., 1993).

Functional neuroimaging procedures are increasingly important in the delineation of brain insult in cases of head injury. For example, while HMPAO (hexamethylpropyleneamine oxime)-SPECT functional neuroimaging does not reveal extraaxial lesions and skull fractures as well as CT, it reveals more intraparenchymal lesions or anomalies in regional cerebral blood flow than CT (Ness et al., 1993). Of more significance for neuropsychological studies of head injury is the fact that brain anomalies identified from functional neuroimaging may have a stronger relationship to patterns of long-term neuropsychological outcome than do structural changes on CT or MR (Levin, 1993). In survivors of head injury, long-term neuropsychological outcome is correlated with regional cerebral blood flow rate on HMPAO-SPECT functional imaging (Goldenberg et al., 1992).

More recent studies have attempted to determine how disordered attention in head-injured children is related to particular medical features of their head injuries, such as injury severity. The data relating severity of childhood head injury to problems in attention is complex. Severe head injuries produce more deficits on continuous performance tests of attention than do mild or moderate injuries (Kaufmann et al., 1993), and the severity of head injury as identified by MRI is correlated with a range of persisting cognitive deficits in head-injured children (Levin et al., 1993). However, it has also been claimed that attention and memory are impaired in children after head injuries that leave no obvious neurological defect (Boll, 1983; Doronzo, 1990).

In childhood, a younger age at head injury is associated with increased risk for poorer outcome. Children under 2 years of age probably have a higher proportion of intentional injuries (Levin, 1993), which may compromise their survival. Certainly, the etiology and pathophysiology of head injury in children under age 2 may be different from that of older children (Duhaime et al., 1992). But throughout the age range of childhood, not just in children under 2 years of age, increasing evidence suggests a relationship between age at injury and both mortality and morbidity.

Age at injury is inversely associated with survival after severe head injury in children (Michaud et al., 1992). Within the group of head-injured children, it is clear that a younger age affords no protection from general or specific cognitive morbidity. Even preschoolers show cognitive problems following closed head injury (Ewing-Cobbs et al., 1989b), and general intelligence appears to be more adversely affected by a younger age at head injury within school-aged samples (Brink et al., 1970; Levin et al., 1982b; but for negative results, see Chadwick et al., 1981).

Age effects are even more apparent for specific cognitive skills. Memory impairment seems more severe in head-injured children than in head-injured adolescents (Fletcher et al., 1987). Of those who are tested 3 months after head injury, younger children show more pronounced specific cognitive deficits than do older children or adolescents (Levin et al., 1993). Younger head-injured children have more difficulty with planning and rule-governed behavior than do older head-injured children (Levin et al., 1994).

After head injury, the younger child is more vulnerable than the older child to disorders of attention. Younger head-injured children show more pronounced attention disturbances than do older head-injured children at 6 months postinjury, when each is compared to uninjured age peers (Kaufmann et al., 1993). Younger head-injured children show more difficulties with the response modulation component of attention than do older head-injured children (Levin et al., 1993). Thus, closed head injury is not associated with preferential sparing of attention in younger children.

Even though problems in memory and attention disrupt long-term school achievement and psychosocial function, few studies have investigated the form these difficulties take. The analyses of intratask variables is one step toward understanding variability in cognitive outcome following childhood head injury.

Short-term memory for information is impaired in head-injured children, with the degree of impairment being related to injury severity. Head-injured children appear to have poorer memory than motor skills (Fuld & Fisher, 1977). Childhood head injury populations show deficits in specific memory skills (Ewing-Cobbs & Fletcher, 1987; Levin et al., 1982a; Levin & Eisenberg, 1979). Long-term storage and retrieval of information is impaired relative to age peers in children with head injuries of varying severity (Levin & Grossman, 1976). Severe head injuries in children and adolescents are also associated with particularly poor retrieval skills at 6 months postinjury (Levin & Eisenberg, 1979) and at 1 year postinjury (Levin et al., 1982a).

The retention of newly learned information over longer time periods is also impaired in head-injured children (Donders, 1993), who show excessive forgetting of a complex story after a delay, which suggests that their memory strategies might involve insufficient encoding. The fact that forgetting was enhanced after a delay regardless of injury severity suggests that memory encoding strategies, unlike short-term retention, might be sensitive to head injury of any degree of severity.

Attention is a construct in neuropsychology that has sometimes been poorly defined but which, in more recent years, has come to be operationalized as a series of somewhat separate cognitive functions having to do with alertness, focused attention, divided attention, sustained attention, and supervisory attentional control (Van Zomeren & Brouwer, 1992). Children demonstrate less efficient attention skills in the early stages of recovery after head injury (Johnson & Roethig-Johnson, 1989), and attentional difficulties continue in some head-injured children into the chronic stage of recovery. However, the nature of attention deficits after childhood head injury is as yet imperfectly understood. At 6 months posttrauma, the Wechsler Digit Span measure (Wechsler, 1974) seems unimpaired in head-injured children, in contrast to measures of continuous or sustained attention, for which more severe injuries are associated with poorer sustained attention (Kaufmann et al., 1993). Severely head-injured children can extract features and identify stimuli as well as controls but are impaired in response selectivity and motor execution (Murray et al., 1992). Just as do head-injured adults (Trexler & Zappala, 1988), head-injured children appear to have particular problems in selective attention and response modulation.

The research described above suggests that an earlier age at head injury produces greater cognitive morbidity than does an older age. Cognitive deficits occur in the short and medium term after head injury, but it is not clear whether they are permanent features of the head-injured child's cognitive profile. Pertinent to the ongoing investigation of attention deficits after childhood head injury is the study described below, which explores how features of the head injury and task demands are related to long-term attention function.

A Study of Attention after Childhood Head Injury

Head Injury Sample and Tests

The sample consists of 83 children and adolescents (43% female, 84% right-handed) who had sustained closed head injury, defined as a blow to the head of sufficient severity to warrant hospital admission (Dennis et al., 1993). Information about the nature and severity of the head injury as well as its physiological, neurological, and cognitive consequences was obtained from medical records; in addition, neuroradiological reports, parent interviews, and a clinical examination were employed. Sample characteristics are shown in Table 9-1.

A standard test of intelligence (Wechsler, 1974; 1991) was administered, and subjects in the study were selected to have either or both of Verbal IQ or Performance IQ above 70. Each subject was administered the Gordon Diagnostic System (GDS) (Gordon, 1983; 1988), which is a portable electronic device with an internal microprocessor that generates three tasks and records qualitative and quantitative measures of performance over time. Because neuropsychological testing of intelligence and attention was conducted an average of 3 1/2 years from the time of head injury, the data bear on long-term cognitive function after childhood head injury.

The data set consists of six sets of outcome measures, concerned, respectively, with intelligence, focused attention, selective attention, distractor interference (the comparison of focused and selective attention within the same individuals), response modulation, and overall attention. Results are described in terms of the characteristics of performance in the childhood head-injury sample as a whole and also in terms of how well outcome measures could be predicted from intrasubject

TABLE 9-1.   Childhood Head Injury Sample (*N* = 83)

	Mean	Standard Deviation	Range
Age at head injury (yr)	7.6	3.5	0.8–15.7
Age at test (yr)	11.0	3.2	5.2–18.0
Head injury duration (yr)	3.4	2.4	0.5–14.3
Glasgow Coma Scale (GCS)	11.1	4.0	3–15
Verbal IQ	92.7	12.5	51–122
Performance IQ	95.2	15.5	55–127
Full-scale IQ	93.3	13.0	65–123

variables. Multiple regressions were conducted to predict the quantitative outcome measures from the quantitative independent variables of age of the child at head injury, the time elapsed since head injury, and GCS rating of severity of head injury. For some quantitative outcome measures, analyses of variance (ANOVAs) were also conducted, using the age of child at head injury as a categorical variable (defined as head injury before or after 7 years of age). The two age-at-injury groups had similar GCS scores. The younger age-at-injury group, despite being younger at test (9.0 versus 12.9 years, p <0.0001), had experienced a longer recovery time since head injury than had the older age-at-injury group ($p = 0.005$).

Intelligence

Verbal intelligence (Verbal IQ), nonverbal intelligence (Performance IQ), and general intelligence (Full Scale IQ) were all average in comparison to age peers. Bearing in mind that the children in the study were selected to have at least one IQ score above the traditional mental retardation cutoff point of 70, it appears that intellectual function is within normal limits in this large sample tested in the long term after childhood head injury. What is not clear, of course, is whether the measured IQ scores represent a decline from premorbid levels.

In the multiple regression model, the three predictor variables were not related to Verbal IQ or Performance IQ. In the ANOVAs, however, the younger age-at-injury group tended to have lower Verbal IQ scores ($p = 0.07$) than the older age-at-injury group.

Visual Monitoring: Focused Attention

"Focused attention" refers to the ability to monitor a target over a stretch of time in the absence of reward or feedback about ongoing performance. In the 9-minute GDS Vigilance Task, an electronic display flashes a series of digits in the central column of the computer screen at the rate of 1 per second. The stimulus is presented for 200 milliseconds, with an 800-millisecond interval between stimuli. The child is required to press a button every time a 1 is followed by a 9 and also to inhibit responding to the alerting stimulus, to nontarget numbers that follow the alerting stimulus, and to non-hot-target numbers, such as a 9 occurring after a 2.

A *focused attention accuracy index* was calculated as follows: Number of correct responses minus number of commission errors (responses to stimuli other than hot targets) divided by number of possible correct responses. The index was then converted to a Z score using supplementary normative data. *Focused attention variability* was a measure of the overall level of consistency across the session, calculated from standard deviations within time blocks that were compared to age-norm tables. *Focused attention response latency* was the average response latency over the session, considered both as raw scores and as converted Z scores from supplementary normative data. A *focused attention task score* was calculated to express overall task performance in numerical terms. It included correct responses, commission errors, and consistency of performance, each component categorized as abnormal, borderline, or normal from age norms.

Considered as a whole, the childhood head-injury sample showed poor focused attention. Sixty-four percent had a focused attention task score that was at an abnormal or borderline level for age. Nine percent made an abnormal level of commission errors, that is, responses to nontargets, and 36% made an abnormal or borderline level of commission errors. Thirty-six percent of the sample had a focused attention variability score that was at an abnormal or borderline level. The focused attention accuracy index for the sample, expressed as a Z score, was below the mean of zero but within normal limits ($M = -0.76$) but ranged widely (SD 2.44, range from -17.61 to 1.15). Time required for a correct response was slightly less than half a second ($M = 0.46$), which was within the Z-score limits for age ($M = -0.61$).

The predictor variables of age at head injury, time since head injury, and GCS scores were not related to either the focused attention accuracy index or to the Z scores for focused attention response latency.

Visual Monitoring with Distractors: Selective Attention

This task measures the ability to maintain visual monitoring over time in the absence of reward or feedback about ongoing performance and in the presence of distractor interference. The GDS Distractibility Task is identical to the Vigilance Task with the addition of distraction in the form of random digits flashing at random intervals on the left and right sides of the central positions of the electronic display. The child must still press the button every time a 1 is followed by a 9 in the center, while ignoring the digits in the outer columns of the display.

Selective attention was scored in the same manner as focused attention. A *selective attention accuracy index* was calculated as follows: number of correct responses minus number of commission errors (responses to stimuli other than hot targets) divided by number of possible correct responses. The index was then converted to a Z score using supplementary normative data. *Selective attention variability* was a measure of the overall level of consistency across the session calculated from standard deviations within time blocks that were compared to age-norm tables. *Selective attention response latency* was the average response latency over the session, considered both as raw scores and as converted Z scores from supplementary normative data. A *selective attention task score* was calculated to express overall task performance in numerical terms. It included correct responses, commission errors, and consistency of performance, each component categorized as abnormal, borderline, or normal from age norms.

The childhood head injury sample showed poor selective attention. Eighty percent had a selective attention task score that was at an abnormal or borderline level for age. Twenty-five percent made an abnormal number of commission errors—that is, responses to nontargets, and 53% made an abnormal or borderline number of commission errors. Fifty-one percent of the sample had a selective attention variability score that was at an abnormal or borderline level. The selective attention accuracy index for the sample, expressed as a Z score, was below normal limits ($M = -1.33$) but ranged widely (SD 2.07, range from -8.49 to 0.85). Time required for a correct response was more than $1/2$ second ($M = 0.57$), which was well below the Z-score limits for age ($M = -1.75$).

The predictor variables of age at head injury and time since head injury were related to the selective attention accuracy index. A younger age at head injury ($p = 0.003$) and a shorter time since head injury ($p = 0.08$) were each associated with less accurate target detection in the presence of distractors. Time since head injury was the significant predictor of Z scores for selective attention response latency ($p = 0.02$). A shorter time since head injury was associated with slower detection of visual targets in the presence of distractors.

Distractor Interference Effects within Subjects

In the analyses of focused and selective attention described above, comparisons were made with published norms. A more direct method of looking at the extent to which distractors interfere with visual monitoring and the extent to which any relationship depends on age at head injury is to compare accuracy and speed of response within the same subjects under conditions of focused and selective attention.

For accuracy of response, an ANOVA was carried out with age at injury (children with injury before age 7, children with injury after age 7) as the between-subjects variable and accuracy index (focused attention accuracy index, selective attention accuracy index) as the within-subject variable. The age-at-injury effect approached significance ($p = 0.06$), congruent with the age-at-injury effects in the multiple regression, and the effect for accuracy index was significant ($p = 0.04$). For both age-at-injury groups, selective attention was poorer than focused attention, and the younger age-at-injury group tended to perform more poorly, in relation to normal-age norms, than the older age-at-injury group.

For latency of response, a score was calculated that reflected, within each subject, how much additional time was required to perform the visual monitoring task under conditions of distraction. The score was calculated as follows: Average time for a correct response in selective attention minus average time for a correct response in focused attention divided by average time for a correct response in focused attention, converted to a proportion. An ANOVA was carried out on these scores, with age at injury as the between-subjects variable. The age-at-injury effect was significant ($p = 0.03$), such that the younger age-at-injury group required proportionally more time (0.32) than the older age-at-injury group (0.16). Thus, the distractors served to extend the time required to make a correct response, and this effect was twice as pronounced in the younger age-at-injury group.

For both age-at-injury groups, selective attention was poorer than focused attention, and the younger age-at-injury group performed more poorly, in relation to normal-age norms, than the older age-at-injury group. Children injured at a younger age appeared more disrupted from a visual monitoring task by the presence of distractors than were children injured at an older age: a younger age at head injury tended to be associated with less accurate detection of visual targets and also with significantly longer response times for successful target detection.

Response Modulation

The GDS Delay Task measures the ability to use external feedback to generate an internal schedule for suppressing a dominant response. During the 8-minute session, subjects are rewarded by brief illumination of a red light and an incremental counter on the screen showing points achieved for each button press that follows an interval of 6 seconds. The duration of the critical interval is not mentioned to the subject, who must discover the minimum time to refrain from responding and thus develop a strategy for estimating the interresponse interval that best paces responding and maximizes the number of points obtained. The constant feedback provided by seeing the red light and point increment on the screen must be used to develop and sustain a self-paced response strategy (which may involve counting, motor activity, or some other internal, self-generated system for response pacing). After the initial strategy is established, the subject must continue to modulate responding for the duration of the task. The automatic, unmodulated response would be to press the button as often as possible; the controlled response would be to pace it according to an internal, self-generated schedule.

Response modulation was measured by the *response modulation efficiency ratio,* which was calculated as correct responses/total responses. The efficiency ratio was then converted to a Z score using supplementary normative data. *Response modulation variability* was a measure of the overall level of consistency across the session, calculated from standard deviations within time blocks that were compared to age-norm tables. A *response modulation task score* was calculated to review overall task performance derived from total responses, efficiency ratio scores, and consistency of performance, each component categorized as abnormal, borderline, or normal on the basis of age norms.

The childhood head injury sample showed poor response modulation. Sixty-three percent had a response modulation task score that was at an abnormal or borderline level for age. The response modulation efficiency ratio score for the sample, expressed as a Z score, was within normal limits ($M = -0.31$) but ranged widely (SD 1.36, range from -5.27 to 1.23). Forty-eight percent of the sample had a response modulation variability score that was at an abnormal or borderline level.

The predictor variable of time since head injury was related to the response modulation efficiency ratio Z score ($p = 0.02$). A shorter time since head injury was associated with less efficient response modulation.

Attention in Childhood Head Injury Sample

To reflect overall test performance, we calculated a composite score. A rating of "intact" meant that the child was at or above the 26th age percentile on all three attention tasks; a rating of "impaired" meant that the child was below the 26th age percentile on one or more attention tasks. Only 3.8% of the sample was rated as intact, which shows that consistently age-appropriate attention skills are rare in this sample of chronic-stage head-injured children.

Discussion

Attention is important because it affects how information is made available to conscious awareness. Information that becomes conscious is more readily amenable to change through education or other less formal learning situations. Attention, then, is a regulator of cognitive activities needed for everyday function and for academic tasks. It is also important for social interactions such as those involved in turn taking and conversations.

Persisting problems in a variety of attention skills are evident in children and adolescents several years after head injury. While the data provide no evidence for generalized sparing of core attention skills in children after head injury, attention varied according to factors within the children and factors in the tasks; specifically, the age of the child at head injury, the time elapsed since head injury, and the processing requirements of particular tests of attention.

Attention was not related to coma scale ratings of injury severity, however, showing that intact attentional skills in the long term after childhood head injury are not guaranteed by intact coma scale ratings at the time of hospital admission. While the GCS is a widely used measure of coma, it taps only a single dimension of head injury, that concerned with impaired consciousness; as a result, GCS ratings may be impaired after head injuries that involve short-term losses of consciousness but no major intracranial injury, or, conversely, they may be unimpaired after major intracranial injuries that entail no loss of consciousness. Although clearly valuable as a marker of coma in the acute phase of head injury, the admitting GCS score is not consistently predictive of chronic-stage global cognitive outcome. When head-injured children do not have low GCS ratings, the traditional measure of a severe head injury, they may be deemed to require no neuropsychological assessment or follow-up. In that case, some children at risk for significant cognitive morbidity may be left without remediation for impairments of attention.

To be sure, the interaction between coma scale ratings and other features of head injury is not fully understood. Levin (1993) has suggested that severity of head injury may affect younger children more than older children, in which case GCS scores may be more predictive for younger samples than for a broad age spectrum. Ongoing work in this area concerns how GCS ratings are related to other measures of head injury severity, such as the focal contusions and diffuse axonal injury revealed by structural and functional brain neuroimaging, and also how both GCS and neuroimaging indices of severity are related to global and discrete measures of neuropsychological function (e.g., Levin et al., 1994).

Even when head-injured children were assessed in the chronic stage of recovery, an average of more than 3 years postinjury, a longer recovery time was associated with better performance on some indices of attention. Thus, while poor attention is evident in the head-injury sample as a whole, a longer recovery time appears to enhance attention skills. Despite having a longer recovery time than children who were older at the time of head injury, however, children who were younger at the time of head injury showed poorer attention and had particular difficulty attending successfully in the presence of distractors.

To understand attention after childhood head injury, it is important to understand the nature of the cognitive processes required for successful attention as well as how these processes develop. Normal adults are able to attend selectively despite distraction, and they can even adjust their selective attention strategies to different conditions (Brown & Fera, 1994). These skills develop only gradually. Normally developing children produce longer interference effects from irrelevant distractors than do adults (Davies et al., 1984) and are thought to show more interference because their inhibitory mechanisms are immature (Tipper et al., 1989). Even when successfully produced, selective attention strategies are effortful for young children (DeMarie-Dreblow & Miller, 1988).

Two mechanisms of selective attention have been identified: (1) an activation process and (2) an inhibitory process by which ignored distractors are actively inhibited (Tipper et al., 1988). Earlier "spotlight" models of attention stressed the enhancement of to-be-attended information; more recent models of attention have concerned the role of inhibitory mechanisms as they are revealed by the fate of the unattended material.

The question of attention in childhood head injury was approached here with a particular focus on two types of inhibitory processes, those concerned with the inhibition of distracting stimulus information, and those concerned with the inhibition of prepotent or dominant response tendencies. The ability to monitor a target in the presence of target-related distractors and the ability to modulate responses to meet an internally-generated schedule both reveal how well an individual can use controlled cognitive processes to override automatic processes or operations. By studying attention within this framework, we aimed to learn more about the balance of controlled and automatic cognitive processes in head-injured children, and thereby gain a better understanding of some of the intratask variables that account for variability in attention outcome after childhood head injury.

With respect to the deployment of controlled cognitive processes, children with head injury had difficulty both in the suppression of irrelevant input and in the modulation of output. The finding of poor response modulation is consistent with the idea that childhood head injury is associated with difficulty in self-regulatory functions. But it is the analysis of head-injured children's difficulty in selective attention that bears on the nature of defective processing of information following childhood head injury.

The intuitively appealing idea that head-injured children cannot activate attentional resources to focus on what is relevant is not supported by the finding that, while they had difficulty in sustaining focused attention over time, they showed a more marked and consistent deficit in selective attention involving the inhibition of distracting information. As a group, they appear deficient in an inhibitory mechanism that prevents them from processing irrelevant information. In this connection, even severely head-injured children can attend to target features as well as controls (Murray et al., 1992), although they produce a high proportion of false positives to distractor stimuli (Levin & Eisenberg, 1979), suggesting that they lack an efficient mechanisms for distractor inhibition.

Distractor inhibition appears to be a limited resource in our childhood head injury sample, sometimes not used successfully but actively maintained, when in use, at the cost of slower responding. In particular, children who sustained head injury at a younger age showed more distractor interference and were slower to inhibit distracting information even when they successfully detected a target, suggesting that a younger age at head injury has resulted in a very poor mechanism for distractor inhibition, a mechanism that is frequently unsuccessful as well as being time-consuming when successfully applied. The mechanism in children who were older at the time of their head injury is more often successful and more fully automatized.

Head-injured children, it appears, are unable to apply low-level inhibitory skills. What ought to be an automatic process is for them less automatic, more effortful, and time-consuming, so that irrelevant material is actively and effortfully processed. The practical implications of these findings are that head-injured children may be operating on a day-to-day basis under a condition of chronic divided attention that constantly taxes their attentional resources and that causes them to overprocess information. This is particularly true for children whose head injury occurred earlier rather than later in childhood.

What are the broader consequences of an early head injury for cognitive function? Head injury early in life may result in delayed vulnerability of information processing skills like attention (Kaufmann et al., 1993) but also in more general cognitive deficits. Consistent with this idea, verbal intelligence tended to be lower in the younger than in the older age-at-injury group. These data suggest that domains like verbal intelligence, which depend on the acquisition and retention of a complex knowledge base, are not preferentially spared with head injury early in life. Congruent with recent findings, our data suggest that children who were younger at the time of head injury may be at risk for developing a limited knowledge base, which would have implications for the whole course of their learning. If the sequelae of an early head injury involve a failure to develop both a normal knowledge base and a normal distractor inhibition mechanism, then the results of early head injury on future academic functioning will be debilitating. It is clear that cognitive processing in the child with head injury under age 7 requires intensive analysis, particularly because these are often the children typically receiving no cognitive rehabilitation.

To study the consequences of attention deficits after head injury early in life for the acquisition of a knowledge base, it is important to plot what is known and to project what has not been directly observed. Recent individual change models have formalized the idea of developmental change into series of procedures that plot the entire developmental trajectories of different cognitive functions for an individual over time (Burchinal & Appelbaum, 1991; Fletcher et al., 1991). Developmental change within childhood head-injury samples measured longitudinally at several time points would allow evaluation of the effects of different medical and environmental variables on the developmental timing of the components of attention, particularly the component processes of selective attention.

In normally developing individuals, the nature of the cognitive processes required for the inhibition of distracting information is a topic of active current research in relation to questions such as: Are individual stimuli selected for attention or conscious awareness on the basis of elementary physical features or of meaning? Does inhibition occur early or late—that is, before or after stimulus identification? Is inhibition a passive and automatic process or an active, effortful, and time-consuming operation? The evidence suggests that unattended items are processed for meaning even when the relevant and irrelevant stimuli are physically separated (Fuentes & Ortells, 1993) and also that the selective attention inhibitory mechanism is active rather than passive, an idea that has emerged from studies of negative priming (e.g., Tipper et al., 1988), showing that an object ignored at one point in time takes longer to respond to when it later becomes a target. In light of this new information about the nature of selective attention, the finding of increased distractor inhibition in head-injured children, particularly in children who were injured at a younger age, is of some theoretical interest.

If distractors interfere with target detection in a visual monitoring task, then they have been processed, which is evidence that unintended processing affects concurrent target detection. If, in addition, the distracting information itself is preferred to the target, then it has been processed to some level of meaning; that is, if poorer performance under conditions of distraction is associated not only with a failure to detect correct targets but also with a tendency to confuse the target and the distractor, then the distractor has become a meaningful target.

Target detection is more difficult in situations—such as our distractor condition—where the same numbers are both targets to be activated and distractors to be suppressed or inhibited. Head-injured children not only failed to detect the target but also detected the wrong target, which was often the distractor to be inhibited. The fact that distractors not only interfered with concurrent processing but were reacted to as if they were targets suggests that irrelevant or nonattended material has been analyzed by head-injured children to some level of meaning. The fact that distractors were successful in competing for attention in this manner is consistent with the idea that distractor inhibition acts on some representation of the target that involves its meaning, not just its physical properties.

It has long been observed that head-injured individuals have slowed reaction times. The consequences of this are probably more debilitating than has been realized. A slowing of response time so that a target is detected some milliseconds later than normal would of itself have few consequences for everyday cognitive function. Most things can wait for a few milliseconds. If, however, the slowed reaction time is also associated with detecting the wrong target in rapidly changing arrays of the kind encountered daily by head-injured children, then the consequences are more serious because the slowing of reaction time means that responses become asynchronous with the surrounding world, with devastating consequences for the performance of many everyday tasks. To determine the extent to which slowed reaction time and a failure to inhibit irrelevant material are separate, conjoint, or causally connected is an important next step in the study of attention after childhood head injury.

Conclusion

The substrate of neuropsychological studies of childhood head injury must include time-tested measures of mental functions. Without this base, there is no method of comparing neuropsychological information across populations. If we are to describe processes and not just test scores, however, it is important that neuropsychological studies also draw on advances in cognitive psychology designed to create theoretical models of the processes to be studied. Only by understanding the putative defective process can we identify what should be remediated and establish whether the same component processes are operative across head-injured and normally developing populations.

Head-injured children have difficulty with the controlled cognitive processes that are the basis of successful attention. The research described here suggests two avenues for further exploration of attention in childhood head-injury populations, one concerning the comparison of attended and unattended processing of the same material and the other concerning the mechanism by which processing of unattended material impairs selective attention. As clinical research proceeds in this manner, the study of attention after childhood head injury becomes both a practical and a theoretical endeavor. Data of this kind not only add to the accumulating evidence for significant cognitive morbidity after childhood head injury but also address theoretical questions about the nature of attention.

Acknowledgment

This research was supported by a project grant to the first and fourth authors from The Physicians' Services Incorporated Research Foundation.

References

Aram, D. M., & Eisele, J. A. (1994). Intellectual stability in children with unilateral brain lesions. *Neuropsychologia 32*, 85–95.

Aram, D. M., & Ekelman, B. (1986). Cognitive profiles of children with early onset unilateral lesions. *Dev. Neuropsychol., 2*, 155–172.

Banich, M. T., Levine, S. C., Kim, H., & Huttenlocher, P. (1990). The effects of developmental factors on IQ in hemiplegic children. *Neuropsychologia, 28*, 35–47.

Binder, L. M. (1986). Persisting symptoms after minor head injury: A review of the post-concussive syndrome. *J. Clin. Exp. Neuropsychol., 8,* 323–346.

Boll, T. J. (1983). Minor head injury in children—out of sight, but not out of mind. *J. Clin. Child Psychol., 12,* 74–80.

Brink, J. D., Garrett, A. L., Hale, W. R., Wo-Sam, J., & Nickel, V. L. (1970). Recovery of motor and intellectual function in children sustaining severe head injuries. *Dev. Med. Child Neurol., 12,* 565–571.

Brown, P., & Fera, P. (1994). Turning selective attention failure into selective attention success. *Can. J. Exp. Psychol., 48,* 25–57.

Burchinal, M., & Appelbaum, M. I. (1991). Estimating individual developmental functions: Methods and their assumptions. *Child Dev., 62,* 23–43.

Chadwick, O., Rutter, M., Shaffer, D., & Shrout, P. E. (1981). A prospective study of children with head injuries: IV. Specific cognitive deficits. *J. Clin. Neuropsychol., 3,* 101–120.

Danoff, B. F., Cowchock, F. S., Marquette, C., Mulgrew, L., & Kramer, S. (1982). Assessment of the long-term effects of primary radiation therapy for brain tumors in children. *Cancer, 49,* 1580–1586.

Davies, D. R., Jones, D. M., & Taylor, A. (1984). Selective and sustained-attention tasks: Individual and group differences. In R. Parasuraman, R. Davies, & J. Beatty (Eds.), *Varieties of attention* (pp. 395–447). New York: Academic Press.

DeMarie-Dreblow, D., & Miller, P. H. (1988). The development of children's strategies for selective attention: Evidence for a transitional period. *Child Dev., 59,* 1504–1513.

Dennis, M., & Barnes, M. A. (1990). Knowing the meaning, getting the point, bridging the gap, and carrying the message: Aspects of discourse following closed head injury in childhood and adolescence. *Brain Lang., 3,* 203–229.

Dennis, M., & Barnes, M. A. (1994). Developmental aspects of neuropsychology: Childhood. In D. Zaidel (Ed.), *Handbook of perception and cognition: Neuropsychology* (Vol. 15, pp. 219–246). New York: Academic Press.

Dennis, M., Koski, L., Wilkinson, M. J., & Humphreys, R. P. (1993). Sustained attention, selective attention, and impulsivity after childhood head injury. *Clin. Neuropsychol., 7,* 326.

Donders, J. (1993). Memory functioning after traumatic brain injury in children. *Brain Inj., 7,* 431–437.

Doronzo, J. F. (1990). Mild head injury. In E. Lehr (Ed.), *Psychological management of traumatic brain injuries in children and adolescents* (pp. 207–224). Rockville, MD: Aspen Publishers.

Duhaime, A. C., Alario, A. J., Lewander, W. J., Schut, L., Sutton, L. N., Seidl, T. S., Nudelman, S., Budenz, D., Hertle, R., Tsiaras, W., & Loporchio, S. (1992). Head injury in very young children: Mechanisms, injury types, and ophthalmologic findings in 100 hospitalized patients younger than 2 years of age. *Pediatrics, 90,* 179–185.

Ewing-Cobbs, L., & Fletcher, J. M. (1987). Neuropsychological assessment of head injury in children. *J. Learning Disabil., 20,* 526–535.

Ewing-Cobbs, L., Fletcher, J. M., Landry, S. H., & Levin, H. S. (1985). Language disorders after pediatric head injury. In J. K. Darby (Ed.), *Speech and language evaluation in neurology: Childhood disorders* (pp. 97–111). San Diego, CA: Grune & Stratton.

Ewing-Cobbs, L., Levin, H. S., Fletcher, J. M., Miner, M. E., & Eisenberg, H. M.

(1989a). Post-traumatic amnesia in children: Assessment and outcome. *J. Clin. Exp. Neuropsychol., 11,* 58.

Ewing-Cobbs, L., Miner, M. E., Fletcher, J. M., & Levin, H. S. (1989b). Intellectual, motor, and language sequelae following closed head injury in infants and preschoolers. *J. Pediatr. Psychol., 14,* 531–547.

Finger, S., & Stein, D. G. (1982). *Brain damage and recovery: Research and clinical perspectives.* New York: Academic Press.

Fletcher, J. M., Francis, D. J., Pequegnat, W., Raudenbush, S. W., Bornstein, M. H., Schmitt, F., Brouwers, P., & Stover, E. (1991). Neurobehavioral outcomes in diseases of childhood: Individual change models for pediatric human immunodeficiency viruses. *Am. Psychol., 6,* 1267–1277.

Fletcher, J. M., Levin, H. S., & Landry, S. H. (1984). Behavioral consequences of cerebral insult in infancy. In C. R. Almi & S. Finger (Eds.), *Early brain damage: Research orientations and clinical observations* (pp. 189–213). New York: Academic Press.

Fletcher, J. M., Miner, M. E., & Ewing-Cobbs, L. (1987). Age and recovery from head injury in children. In H. Levin, J. Grafman, & H. Eisenberg (Eds.), *Neurobehavioral recovery from head injury* (pp. 279–291). New York: Oxford University Press.

Fletcher, J. M., & Satz, P. (1983). Age, plasticity, and equipotentiality: A reply to Smith. *J. Consult. Clin. Psychol. 51,* 763–767.

Fuentes, L. J., & Ortells, J. J. (1993). Facilitation and interference effects in a Stroop-like task: Evidence in favor of semantic processing of parafoveally-presented stimuli. *Acta Psychol., 84,* 213–229.

Fuld, P. A., & Fisher, P. (1977). Recovery of intellectual ability after closed head-injury. *Dev. Med., Child Neurol., 25,* 495–502.

Gaidolfi, E., & Vignolo, L. A. (1980). Closed head injuries of school aged children: Neuropsychological sequelae in early adulthood. *J. Neurol. Sci., 1,* 65–73.

Goldenberg, G., Oder, W., Spatt, J., & Podreka, J. (1992). Cerebral correlates of disturbed executive function and memory in survivors of severe closed head injury: A SPECT study. *J. Neurol. Neurosurg. Psychiatry, 55,* 362–368.

Goldman, P. S. (1972). Developmental determinants of cortical plasticity. *Acta Neurobiol. Exp. 32,* 495–511.

Gordon, M. (1983). *The Gordon Diagnostic System.* DeWitt, NY: Gordon Systems.

Gordon, M. (1988). *The Gordon Diagnostic System: Model III Instruction Manual.* DeWitt, NY: Gordon Systems.

Gulbrandsen, G. B. (1984). Neuropsychological sequelae of light head injuries in older children six months after trauma. *J. Clin. Neuropsychol., 6,* 257–268.

Halberg, F. E., Kramer, J. H., Moore, I. M., Wara, W. M., Matthay, K. K., & Ablin, A. R. (1991). Prophylactic cranial irradiation dose effects on late cognitive function in children treated for acute lymphoblastic leukemia. *Int. J. Radiat. Oncol. Biol. Phys., 22,* 13–16.

Han, J. S., Kaufman, B., Alfidi, R. J., Yeung, H. N., Benson, J. E., Haaga, J. R., El Yousef, S. J., Clampitt, M. E., Bonstelle, C. T., & Huss, R. (1984). Head trauma evaluated by magnetic resonance and computer tomography: A comparison. *Radiology, 150,* 71–77.

Hart, K., & Faust, D. (1988). Prediction of the effects of mild head injury: A message about the Kennard Principle. *J. Clin. Psychol., 44,* 780–782.

Jaffe, K. M., Fay, G. C., Polissar, N. L., Martin, K. M., Shurtleff, H., Rivara, J. M.

B., & Winn, H. R. (1992). Severity of pediatric traumatic brain injury and early neurobehavioral change: A cohort study. *Arch. Phys. Med. Rehabil., 73,* 540–547.

Jane, J. A., Rimel, R. W., Alves, W. M., Wayne, M. A., Dacey, R. G., Winn, H. R., & Colohan, A. R. (1985). Minor and moderate head injury: Model systems. In R. G. Dacey, H. R. Winn, R. W. Rimel, & J. A. Jane (Eds.), *Seminars in neurological surgery* (pp. 27–33). New York: Raven Press.

Jennett, B. & Teasdale, G. (1981). *Management of head injuries.* Philadelphia, PA: Davis.

Johnson, D. A., & Roethig-Johnston, K. (1989). Life in the slow lane: Attentional factors after head injury. In D. A. Johnson, D. Uttley, & M. Wyke (Eds.), *Children's head injuries: Who cares?* (pp. 96–110). New York: Taylor & Francis.

Johnson, D. A., Uttley, D., & Wyke, M. (Eds.) (1989). *Children's head injuries: Who cares?* New York: Taylor & Francis.

Kaufmann, P. M., Fletcher, J. M., Levin, H. S., Miner, M. E., & Ewing-Cobbs, L. (1993). Attentional disturbance after closed head injury. *J. Child Neurol., 8,* 348–353.

Kennard, M. A. (1940). Relation of age to motor impairment in man and in subhuman primates. *Arch. Neurol., Psychiatry, 44,* 377–397.

Kennard, M. A. (1942). Cortical reorganization of motor function: Studies on series of monkeys of various ages from infancy to maturity. *Arch. Neurol., Psychiatry, 47,* 227–240.

Kleinman, S. N., & Waber, D. P. (1992). Neurodevelopmental bases of spelling acquisition in children treated for acute lymphoblastic leukaemia. *Cogn. Neuropsychol., 9,* 403–425.

Kraus, J. F., Fife, D., & Conroy, C. (1987). Pediatric brain injuries. *Pediatric, 79,* 501–507.

Lehr, E. (Ed.) (1990). *Psychological management of traumatic brain injuries in children and adolescents.* Rockville, MD: Aspen.

Lenneberg, E. H. (1967). *Biological foundations of language.* New York: Wiley.

Levin, H. S. (1993). Head trauma. *Curr. Opin. Neurol., 6,* 841–846.

Levin, H. S., Amparo, E., Eisenberg, H. M., Williams, D., High, W. M., McArdle, C. B., & Weiner, R. L. (1987). Magnetic resonance imaging and computerized tomography in relation to the neurobehavioral sequelae of mild and moderate head injuries. *J. Neurosurg. 66,* 706–713.

Levin, H. S., Benton, A. L., & Grossman, R. G. (1982a). *Neurobehavioral consequences of closed head injury.* New York: Oxford University Press.

Levin, H. S., Culhane, K. A., Mendelsohn, E., Lilly, M. A., Bruce, D., Fletcher, J. M., Chapman, S. B., Harward, H., & Eisenberg, H. M. (1993). Cognition in relation to magnetic resonance imaging in head-injured children and adolescents. *Arch. Neurol., 50,* 897–905.

Levin, H. S., & Eisenberg, H. M. (1979). Neuropsychological outcome of closed head injury in children and adolescents. *Childs Brain, 5,* 281–292.

Levin, H. S., Eisenberg, H. M., Wiig, N. R., & Kobayashi, K. (1982b). Memory and intellectual ability after head injury in children and adolescents. *Neurosurgery, 11,* 668–673.

Levin, H. S., Ewing-Cobbs, L., & Fletcher, J. M. (1989). Neurobehavioral outcome of mild head injury in children. In H. S. Levin, H. M. Eisenberg, & A. L. Benton (Eds.), *Mild head injury* (pp. 189–213). New York: Oxford University Press.

Levin, H. S., & Grossman, R. G. (1976). Effects of closed head injury on storage and retrieval in memory and learning of adolescents. *J. Pediatr. Psychol., 1,* 38–42.

Levin, H. S., Mendelsohn, D., Lilly, M., Fletcher, J. M., Culhane, K. A., Chapman, S. B., Harward, H., Kusnerik, L., Bruce, D., & Eisenberg, H. M. (1994). Tower of London performance in relation to magnetic resonance imaging following closed head injury in children. *Neuropsychology, 8,* 171–179.

Lieh-Lai, M. W., Theodorou, A. A., Sarniak, A. P., Meert, K. L., Moylan, P. M., & Canady, A. I. (1992). Limitations of the Glasgow Coma Scale in predicting outcome in children with traumatic brain injury. *J. Pediatr., 120,* 195–199.

Luerssen, T. G., Hesselink, J. R., Ruff, R. M., Healy, M. E., & Grote, C. A. (1987). Magnetic resonance imaging of craniocerebral injury. In A. E. Marlin (Ed.), *Concepts in pediatric neurosurgery* (pp. 190–208). Basel: Karger.

Meadows, A. T., Massari, D. J., Fergusson, J., Gordon, J., Littman P., & Moss, K. (1981). Declines in IQ scores and cognitive dysfunctions in children with acute lymphocytic leukemia treated with cranial irradiation. *Lancet, 2,* 1015–1018.

Mendelsohn, D., Levin, H. S., Bruce, D., Lilly, M., Harward, H., Culhane, K. A., & Eisenberg, H. M. (1992). Later MRI after head injury in children: Relationship to clinical features and outcome. *Child Nerv. Syst., 8,* 445–452.

Michaud, L. J., Rivara, G. P., Grady, M. S., & Reay, D. T. (1992). Survival and severity of disability after severe brain injury in children. *Neurosurgery, 31,* 254–264.

Mulhern, R. K., Hancock, J., Fairclough, D., & Kun, L. (1992a). Neuropsychological status of children treated for brain tumors: A critical review and integrative analysis. *Med. Pediatr. Oncol., 20,* 181–191.

Mulhern, R. K., Kovnar, E., Langston, J., Carter, M., Fairclough, D., Leigh, L., & Kun, L. E. (1992b). Long-term survivors of leukemia treated in infancy: Factors associated with neuropsychological status. *J. Clin. Oncol., 10,* 1095–1102.

Mulhern, R. K., Ochs, J., & Fairclough D. (1992c). Deterioration of intellect among children surviving leukemia: IQ test changes modify estimates of treatment toxicity. *J. Consult. Clin. Psychol., 60,* 477–480.

Murray, R., Shum, D., & McFarland, K. (1992). Attentional deficits in head-injured children: An information processing analysis. *Brain Cogn., 18,* 99–115.

Nass, R., Peterson, H., & Koch, D. (1989). Differential effects of congenital left and right brain injury on intelligence. *Brain Cogn., 9,* 258–266.

Ness, K., Sfakianakis, G., Ganz, W., Uricchio, B., Vernberg, D., Villanuevas, P., Jabir, A. M., Bartlett, J., & Keena, J. (1993). ^{99m}Tc-HMPAO SPECT of the brain in mild to moderate traumatic brain injury patients: Compared with CT-a prospective study. *Brain Inj., 7,* 469–479.

Papinacolau, A. C., Loring, D. W., Eisenberg, H. M., & Contreras, F. L. (1985). Brain stem potentials in comatose head-injury patients. *Proceedings of the European Meeting of the International Neuropsychological Society.* Copenhagen.

Povlishock, J. T., & Coburn, T. H. (1989). Morphopathological change associated with mild head injury. In H. S. Levin, H. M. Eisenberg, & A. L. Benton (Eds.), *Mild head injury* (pp. 37–53). New York: Oxford University Press.

Rimel, R. W., Giordani, F., Barth, J. T., Boll, T. J., & Jane, J. A. (1981). Disability caused by minor head injury. *Neurosurgery, 9,* 221–228.

Ris, M. D., & Noll, R. B. (1994). Long-term neurobehavioral outcome in pediatric brain-tumor patients: Review and methodological critique. *J. Clin. Exp. Neuropsychol., 16,* 21–42.

Salcman, M., & Pevsner, P. H. (1992). The value of MRI in head injury comparison with CT. *Neurochirurgie, 38,* 329–332.

Sekino, H., Nakamura, N., Yuki, K., Satoh, J., Kiduchi, K., & Sanada, S. (1981). Brain lesions detected by CT scans in cases of minor head injuries. *Neurol. Med. Chir.,* *21,* 667–683.

Siegel, A. W., Bisanz, J., & Bisanz, G. L. (1983). Developmental analysis: A strategy for the study of psychological change. *Contr. Hum. Dev., 8,* 53–80.

Snoek, J. W. (1989). Mild head injury in children. In H. S. Levin, H. M. Eisenberg, & A. L. Benton (Eds.), *Mild head injury* (pp. 102–132). New York: Oxford University Press.

Spunberg, J. J., Chang, C. H., Goldman, M., Auricchio, E., & Bell, J. J. (1981). Quality of long-term survival following irradiation for intracranial tumors in children under the age of two. *Int. J. Radiat. Oncol., 7,* 727–736.

Stuss, D. T., Hugenholtz, H., Richard, M. T., LaRochelle, S., Poirier, C. A., & Bell, I. (1985). Subtle neuropsychological deficits in patients with good recovery after closed head injury. *Neurosurgery, 17,* 41–47.

Tipper, S. P., Bourque, T. A., Anderson, A. H., & Brehaut, J. C. (1989). Mechanisms of attention: A developmental study. *J. Exp. Child Psychol., 48,* 353–378.

Tipper. S. P., MacQueen, G. M., & Brehaut, J. C. (1988). Negative priming between response modalities: Evidence for the central locus of inhibition in selective attention. *Percept. Psychophys., 43,* 45–72.

Trexler, L. E., & Zappala, G. (1988). Re-examining the determinants of recovery and rehabilitation of memory defects following traumatic brain injury. *Brain Inj., 2,* 187–203.

Van Zomeren, A. H., & Brouwer, W. H. (1992). Assessment of attention. In J. R. Crawford, D. M. Parker, & W. W. McKinlay (Eds.), *A handbook of neuropsychological assessment* (pp. 241–266). Hillsdale, NJ: Erlbaum.

Van Zomeren, A. H., & Deelman, B. G. (1978). Long-term recovery of visual reaction time after closed head injury. *J. Neurol. Neurosurg. Psychiatry, 41,* 452–457.

Vogenthaler, D. R. (1987). An overview of head injury: Its consequences and rehabilitation. *Brain Inj., 1,* 113–127.

Waber, D. P., Bernstein, J. H., Kammerer, B. L., Tarbell, N. J., & Sallan, S. E. (1992). Neuropsychological diagnostic profiles of children who received CNS treatment for acute lymphoblastic leukemia: The systemic approach to assessment. *Dev. Neuropsychol., 8,* 1–28.

Wechsler, D. (1974). *Wechsler Intelligence Scale for Children—Revised.* New York: Psychological Corporation.

Wechsler, D. (1991). *Wechsler Intelligence Scale for Children—Third Edition.* New York: Psychological Corporation.

Winogron, H. W., Knights, R. M., & Bawden, H. N. (1984). Neuropsychological deficits following head injury in children. *J. Clin. Neuropsychol., 6,* 269–286.

Wohlwill, J. (1973). *The study of behavioral change.* New York: Academic Press.

Zappala, G., & Trexler, L. E. (1992). Quantitative and qualitative aspects of memory performance after head injury. *Arch. Clin. Neuropsychol., 7,* 145–155.

10

Recovery from Traumatic Brain Injury in Children: The Importance of the Family

H. GERRY TAYLOR, DENNIS DROTAR,
SHARI WADE, KEITH YEATES, TERRY STANCIN,
and SUSAN KLEIN

Families of children with traumatic brain injury (TBI) frequently have difficulties coping with the behavioral and cognitive consequences of injury (Brooks, 1990, 1991; DePompei & Zarski, 1989; Lezak, 1987). Failure to overcome these difficulties may jeopardize continued recovery of function in the child and contribute to longer-term behavior problems (Boll, 1983; Brooks, 1991). Unfortunately, little research has been conducted to determine how TBI in children affects their families. We also know little about the relationship of the family environment to child outcomes post-TBI or about the importance of the family environment, relative to injury severity, as a source of variability in child outcomes. An understanding of how environmental factors influence recovery, therefore, is critical to study of brain-behavior relationships following TBI and to discovery of ways to promote recovery.

The first section of this chapter reviews the impact of the injury on the family, and factors that predict child outcomes. The methodological requirements for meaningful study of post-TBI child and family outcomes are discussed in the second section. The third section describes an ongoing investigation of recovery of function and the family environment in school-age children who have sustained moderate to severe TBI. The conceptualization, aims, and methods of this study are detailed as a means of illustrating research approaches. Although data collection is ongoing and results are incomplete, preliminary findings are presented to document the adverse consequences of injury for families and the relevance of family characteristics to child outcomes. The final section of the chapter provides an overview of progress to date on this topic and highlights methodological limitations, implications of research findings, and useful directions for future research.

Family Outcomes

Serious TBI in a child also has family consequences (DePompei & Zarski, 1989). Families are faced with a heavy burden of care and have to make immediate emotional adjustments. Family financial resources may be stretched and schools usually are ill prepared to respond appropriately to the child's special needs (Telzrow, 1987). Clinical observations suggest that families of children with TBI are susceptible to organizational difficulties, lack of support or communication within the family, and restriction in social involvements and supports outside of the family (Brooks, 1991; DePompei & Zarski, 1989; Zarski et al., 1988). Clinical impressions also indicate that intact and communicative families are able to cope more effectively with the child's trauma than families in which there are higher levels of preexisting stress or less cohesiveness, and that the child's recovery is facilitated by a functional and supportive family environment (DePompei & Zarski, 1989; Fletcher et al., 1990). Interventions advocated to assist family adaptation following childhood TBI—and in this way to promote the child's recovery as well—include professional guidance in understanding and coping with the child's disability, attention to reactions of siblings, educational accommodations, social support, and continuity of care over time (Waaland & Kreutzer, 1988).

More formal support for the assumption that TBI has adverse family consequences comes from a variety of sources. Studies of TBI in adults have documented a high frequency of self-reported psychological symptoms and subjective distress in family members (Brooks, 1990, 1991). Family members' distress increases over time and is predicted by post-TBI behavioral and personality changes in the injured adult as well as by the psychological adjustment of the family member before and immediately after the injury. Although the family system may be affected differently by TBI in a child, behavioral effects of TBI are similar in adults and children. For this reason, TBI is likely to subject families to the same types of stressors, regardless of whether the injured person is an adult or a child (Brooks, 1991).

Studies of the family impact of other health-related conditions in children provide further grounds for anticipating family disruption following pediatric TBI. Problems in the psychological adjustment of parents and siblings, marital difficulties, and self-reported family distress are associated with a number of chronic childhood illnesses and disabilities (Breslau & Prabucki, 1987; Breslau et al., 1982; Crnic et al., 1983; Kazak & Marin, 1984; McCormick et al., 1986; Quittner et al., 1990; Varni & Wallander, 1988; Wallander et al., 1989).

Similar findings are reported in two studies of children with traumatic injuries including but not limited to TBI. Harris and associates (1989) conducted phone interviews with families a minimum of 1 year following serious multisystem pediatric injuries involving blunt trauma. In addition to reporting adverse changes in the behavior and learning abilities of children after injury, many of the parents noted deterioration of their marriages. Sixty percent of the sample indicated that they had new social and financial problems and 66% reported negative behavior changes in siblings of the injured child.

Hu and colleagues (1993) also found evidence of family disruption after severe traumatic injuries in children. In this study, 45% of the parents indicated that family life had not returned to normal by 6 months postinjury. Twenty-three percent reported disruption even a full year after the event. Variables that were related to self-reports of family disruption at 6 months postinjury included the child's functional health status, the presence of a maternal psychological disorder, and a behavior problem in the child. Factors that were related to family disruption at 1 year after the injury included the child's functional health status, the family's out-of-pocket medical expenses, the presence of maternal psychological disorder, and the child's participation in rehabilitation treatment. Families reporting subsequent disruption also were more likely to be single-parent households.

Unfortunately, neither of the latter studies separated children with TBI from children with injuries not affecting the central nervous system (CNS). The consequences of injury for families may have been due to nonspecific factors, such as hospitalization. These studies also failed to take preinjury family status into account and did not include a comparison group without severe injury. It is unclear, therefore, if reports of postinjury changes were due to injury or if they reflected a tendency to attribute problems present prior to injury to the injury event.

To our knowledge, only two studies have focused more specifically on the family consequences of childhood TBI. In a study by Perrott and colleagues (1991), the parents of children with TBI completed self-ratings of parenting stress and family health and psychosocial adjustment. Analysis of the latter measures indicated that parents were more stressed by children with TBI than by their noninjured siblings. Parents also reported somewhat higher levels of depressive symptoms and social isolation than a normative sample of parents, although the latter differences were nonsignificant.

In a second and more comprehensive study, Rivara and associates (1992) followed families of children with mild, moderate, and severe TBI over the first postinjury year. The assessments of family functioning were conducted soon after injury (baseline) to determine preinjury functioning and then again at 3 and 12 months postinjury. The family assessments described in this report were coincident with the child behavior evaluations examined in a companion paper by Rivara and coworkers (1993). Family measures included both standardized rating scales completed by the families and interviewer ratings of family functioning. Preinjury ratings of the child's behavior were also obtained from parents and teachers. The effect of the child's injury on family functioning was evaluated in terms of changes in the family measures over time. Analysis of the interviewer-based ratings indicated a deterioration of family functioning for children with severe TBI relative to children with mild or moderate TBI. The fact that a substantial proportion of the families reported being distressed by post-TBI behavioral changes in their children—such as memory problems, distractibility, difficulty following through on tasks, and temper outbursts—provided further evidence for adverse effects of injury on families. An additional finding reported by Rivara and colleagues was that pre- to postinjury changes in family functioning were related to the child's behavior before the injury and to preinjury family functioning. Even after taking injury severity into account, ratings of preinjury family coping and global functioning, together with a teacher rating of the child's preinjury adaptive behavior, predicted which families would show the greatest deterioration in functioning following the injury.

Existing data have clearly substantiated the relevance of the child's preinjury functioning and the family environment to postinjury outcomes. In their 2¼-year prospective study of children with head and orthopedic injuries, Brown and colleagues (1981) found that children with preinjury behavioral abnormalities, even if regarded as "trivial" or "dubious," were more likely to develop a psychiatric disorder following injury than were children without any prior behavior problems. Consistent with earlier observations by Harrington and Letemendia (1958), children from problematic family backgrounds also were at high risk for developing new psychiatric disorders following the injury.

A study by Rivara and coworkers (1993) yielded similar findings. Child behavior ratings obtained 1 year after TBI correlated with preinjury ratings of both family functioning and child behavior. According to the results of regression analysis, high ratings of children's adaptive functioning, global functioning, and social competence were associated with low levels of parental control and with high ratings of global family functioning, family cohesion, and positive family relationships. Ratings of preinjury adaptive behavior also were associated with more positive child outcomes. Each of these associations was observed even after controlling for injury severity.

In one of the only studies that examined the relationship of estimates of preinjury skills to postinjury functioning, Levin and Eisenberg (1979) obtained the results of group tests of ability administered prior to injury for a subset of the children and adolescents they were following post TBI. The investigators compared these results to Wechsler IQ scores obtained a minimum of six months post injury. Correlations between performances before and after injury were significant for Wechsler Intelligence Scale for Children—Revised (WISC-R) Verbal IQ, and approached significance for WISC-R Performance IQ.

The importance of the family environment has been demonstrated in numerous studies linking child behavior problems to family stress, negative life events, and parental psychological symptoms (Berden et al., 1990; Blanz et al., 1991; Campbell & Ewing, 1990; Cohen & Brook, 1987; Egeland et al., 1990; Esser et al., 1990; Prior et al., 1992; Wallander, et al., 1989). Social and family factors also account for variability in the outcomes of neurologic disorders other than TBI, even after taking disease severity into account (Taylor et al., 1992; Taylor & Schatschneider, 1992). It is not surprising, therefore, that this same relationship would hold for children with TBI.

The findings of studies by Rutter and his associates (Brown et al., 1981; Chadwick et al., 1981) and by Perrott and coworkers (1991) provide additional justification for considering family factors as potential predictors of post-TBI outcomes. In both studies, children with TBI exhibited long-term behavior problems in spite of cognitive recovery. According to Perrott and colleagues, (1991), cognitive impairments and behavior changes exhibited by children earlier in the postinjury period may have disrupted family life and had a negative impact on parent adjustment and the parent-child relationship. These circumstances, in turn, may have had adverse effects on subsequent child behavior and adaptation in spite of continuing cognitive recovery. The suggestion that family dysfunction may lead to persistent behavior and learning problems in spite of cognitive recovery echoes speculations by other researchers (Boll, 1983; Brooks, 1991; Brown et al., 1981; Fletcher et al., 1990; Perrott et al., 1991; Rutter, 1981). Observations that the severity of TBI is more closely related to cognitive functioning than to behavioral outcomes are consistent with this interpretation (Fletcher et al., 1990). As summarized by Brooks (1990), "The greater the severity of the injury, the greater the deficit, but factors other than organic brain damage are important in leading to and maintaining behaviour deficits" (p. 86).

A final rationale for considering family and psychosocial factors as predictors of child outcomes following TBI is provided by data showing environmentally related influences on recovery of function in animal research (Goldman & Lewis, 1978; Kolb, 1989; Stein, 1987). Animal studies also indicate that the condition of the brain following injury is determined not only by the primary injury but also by secondary degenerative and regenerative processes (Finger et al., 1989). If the environmental context in which injury occurs affects these processes, as some researchers believe (Stein, 1987), it is reasonable to hypothesize that human recovery of function may be related in part to social and family factors. Evidence that motivation enhances the responses of persons with brain injuries to rehabilitation efforts offers some support for this possibility (Prigatano, 1989).

Methodological Critique and Research Demands

Despite these several reasons for considering family and social factors as determinants of outcome after TBI in children, research in this area has been sparse. The follow-up project described earlier by Rivara and her colleagues (Rivara et al., 1992; Rivara et al., 1993) is the only one to date that has incorporated systematic assessments of the impact of the child's injury on the family and the relationship of family functioning to child outcomes. Among this project's several strengths are the collection of data on preinjury child and family status, systematic follow-up of children and their families for a full year postinjury, and examination of pre-post changes in children's behavior. Findings from this groundbreaking project also underscore the importance of broadening the scope of studies in this area to include evaluations of the context in which the child lives before and after injury.

Nevertheless, methodological limitations raise some questions with regard to interpretation of the findings. To begin with, the family measures that showed relative deterioration over follow-up for the group with severe TBI were based on

interviewer impressions of the family. The basis of the interviewer ratings is unclear; the ratings could have been biased by the interviewer's knowledge of the
injury. Parent ratings of family functioning were administered, but changes in
these measures over the follow-up interval were not reported. Second, failure to
compare children with TBI to children with other serious traumatic injuries pre-
cluded isolation of the effects of the child's head injury from the effects of accompanying non-CNS injuries. Finally, in conducting analyses of the child outcomes,
the investigators did not enter the child's preinjury status into the regression analyses prior to inclusion of other predictor variables. For this reason, the extent to
which measures of preinjury family and child functioning were related to changes
in the child following injury was unclear. The results of the regression analyses
may merely have reflected associations of child and family functioning prior to
injury to child status at a later point in time.

   Further studies of the contribution of environmental factors to outcomes of TBI
in children are therefore needed. In general, methodologically sound approaches to
research in this area must fulfill the following five criteria: (1) consideration of
factors that may be confounded with injury outcomes, (2) measurement of injury
severity, (3) assessment of environmental influences on recovery, (4) comprehensive measurement of outcomes, (5) longitudinal follow-up.

An Example of Research Methods

Background and Aims

An ongoing 5-year study, entitled *Recovery from Traumatic Brain Injury in Children,* represents one attempt to meet these methodological challenges. This project
was first funded late in 1990 and is currently in its third year. Participating sites
include Rainbow Babies and Childrens Hospital and MetroHealth Medical Center
in Cleveland, Ohio; Columbus Children's Hospital in Columbus, Ohio; and Children's Hospital Medical Center of Akron in Akron, Ohio. One of the major aims
of the project is to examine the relative impact on families of two types of traumatic injuries in children: moderate to severe TBI and orthopedic injuries not
involving insult to the central nervous system (CNS). A second objective is to
determine the extent to which postinjury family characteristics predict cognitive,
behavioral, and educational outcomes in children with TBI compared to children
with orthopedic injuries. Our central interest in undertaking this project is to examine the possibility that both the initial brain insult and environmental factors
contribute to the adverse consequences of childhood TBI.

Conceptual Framework

The conceptual framework for the study is depicted in Figure 10-1. The basis of
this conceptualization is the assumption that outcomes of TBI for the child are
determined by direct effects of the injury as well as indirect effects mediated by

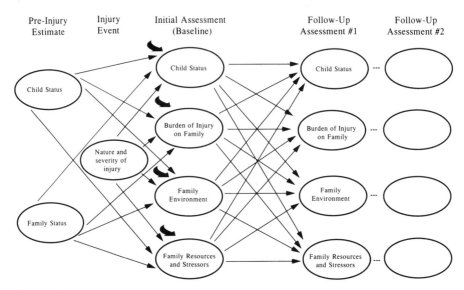

Figure 10-1. Conceptual framework for study of the consequences of childhood traumatic brain injury on children and their families.

the impact of the injury event on the family. Child outcomes include health status, neuropsychological functioning, academic achievement, behavioral adjustment and social competence, school performance and educational treatment, and adaptive behavior. Family variables include: (1) the burden of the injury on the family due, for example, to worry about the child, changes in child behavior due to injury, or to efforts to accommodate to injury-related needs of the child or others; (2) the family environment, which entails family functioning (i.e., organization, communication, and interaction within the family system), parent psychological distress, and parent-child interactions; and (3) family resources and stressors such as support from relatives and friends, coping strategies, and positive and negative life events.

According to this conceptualization, the injury event exerts its most direct impact on families via injury-related family burden. Specific aspects of the family environment (e.g., parent psychological distress) may also be affected directly by the injury event or via the burden of injury on the family. The emphasis that the model places on the burden of injury addresses the need to consider context-specific stressors in evaluating family outcomes (Coyne & Downey, 1991). Quittner and her colleagues have demonstrated that stresses specific to the child's health condition are better predictors of family adaptation than global ratings of parenting stress (Quittner et al., 1990; Quittner et al., 1992).

Family resources and stressors are included in the model to allow for the possibility that the effects of injury, like the effects of chronic illness, may be determined by a wide range of "risk and resistance" factors (Crnic et al., 1983; Varni & Wallander, 1988; Wallander et al., 1989). To further broaden the model, potential influences on child outcomes could be extended to include circumstances of schooling, peer interactions, and the child's relationships with the broader community (Crnic et al., 1983).

Although not represented in Figure 10-1, we assume that child and family characteristics are correlated at any given point in time. In accordance with models of reciprocal influence or bidirectionality, both child and family outcomes are assumed to change over time from assessments conducted initially postinjury (baseline) to later follow-up assessments. A further assumption is that child outcomes in the early postinjury period have the potential to alter later family characteristics and vice versa (Crnic et al., 1983; Sameroff & Chandler, 1975; Waaland & Raines, 1991). The pattern of potential relationships between variables across time is illustrated in Figure 10-1 by the arrows connecting the first two postinjury assessments. A similar pattern of connections is assumed between any two consecutive assessments (omitted from Figure 10-1 for the sake of simplicity).

A final feature of our conceptual framework is the hypothesis that postinjury characteristics of the child and family are influenced not only by the injury itself but also by preinjury child and family status (estimates of preinjury child and family status are represented in the model by the ovals in the left-hand column of Figure 10-1). The effects of preinjury status on postinjury outcomes is represented by the arrows connecting these variable sets to factors measured at baseline. Other undetermined influences on postinjury child and family characteristics, such as aspects of preinjury status that cannot be assessed postinjury, are represented by the downward-pointing arrows positioned next to the baseline measures.

The framework depicted in Figure 10-1 is intended more as a conceptualization of relevant variables and of potential associations than as a testable statistical model. Hypothesized relationships between certain variable sets and others can be tested without the need for omnibus testing of all potential relationships. Nevertheless, given sufficient statistical power and validated summary measures of model constructs, statistical modeling procedures could be applied to the wider set of determinants of child outcomes. The primary purpose of the conceptual framework is to emphasize the possible role of family factors as determinants of child outcomes and to acknowledge the complexity of the recovery process from a longitudinal perspective.

Hypotheses and Rationale

Two major hypotheses follow from this conceptualization. *Hypothesis 1* is that moderate to severe TBI will adversely affect the family social environment and will result in more parental burden and psychological distress than orthopedic injuries not involving CNS insult. A corollary to this first hypothesis is that the impact of both types of injuries on families will vary with sociodemographic status, concurrent family stressors and resources, and parental coping strategies. *Hypothesis 2* is that postinjury family characteristics will predict behavioral, educational, and neuropsychological outcomes in the TBI group even after injury severity and estimates of preinjury child status are taken into account. Family variables also are hypothesized to predict changes in outcomes over time after TBI.

Hypothesis 1 will be tested by comparing the TBI and orthopedic injury groups on measures of the perceived impact or burden of the injury on the family and on postinjury parent and family functioning. We hypothesize that families will be more adversely affected by TBI than by orthopedic injury, at least once families have begun to experience the burden of the cognitive and behavioral consequences of TBI for the child. We further anticipate that, whereas the negative effects of the injury on families of children with TBI will become more pronounced over time, the impact on families of children with orthopedic injuries will either remain unchanged or diminish across follow-up. Finally, we expect that the effects of traumatic injury on families will vary with injury severity, baseline neuropsychological impairment, and family resources and stressors (Cohen & Wills, 1985; Rutter, 1983).

Hypothesis 2 focuses on the validity of family variables as predictors of child outcome post-TBI. Our essential aim is to determine whether any of a broad set of family variables predicts outcomes of TBI even after injury severity and estimates of preinjury child status have been taken into account. Long-term outcomes are expected to be more favorable the more advantageous the family circumstances at follow-up (e.g., more functional family environment, fewer symptoms of parental distress, less family adversity, more social resources, fewer concurrent stressors, more positive parent coping) (Cohen & Brook, 1987; Wallander et al., 1989). Although both TBI and orthopedic injuries may have adverse child and family consequences, we hypothesize that TBI will have a more negative family impact. More negative consequences for families, in turn, are hypothesized to add to group differences in child outcomes (i.e., over and above effects attributable to injury type or severity alone).

Sample

Our sample quota for the study is approximately 100 children in each of the two groups. The TBI group consists of children admitted to one of our hospital sites with moderate to severe TBI. Eligibility criteria are documentation of moderate to severe TBI, age between 6 and 12 years at time of injury, no evidence of child abuse or a previous history of neurological disease or neurosensory impairment, and English as the primary language spoken at home. Children with types of TBI not falling into the general category of closed head injuries are excluded (e.g., brain injury due to near drowning or toxins, projectile wounds, stroke). Consistent with previous work in the area, severe injuries are defined as those in which the initial GCS is 8 or less (Fletcher et al., 1990; Kraus et al., 1986; Levin et al., 1988). Moderate injuries are defined as those in which the initial GCS falls within the range of 9 to 12 on or shortly after admission, or in which a higher GCS rating is accompanied by seizures or other signs of neurological dysfunction, skull fracture, intracranial mass lesion, diffuse cerebral swelling, or documented loss of consciousness >15 minutes.

TABLE 10–1.   Study Design

Group	Assessment			
	Hospitalization	Baseline	6-Month Follow-up	12-Month Follow-up
Traumatic brain injury (sample goal, $n = 100$)	Assessment of burden of injury on family, ratings of preinjury child, and family status	Assessment of child outcomes, burden of injury on family, and preinjury family resources and stressors	Reassessment of child outcomes and postinjury family characteristics	Reassessment of child outcomes and postinjury family characteristics
Orthopedic injury (sample goal, $n = 100$)	Assessment of burden of injury on family, ratings of preinjury child, and family status	Assessment of child outcomes, burden of injury on family, and preinjury family resources and stressors	Reassessment of child outcomes and postinjury family characteristics	Reassessment of child outcomes and postinjury family characteristics

Criteria for inclusion in the orthopedic group are documentation of fracture requiring at least one night's hospital stay, no evidence of loss of consciousness, postconcussion symptoms, or other findings that would raise question as to possible brain injury, age between 6 and 12 years, no evidence of child abuse or of a history of neurological disease or neurosensory impairment, and English as the primary language spoken at home.

Design

As shown in Table 10-1, the study employs a concurrent cohort/prospective design involving repeated postinjury assessments of family functioning and child outcomes. To balance the groups as closely as possible on background factors associated with proneness to accidental injury and the hospitalization experience, we are comparing children with TBI to a group of children hospitalized for orthopedic injuries not involving insult to the CNS. Assessments are conducted during the child's hospitalization, at a baseline assessment soon after discharge, and at 6 and 12 months following the baseline evaluation.

Procedures

The first step in recruiting children and their families into the study involves the tracking of age-appropriate admissions for potential eligibility. As soon as children who meet eligibility criteria are medically stable and informed consent has been granted, the child's mental status is monitored (if a TBI case). Other procedures carried out during the child's hospitalization include (1) parent interviews; (2) parent ratings of the child's preinjury behavior; (3) mailing of forms to schools to obtain teacher ratings of preinjury behavior and school performance, copies of

TABLE 10-2.   Data Collected at Hospitalization

Area Assessed	Measure	Source	Reference
Nature of injury/both groups	Modified Injury Severity Scale	Hospital chart	Mayer et al. (1980)
	Injury circumstances	Parent interview	Authors
	Days hospital/surgery intervention/ medication status	Hospital chart	Authors
Nature of traumatic brain injury	Glasgow Coma Scale	Hospital chart	Jennett & Bond (1975)
	Duration of impaired consciousness	Hospital chart	Fletcher & Levin (1988)
	Neurological status (neurological exam/CT scan findings)	Hospital chart	Authors
	Children's Orientation & Amnesia Test	Direct assessment	Ewing-Cobbs et al. (1990)
Preinjury child status	Background, Family and Health Information Form	Parent	Authors
	Child Behavior Checklist	Parent	Achenbach (1991a)
	Child's Schooling Prior to Injury	Parent	Authors
	Child Behavior Checklist-Teacher's Report Form	Teacher	Achenbach (1991b)
	Walker-McConnell Scale of Social Competence	Teacher	Walker & McConnell (1988)
	Teacher Observation of Classroom Communication	Teacher	Blosser & DePompei (1991)
	Teacher Report Child's Education Program	Teacher	Authors
Preinjury family status	Background, Family and Health Information Form	Parent	Authors
	Family Assessment Device	Parent	Miller et al. (1985)
	Dyadic Adjustment Scale	Parent	Spanier (1976)
Postinjury family status	Family Burden of Injury Interview	Parent	Authors

school records or previous test results and grades if available, and information regarding preinjury special placements or classroom accommodations; and (4) review of the child's medical chart. Although mothers serve as the primary informants, both parents are asked to complete some of the questionnaires to determine parental consistency in ratings of the child and family.

Areas assessed during hospitalization include the nature and circumstances of the injury, the child's acute medical status, the preinjury behavioral status of the child, and preinjury family functioning. The measures employed to assess each of these areas are listed in Table 10-2. The Background, Family, and Health Information Form, completed via parent interview, requests information on sociodemographic status and the child's medical history. Information collected in this form is used to calculate indices of social status, such as the Hollingshead Four Factor Index of Social Status (Hollingshead, 1975). To determine the perceived burden of injury on the family during the hospitalization period, the child's parent is interviewed using the questions given in Table 10-3. For each area of concern, the parent is asked to rate the level of stress caused by this concern.

Baseline assessments are conducted as soon as can be arranged following hospital discharge but not prior to resolution of posttraumatic amnesia (PTA). (Resolution of PTA is defined as two consecutive days in which the measure of PTA falls in the normal range for age, using norms provided by Ewing-Cobbs et al., 1990). Tests administered to the child include measures of achievement and neuropsychological abilities (see Table 10-4). The Children's Depression Inventory (Kovacs, 1981) is also administered to obtain the child's self-perceptions of mood. These same measures are readministered at each of the two follow-up assessments. The tests are divided into three clusters, and the clusters given in counterbalanced order across children to control for fatigue effects. As much as possible, the psychometrist conducting the testing is kept blind to the status of the child being assessed (TBI or orthopedic injury). Even with breaks, the testing typically is

TABLE 10-3.   Questions on Family Burden of Injury Interview: Hospital Assessment[a]

1. Has the medical treatment your child required been distressful to you?
2. Have you had difficulty getting information from medical staff about your child's condition?
3. Has there been any change in how your child reacts or relates to you or your spouse?
4. Have you or your spouse had any difficulties managing your child's behavior since the accident?
5. If you have other children at home, have you had difficulty arranging for your family members or other persons to take care of them?
6. Have you had difficulties paying for their care?
7. Have you or your spouse had difficulties in disciplining or managing your other children's behavior since the accident?
8. Are you concerned about how your other children are reacting to or accepting your child's injury or hospitalization?
9. Have you noticed any changes in the behavior of your other children?
10. Are you concerned about your child's recovery or any possible problems in the future?
11. Has it been difficult to be separated from other family members during your child's hospitalization?
12. Have job or school schedules been affected in any way?
13. Is either parent missing work or school?
14. Are you having difficulty keeping up with daily chores, such as shopping or household tasks?
15. Have any family routines been affected or changed as a result of your child's injury?
16. If you have a spouse/partner, are you concerned about their reaction to your child's injury?
17. Do you and your spouse/partner disagree since the injury about how to best care for your child and family?
18. Has it been difficult in any way for you and your spouse to talk about your child's injury?
19. Are you concerned about how other family members or persons outside the family are reacting to your child's injury?
20. Do you disagree with other family members or persons outside the family about how to best care for your child and family?
21. Is it difficult for you to talk to other family members or persons outside the family about your child's injury or what has happened since?

[a]If answer is yes, parent asked to rate level of stress caused by this concern on following scale: 0 = not at all; 1 = a bit; 2 = fairly; 3 = quite; 4 = extremely.

TABLE 10-4. Children's Test Battery at Baseline and Follow-up

Skill Area	Test	Reference
Academic achievement	Woodcock Johnson Tests of Achievement-Revised (Letter/Word Identification, Passage Comprehension, Dictation, Writing Sample, Calculation, Applied Problems)	Woodcock & Mather (1989)
Intelligence	Wechsler Intelligence Scale for Children-III (Similarities, Vocabulary, Block Design, Object Assembly)	Wechsler (1991)
Language abilities	Photo Articulation Test	Pendergast et al., (1969)
	Boston Naming Test	Kaplan et al., (1983)
	Controlled Oral Word Association	Gaddes & Crockett (1975)
	Token Test, Part V	DiSimoni (1978)
	Clinical Evaluation of Language Fundamentals-Revised (Sentence Structure, Recalling Sentences)	Semel et al. (1987)
Psychomotor skills	Developmental Test of Visual Motor Integration	Beery (1989)
	Grooved Pegboard	Knights & Norwood (1980)
Memory	California Verbal Learning Test	Delis et al. (1986)
Attention	Continuous Performance Test 3	Lindgren & Lyons (1984)
	Underlining Subtests 2, 4, 9	Rourke & Orr (1977)
	Contingency Naming Test	Taylor et al. (1987)
Abstract reasoning	Test of Nonverbal Intelligence, 2nd ed.	Brown et al. (1990)
Emotional status	Children's Depression Inventory	Kovacs (1981)
	Child's Post-Traumatic Stress Reaction Index (Child Interview)[a]	Frederick et al. (1992)

[a] Administered only at follow-ups.

completed in half a day. Although the vast majority of children are assessed on an outpatient basis, children who remain in the hospital for extended periods are assessed in that setting. Children who remain untestable after 3 months postinjury are not excluded from the study but are considered outliers in conducting data analysis.

While the child is being tested, parents are interviewed and parent questionnaires are completed. The Vineland Adaptive Behavior Scales are administered to parents to obtain preinjury estimates of adaptive behavior (Sparrow et al., 1984). Aspects of the preinjury family environment not assessed during hospitalization are evaluated at this time. The latter assessments include measures of family resources and stressors; the extent to which family members share household tasks, have disagreements, and participate in common activities; social supports; and parenting style. Postinjury measures collected at the baseline assessment include parent reports of the child's postinjury health status, self-reports by parents of psychological distress and of coping behaviors, and parent perceptions of the impact or burden of the injury on the family. The measures employed to assess each of these areas are listed in Table 10-5, and the questions included in the Family Burden of Injury Interview are given in Table 10-6. As indicated in Table 10-5, the parent and teacher measures obtained during hospitalization or at the baseline assessment are readministered at each follow-up. Brief assessments of posttrau-

TABLE 10-5.   Data Collected from Parents and Teachers at Baseline and Follow-up Assessments

Area Assessed	Measure	Source	Reference
Postinjury health status	Continuing medical problems/post-concussion symptoms	Parent	Authors
	Health Status[a]	Parent	Rivara et al. (1991)
	Restriction in Activities Scale[b]	Parent	National Center for Health Statistics (1981)
	Health Care Utilization Form[b]	Parent	Authors
Postinjury child behavior	Vineland Adaptive Behavior Scales[b]	Parent	Sparrow et al. (1984)
	Child Behavior Checklist[c]	Parent	Achenbach (1991a)
	Child Behavior Checklist-Teacher's Report Form[c]	Teacher	Achenbach (1991b)
	Child's Schooling Following Injury[c]	Parent	Authors
	Walker-McConnell Scale of Social Competence[c]	Teacher	Walker & McConnell (1988)
	Teacher Observation of Classroom Communication[c]	Teacher	Blosser & DePompei (1991)
	Child's Post-Traumatic Stress Reaction Index[d]	Parent	Frederick et al. (1992)
Postinjury family status	Family Burden of Injury Interview	Parent	Authors
	Impact on Family Scale	Parent	Stein & Jessop (1985)
	Brief Symptom Inventory	Parent	Derogatis & Spencer (1982)
	COPE	Parent	Carver et al. (1989)
	Iowa Parent Behavior Inventory[b]	Parent	Crase et al. (1977)
	Life Stressors & Social Resources Inventory[b]	Parent	Moos & Moos (1988)
	Health & Daily Living Form Scales[b] (Family Task Sharing, Disagreements and Social Activities)	Parent	Moos et al. (1987)
	Quality of Relationships Interview[b]	Parent	Pierce et al. (1991)
	Background, Family and Health Information Form[c]	Parent	Authors
	Family Assessment Device[c]	Parent	Miller et al. (1985)
	Dyadic Adjustment Scale[c]	Parent	Spanier (1976)
	Vulnerable Child Scale[d]	Parent	Perrin et al. (1989)

[a]Baseline assessment separately evaluates current status and status over 6-month period prior to injury.

[b]Baseline assessment covers period prior to injury.

[c]Excluded from baseline assessment due to administration during child's hospitalization.

[d]Administered only at follow-ups.

TABLE 10-6.   Questions Included on Family Burden of Injury Interview: Baseline and Follow-up Assessment[a]

1. Has there been any change in how your child reacts or relates to you or your spouse/partner?
2. Have you or your spouse/partner had difficulties in disciplining or managing your child's behavior since the accident?
3. Have you noticed changes in the behavior of your other children?
4. Have you or your spouse/partner had difficulties in disciplining or managing your other children's behavior since the accident?
5. If you have other children, are you concerned about how they are reacting to or accepting your child's injury
6. Are you concerned about your child's recovery or any possible problems in the future?
7. Has day-to-day life changed for you and your family since we last saw you?
8. Is either parent still missing work or school?
9. Have job or school schedules been affected in any way?
10. If you have other children, has your child's injury made it difficult for you to take care of them?
11. Are you having difficulty keeping up with daily chores, such as shopping or household tasks?
12. Have any family routines been affected or changed as a result of your child's injury?
13. Have any long-term goals been affected by your child's injury, i.e., career, financial, or educational goals?
14. Has it been difficult for you to accept and deal with your child's injury?
15. If you have a spouse/partner, are you concerned about their reaction to your child's injury?
16. Has it been difficult for your spouse/partner to accept and deal with your child's injury?
17. Are you concerned about how your child is being accepted by his/her peers?
18. If you have a spouse/partner, do you disagree about how to take care of problems with your child and family that have resulted from the injury?
19. Has it been difficult in any way for you and your spouse/partner to talk about your child's injury?
20. Are you concerned about how other family members of persons outside the family are reacting to your child's injury?
21. Do you disagree with other family members or persons outside the family about how to best care for your child and family?
22. Are you concerned about what other persons think about how you are disciplining your child, or the kinds of things you allow your child to do or not do?
23. Is it difficult in any way for you to talk to other family members or persons outside the family about your child's injury or what has happened since?
24. Are you having difficulty finding time for your own activities?
25. Is your spouse/partner having difficulty finding time for his/her own activities?
26. Are you having difficulty finding time to be together and doing things together with your spouse/partner?
27. Are you having difficulty finding time to do things with your other children?

[a]If answer is yes, parent asked to rate level of stress caused by this concern on following scale: $0 =$ not at all; $1 = $ a bit; $2 = $ fairly; $3 = $ quite; $4 = $ extremely.

matic stress and of parent perceptions of child vulnerability to health problems are also carried out at each follow-up.

Preliminary Findings

Sample Description and Goals of Preliminary Analysis. To date, baseline child and family data are available for about half of the intended samples of children with TBI and orthopedic injuries. Six-month follow-up data are available for only a portion of these children. Sample sizes and mean ages for the two groups at each assessment, together with sex and race distributions, are reported in Table 10-7. Because too few 12-month follow-ups have been completed and coded to allow for meaningful analysis, only data from the hospitalization, baseline, and 6-month follow-up assessments will be considered in presenting preliminary findings. It is important to emphasize that statistical power is compromised by analysis of only a subset of the data. Equating groups on important variables such as sex, race, and age is incomplete, as is coding of indices of injury severity. Results will no doubt be different once the full data set is available, our groups are better matched on background variables, and analysis of outcomes by injury severity is possible. Given these limitations, the results summarized in this section are reported primarily to illustrate the promise of our approach and the need to consider family factors.

The goals of preliminary data analysis were to explore group differences in family and child outcomes and to investigate factors associated with postinjury child outcomes. Analysis was restricted to measures representing child functioning in four major developmental domains: (1) behavior adjustment at the 6-month follow-up as assessed by the Child Behavior Checklist (parent version) behavior problems T score; (2) adaptive behavior at the 6-month follow-up as measured by the Vineland Adaptive Behavior Composite; (3) academic achievement at the baseline and 6-month follow-up assessments as measured by the Woodcock-Johnson Tests of Achievement—Revised Skills Cluster (composite of performances on subtests of reading, spelling, math); and (4) neuropsychological performance at the baseline and 6-month follow-up assessments as indexed by prorated Performance IQ from the Wechsler Intelligence Scale for Children, third edition (WISC-III; see Table 10-4). Performance IQ was selected as a summary neuropsychological measure based on previous data indicating its special sensitivity to brain disorders in children (Taylor, 1984).

Three categories of predictor variables were related to these outcomes. The first predictor set included measures of the child's preinjury status. Although sev-

TABLE 10-7. Injury Groups Considered in Preliminary Data Analysis

Measure	Traumatic Brain Injury	Orthopedic Injury
Baseline assessment		
Sample size	54	44
Mean age at injury (SD)	9.7 (2.0)	9.2 (1.8)
Males(%) / Females(%)	78% / 22%	64% / 36%
White(%) / Minority(%)	73% / 27%	52% / 48%
6-Month follow-up assessment		
Sample size	42	27
Mean age at injury (SD)	9.8 (2.0)	9.1 (1.6)
Males(%) / Females(%)[a]	86% / 14%	56% / 44%
White(%) / Minority(%)	66% / 34%	63% / 37%

[a] χ^2 significant, $p < 0.05$.

eral indices of preinjury status deserve further study (e.g., school records, educational history, and teacher ratings of preinjury school performance and behavior), the measures chosen for the present analysis were limited to two formal parent-based measures of preinjury behavior: the Child Behavior Checklist behavior problems T score and the Vineland Adaptive Behavior Composite (see Table 10-5). The second predictor set included measures of the preinjury family environment, and the third set included measures of the postinjury family environment and of parent perceptions of the effect of injury on the family (see Tables 10-2 and 10-5).

Group Differences in Child Outcomes and Post-Injury Family Characteristics. The results of t-test comparisons of the TBI and orthopedic injury groups on the four child-outcome measures are summarized in Table 10-8. Due to the exploratory nature of the analyses, both significant ($p <0.05$) and marginally significant ($p <0.10$) differences are noted. Findings indicate higher rates of postinjury behavior problems in the TBI group. A marginally significant difference is found in academic skills at the baseline assessment, with a lower mean score in the TBI group. Although group differences are not significant for prorated WISC-III performance IQ at the two assessments, they are in the expected direction. Furthermore, analyses of other neuropsychological tests, including those assessing memory and attention, reveal significantly lower scores for the TBI group. Group differences change very little when sociodemographic factors (marital status of parent, mother's education, and race) are taken into account via analysis of covariance.

Preliminary t-test comparisons also show group differences in postinjury family characteristics (see Table 10-9). Group differences are significant for the Reasoning Guidance and Intimacy scales of the Iowa Parent Behavior Inventory and the Family Disagreements scale of the Health and Daily Living Form, and margin-

TABLE 10-8. Child Outcomes

Measure	Traumatic Brain Injury			Orthopedic Injury		
	n	$\bar{\chi}$	SD	n	$\bar{\chi}$	SD
Child Behavior Checklist, Behavior						
Problems (Follow-up)[a]	42	54.3	10.5	27	48.8	10.9
Vineland Adaptive Behavior Composite						
(Follow-up)	29	94.0	10.4	20	94.3	12.1
Woodcock Johnson Tests of Achievement-						
Revised, Skills Cluster						
Baseline[b]	48	91.0	16.9	32	98.3	16.8
Follow-up	38	95.7	13.9	19	94.2	19.0
Wechsler Intelligence Scale for Children-						
III, Performance IQ						
Baseline	47	92.2	17.9	22	96.1	18.1
Follow-up	40	99.8	20.1	19	103.3	16.6

[a] $p<0.05$.

[b] $p<0.10$.

TABLE 10-9.   Postinjury Family Characteristics

Measure	Traumatic Brain Injury			Orthopedic Injury		
	n	$\bar{\chi}$	SD	n	$\bar{\chi}$	SD
Brief Symptom Inventory, General Severity Index						
Baseline[a]	54	56.93	10.36	40	52.28	12.44
Follow-up	28	54.11	10.42	20	50.75	10.86
Family Burden of Injury Interview[b]						
Hospitalization	53	0.46	0.16	44	0.40	0.17
Baseline	54	0.43	0.18	42	0.39	0.19
Follow-up	28	0.34	0.26	20	0.26	0.17
Iowa Parent Behavior Inventory (follow-up)						
Parental involvement	29	3.14	0.68	20	3.22	0.66
Limit setting	29	3.98	0.58	20	3.96	0.54
Responsiveness	29	4.31	0.49	20	4.14	0.69
Reasoning guidance[c]	29	4.40	0.49	20	4.07	0.56
Free expression	28	2.80	0.74	20	2.55	0.91
Intimacy[c]	29	4.16	0.49	20	3.79	0.50
Family Assessment Device, General Functioning						
(follow-up)	34	3.10	0.41	20	3.15	0.49
Dyadic Adjustment Scale (follow-up)	26	100.69	18.24	10	103.50	22.74
Impact on Family Scale, Total Impact						
Baseline	54	30.28	5.37	44	32.15	6.83
Follow-up	29	29.62	5.12	20	28.65	3.70
Health & Daily Living Form Scales (follow-up)						
Household task sharing[a]	29	3.25	0.60	19	3.54	0.50
Family disagreements[c]	29	0.29	0.21	19	0.18	0.12
Family social activities	29	3.89	2.38	19	2.80	2.00

[a]$p < 0.10$.

[b]Proportion of items rated as stressful.

[c]$p < 0.05$.

ally significant for the Brief Symptom Inventory (General Severity Index) and Family Task Sharing Scale of the Health and Daily Living Form. Specifically, the parents of children with TBI reported listening to and reasoning with their children more frequently than did parents of children with orthopedic injuries. The parents of children with TBI also reported being more intimate in their relationship with the child, more family disagreements, greater parental distress, and a greater distribution of responsibility for household tasks (lower scores on the latter measure indicating that persons other than the informant have more responsibility for tasks). Group differences in family characteristics were similar when sociodemographic factors were taken into account as covariates.

The two groups did not differ on the Family Burden of Injury Interview, at least in terms of the percentages of interview items on which parents indicate injury-related stress. Nevertheless, results clearly document high levels of self-reported family burden for both groups, with families reporting stress in nearly half of the areas assessed. Group differences, moreover, were consistently in the

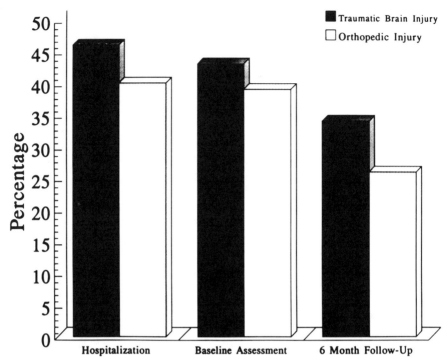

Figure 10-2. Percentages of items rated as stressful on the Family Burden of Injury Interview.

hypothesized direction (see Figure 10-2). Although a repeated measures analysis of variance revealed a significant decline in stress levels across time, this decline did not interact with the group classification (TBI versus orthopedic injury). Further data collection at the 6- and 12-month assessments will be required to more rigorously test the hypothesis that perceived family burden is more enduring for families of children with TBI than for families of children with orthopedic injuries.

To determine if some items from the Family Burden of Injury Interview might be more discriminating than other items, chi-square analyses were used to compare the groups in terms of the frequencies with which parents endorsed individual items as stressful. In general, the two groups reported similar frequencies of stress for many of the items, including those items reflecting general family burden. Items that assessed concern about the child's recovery, sibling behavior, and communication with others about the injury were more discriminating. Significant differences were found for items 7, 10, and 21 from the hospitalization interview; items 4 and 6 from the baseline interview; and items 21 and 22 from the 6-month follow-up interview (see Tables 10-3 and 10-6). These preliminary results suggest that, whereas some sources of family burden were common to both groups of families, other stressors were more specific to the TBI group.

Predictors of Postinjury Child Outcomes. Relationships between preinjury factors and postinjury child functioning were explored by regressing the four major 6-month child outcomes onto estimates of preinjury child behavior and preinjury family characteristics. Due to limited sample size and interests in identifying predictors of outcomes for both groups of children, the two groups were combined for these analyses. The predictor sets included (1) child behavior, as measured by the Child Behavior Checklist Behavior Problems T score and Vineland Adaptive Behavior Composite; (2) the Dyadic Adjustment Scale (marital adjustment); (3) the seven Family Assessment Device scales; (4) the three Health and Daily Living Form scales; and (5) the six Iowa Parent Behavior Inventory scales (see Tables 10-2 and 10-5). Stepwise regression analysis was used to examine relationships between each predictor or set of predictors and outcomes. Associations were evaluated in terms of the total variance accounted for in the dependent measure by the "best" set of predictor variables (R^2).

All significant R^2s are reported in Table 10-10. Regression coefficients indicated that higher behavior problem ratings were associated with higher preinjury ratings on this same measure, poorer family functioning (Behavior Control scale of the Family Assessment Device), and higher scores on the Responsiveness scale of the Iowa Parent Behavior Inventory. Lower adaptive behavior scores were associated with lower preinjury adaptive behavior scores and higher preinjury behavior problem ratings. Lower achievement scores and prorated WISC-III Performance IQs were associated, respectively, with higher scores on the Limit Setting and Reasoning Guidance scales of the Iowa Parent Behavior Inventory.

To estimate the overall strength of associations between preinjury variables and child outcomes, all of the variables that were identified as predictors of each outcome were entered into the regression equation simultaneously. The results of these analyses revealed that the preinjury factors accounted for 57% of the variance in the behavior problem ratings, 37% of the variance in the Vineland scores, 13% of the variance in the achievement scores, and 10% of the variance in prorated WISC-III Performance IQ.

TABLE 10-10.   Variance Accounted for in 6-Month Outcomes by Measures of Preinjury Child and Family Status (R^2 Total) [a]

			W-J Skills	
Measure of Preinjury Status	CBCL	Vineland	Cluster	WISC-III PIQ
Child Behavior: CBCL and Vineland	0.56	0.37	—	—
Dyadic Adjustment Scale	—	—	—	—
Family Assessment Device Scales	0.06	—	—	—
Health/Daily Living Form Scales	—	0.09	—	—
Iowa Parent Behavior Inventory Scales	0.08	—	0.13	0.10

Abbreviations: CBCL = Child Behavior Checklist Behavior Problems T-scores; Vineland = Vineland Adaptive Behavior Composite; W-J = Woodcock-Johnson; WISC-III PIQ = Wechsler Intelligence Scale for Children, 3rd ed., performance IQ.

[a] Variables from multivariate scales are entered in stepwise fashion. Only significant R^2 are reported.

Because the Child Behavior Checklist and Vineland Adaptive Behavior scales were used to estimate preinjury status, it is not surprising that preinjury child behavior was associated with these same measures at the 6-month follow-up. The results do, however, demonstrate the need to take the child's preinjury status into account in assessing postinjury behavioral changes. These findings also underscore the importance of considering preinjury family characteristics in evaluating child outcomes.

Similar analyses for the combined injury groups were carried out to explore relationships between family characteristics at the 6-month follow-up and child outcomes at that time. Predictor sets included (1) the proportion of items rated as stressful from the Family Burden of Injury Interview; (2) the four types of family impact measured on the Impact on Family Scale; (3) the nine subscales of the Brief Symptom Inventory; (4) the Dyadic Adjustment Scale; (5) the seven Family Assessment Device scales; (6) the three Health and Daily Living Form scales; and (7) the six scales of the Iowa Parent Behavior Inventory (see Tables 10-2 and 10-5).

According to results summarized in Table 10-11, postinjury family characteristics predicted three of the 6-month child outcomes. Higher ratings of behavior problems at follow-up were associated with greater injury-related family disruption as assessed on the Impact on Family Scale, greater parental psychological distress (Psychoticism scale of the Brief Symptom Inventory), and poorer family functioning (Roles scale of the Family Assessment Device). Lower scores on the Vineland Adaptive Behavior Composite were associated with greater parental distress (Interpersonal Sensitivity scale of the Brief Symptom Inventory), poorer family functioning (Affective Responsiveness scale of the Family Assessment Device), and more disagreements among family members. Lower prorated WISC-III Performance IQs were associated with more frequent family social activities, greater responsibility of the informant for household tasks, and higher scores on the Reasoning Guidance scale of the Iowa Parent Behavior Inventory.

TABLE 10-11. Variance Accounted for in 6-Month Outcomes by 6-Month Postinjury Measures of Family Status (R^2 Total) [a]

| | | W-J Skills | | |
Measure of Postinjury Status	CBCL	Vineland	Cluster	WISC-III PIQ
Family Burden of Injury Interview (proportion of items rated as stressful)	—	—	—	—
Impact on Family Scales	0.11	—	—	—
Brief Symptoms Inventory (General Severity Index)	0.34	0.21	—	—
Dyadic Adjustment Scale	—	—	—	—
Family Assessment Device Scales	0.15	0.14	—	—
Health/Daily Living Form Scales	—	0.18	—	0.20
Iowa Parent Behavior Inventory Scales	—	—	—	0.11

Abbreviations: CBCL = Child Behavior Checklist Behavior Problems T-scores; Vineland = Vineland Adaptive Behavior Composite; W-J = Woodcock-Johnson; WISC-III PIQ = Wechsler Intelligence Scale for Children, 3rd ed., performance IQ.

[a] Variables from multivariate scales are entered in stepwise fashion. Only significant R^2 are reported.

To examine the extent to which the larger set of postinjury family factors were associated with child outcomes, all postinjury family factors that were identified as predictors of a given outcome were entered into the regression equation simultaneously. According to these analyses, the latter family factors accounted for 37% of the variance in behavior problem ratings, 29% of the variance in adaptive behavior scores, and 25% of variance in prorated WISC-III performance IQ.

These findings confirm expectations that child outcomes following injury are related to postinjury family functioning, parental psychological distress, and the perceived impact or burden of the injury on the family. To the extent that the latter family characteristics are attributable to the injury itself (i.e., were not present prior to injury), the results are also consistent with the hypothesis that child outcomes depend in part on how the family has been affected by the injury.

To explore the possibility of relationships of family factors to *changes* in behavior since the injury, behavior problem T scores from the Child Behavior Checklist and the Vineland Adaptive Behavior Composite were subjected to further regression analyses. Family measures obtained at the 6-month assessment were again examined in relation to the four major 6-month child outcomes; but in these analyses, the child's preinjury score on the outcome was entered into the regression equation as a covariate. The results showed that scales from the Brief Symptom Inventory and Impact on Family Scale accounted for variance in behavior problems at the 6-month follow-up even after controlling for preinjury behavior problems. Similarly, even after taking preinjury adaptive behavior into account in the regression equation, adaptive behavior at the 6-month follow-up was predicted by scales from the Brief Symptom Inventory and Health and Daily Living Form. In each instance, more adverse outcomes at the 6-month assessment were associated with greater parental psychological distress, greater impact of injury on the family, and more negative family interactions. The findings, although preliminary in nature, provide some of the strongest support to date for a relationship between the postinjury family environment and the sequelae of childhood injuries.

Further Study Objectives

Because the present study is in many ways incomplete, caution is advised in interpretating these preliminary findings. Increased sample size, more complete group matching and follow-up, and coding of measures of injury severity will enable us to determine the best predictors of child outcomes for each group separately. Continued data collection will also allow us to address other project objectives. One of these objectives is to relate injury type and severity to the full range of outcomes, including the complete battery of neuropsychological and achievement tests, health status and health care utilization, postconcussional symptoms, school performance, and educational reentry. Our focus will be on factors that are associated with postinjury changes in abilities and behavior. These changes will be defined on the basis of postinjury outcomes adjusted for preinjury estimates or in terms of changes in outcomes over the three assessments. Particular attention will be given to associations between these changes and the postinjury family environment. Family resources and other stressors—as assessed by procedures such as the Quality of Relationships Interview (Pierce et al., 1991) and the Life Stressors and Social Resources Inventory (Moos & Moos, 1988)—will be considered as additional predictors of injury sequelae.

A second objective is to examine the effects of injury on families and the factors associated with adverse family consequences. Factors considered will include the nature of the injury itself, the child's level of functioning before and after injury, preinjury family status, postinjury family resources and other stressors, and parental coping strategies. The sequelae of injury for the family will be evaluated in terms of the perceived burden or impact of injury on the family as well as in terms of changes in the family environment over the follow-up period.

Summary and Conclusions

The Current Status of Research on the Role of the Family in Recovery from Childhood Traumatic Brain Injury

Surprisingly few studies of TBI in children have examined the family impact of childhood TBI or the relevance of the family environment to the child's long-term recovery. Rutter and coworkers (1983) summarized observations of families made in the course of their prospective study of children with TBI, noting the parental anxiety aroused by a comatose child or a child with posttraumatic behavior problems. These investigators also observed posttraumatic changes in parent-child relationships, marital tensions, and associations between parental reactions to the injury and the child's psychiatric outcome. But it is unclear from published reports how family factors were assessed, and the sample size was too small to allow for appropriate analysis of family variables.

The impact of pediatric TBI on families was assessed more systematically by Perrott et al. (1991). As summarized earlier, these investigators compared a relatively small sample of school-age children with moderate to severe TBI to their siblings on a variety of outcome measures. Parent and family assessments also were carried out. Findings suggested that long-term behavioral adjustment and school performance are particularly vulnerable following TBI. Consistent with the possibility that injury has negative repercussions for families, parenting stress was higher for the children with TBI than for siblings. The fact that parenting stress was related to measures of child outcome raised the possibility of family influences on recovery of function. The major drawback of the study was the fact that the children and their families were recruited long after the injury event. The children with TBI may have differed from their siblings prior to injury. If so, group differences in parenting stress may not have been precipitated by the injury per se.

In a larger and better-designed study, Rivara and her colleagues (Rivara et al., 1992; Rivara et al., 1993) followed children with TBI and their families prospectively from the time of injury. The sequelae of TBI were evaluated by assessing changes in child and family functioning relative to estimates of preinjury status and by comparing groups of children that varied in injury severity. Analyses of change scores revealed adverse effects of TBI on parent, teacher, and interviewer ratings of child functioning as well as on interviewer-based assessments of family functioning. For the most part, these negative consequences of TBI were confined to children with severe injuries. Measures of family functioning, in turn, predicted later child outcomes. In light of the fact that outcomes were assessed in terms of group comparisons of pre- to postinjury changes in child and family status, it is difficult to attribute injury consequences to preexisting group differences, natural variations in family functioning over time, or family reactivity to study participation. Unfortunately, child outcomes were not broadly assessed; it is not clear how interviewer ratings of child and family functioning were assigned; and it is difficult to determine if family factors were related to changes in child status following TBI. Discovery of associations between interview ratings and child outcomes at a given point in time is not the same as demonstrating that interview ratings predict changes in the child's behavior or abilities subsequent to injury.

One of the goals of our own, ongoing injury follow-up project is to test the hypothesis that families of children with moderate to severe TBI are affected more adversely by the injury event than are families of children with orthopedic injuries. A second aim is to explore the possibility that the consequences of TBI (and perhaps of orthopedic injuries as well) are associated with postinjury family characteristics. As in the study by Rivara and her colleagues, we are assessing preinjury child and family status and are following our sample prospectively from the time of injury.

Preliminary findings offer support for both study hypotheses. Six months after an initial postinjury assessment, parents of children with TBI report more family disagreements than do parents of children with orthopedic injuries. We are also observing group differences in parenting behaviors and in specific areas of injury-related family burden; there is a trend for parents of children with TBI to report higher levels of psychological distress. A considerable amount of the variance in child outcomes at a 6-month follow-up assessment is accounted for by measures of preinjury child and family status as well as by postinjury family characteristics. Most critically, certain postinjury family factors account for variance in 6-month behavior outcomes even after controlling for preinjury scores on the same measures. The latter result constitutes the strongest support to date for an association between the family environment and the behavioral sequelae of traumatic injury in children. More generally, these preliminary findings underscore both the need to take preinjury child and family status into account in evaluating injury sequelae and the potential value of context-specific measures of family burden (Coyne & Downey, 1991; Quittner et al., 1992).

Studies of the families of children with TBI have important clinical benefits. Knowledge of the process of family adaptation and coping following TBI and identification of child and family characteristics that are associated with good long-term outcomes will suggest strategies of intervention. Conversely, discovery of factors that are associated with poor outcomes will indicate which children and families are most in need of counseling or other more intensive therapeutic interventions. If environmental factors do, in fact, predict outcomes of TBI, it may be possible to facilitate children's recovery of function and to avoid or reduce undesirable long-term behavioral sequelae.

Acknowledgments

This work was supported by Grant MCJ-390611, Maternal and Child Health Bureau (Title V, Social Security Act), Health Resources and Services Administration, Department of Health and Human Services. The efforts of Elizabeth Shaver, Madeline Polonia, Barbara Shapero, and Nori Mercury-Minich in data collection and coding are greatly appreciated. We also wish to acknowledge the collaboration of Christine Barry, Ph.D., Duane Bishop, M.D., Jean Blosser, Ph.D., Roberta DePompei, Ph.D., Matthew Likavec, M.D., Timothy Mapstone, M.D., Scott Maxwell, Ph.D., George Thompson, M.D., G. Dean Timmons, M.D., and Dennis Weiner, M.D.

References

Achenbach, T. (1991a). *Manual for the Child Behavior Checklist 4-18 and 1991 Profile.* Burlington, VT: Department of Psychiatry, University of Vermont.

Achenbach, T. (1991b). *Manual for the Teacher's Report Form and 1991 Profile.* Burlington, VT: Department of Psychiatry, University of Vermont.

Beery, K. E. (1989). *Revised Administration, Scoring, and Teaching Manual for the Developmental Test of Visual-Motor Integration.* Cleveland, OH: Modern Curriculum Press.

Berden, G., Althaus, M., & Verhulst, F. (1990). Major life events and changes in the behavioral functioning of children. *J. Child Psychol. Psychiatry, 31,* 949–959.

Blanz, B., Schmidt, C., & Esser, G. (1991). Family adversities and child psychiatric disorders. *J. Child Psychol. Psychiatry, 32,* 939–950.

Blosser, J., & DePompei, R. (1991). *Teacher observation of classroom communication.* Akron, OH: University of Akron.

Boll, T. (1983). Minor head injury in children—Out of sight, but not out of mind. *J. Clin. Child Psychol., 12,* 74–80.

Breslau, N., & Prabucki, K. (1987). Siblings of disabled children. *Arch. Gen. Psychiatry, 44,* 1040–1046.

Breslau, N., Staruch, K., & Mortimer, E. (1982). Psychological distress in mothers of disabled children. *Am. J. Dis. Child., 136,* 682–686.

Brooks, D. N. (1990). Behavioral and social consequences of severe head injury. In B. Deelman, R. Soan, & A. van Zomeren (Eds.), *Traumatic brain injury: Clinical, social and rehabilitational aspects* (pp. 77–88). Amsterdam: Swets & Zeitlinger.

Brooks, D. N. (1991). The head-injury family. *J. Clin. Exp. Neuropsychol., 13,* 155–188.

Brown, G., Chadwick, O., Schaffer, P., Rutter, M., & Traub, M. (1981). A prospective study of children with head injuries: III. Psychiatric sequelae. *Psychol. Med., 11,* 63–78.

Brown, L., Sherbenou, R., & Johnsen, S. (1990). *Test of Nonverbal Intelligence,* 2nd ed. Austin, TX: PRO-ED.

Campbell, S., & Ewing, L. (1990). Follow-up of hard-to-manage preschoolers: Adjustment at age 9 and predictors of continuing symptoms. *J. Child Psychol. Psychiatry, 31,* 871–889.

Carver, C., Scheir, M., & Weintraub, J. (1989). Assessing coping strategies: A theoretically based approach. *J. Pers. Soc. Psychol., 56,* 267–283.

Chadwick, O., Rutter, M., Shaffer, D., & Shrout, P. E. (1981). A prospective study of children with head injuries: IV. Specific cognitive deficits. *J. Clin. Neuropsychol., 3,* 101–120.

Cohen, P., & Brook, J. (1987). Family factors related to the persistence of psychopathology in childhood and adolescence. *Psychiatry, 50,* 332–345.

Cohen, S., & Wills, T. A. (1985). Stress, social support, and the buffering hypothesis. *Psychol. Bull., 98,* 310–357.

Coyne J., & Downey, G. (1991). Social factors and psychopathology: Stress, social support, and coping processes. *Am. Rev. Psychol., 42,* 401–425.

Crase, S. J., Clark, S., & Pease, D. (1977). *Iowa Parent Behavior Inventory.* Ames: Iowa State University Research Foundation.

Crnic, K., Friedrich, W., & Greenberg, M. (1983). Adaptation of families with mentally retarded children: A model of stress, coping, and family ecology. *Am. J. Mental Def., 88,* 125–138.

Crnic, K., Greenberg, M., Ragozin, A., Robinson, N., & Bashan, R. (1983). Effects of stress and social support on mothers and premature and full-term infants. *Child Dev., 54,* 209–217.

Delis, D., Kramer, J., Kaplan, E., & Ober, B. (1986). *The California Verbal Learning Test: Children's version.* San Antonio, TX: Psychological Corporation.

DePompei, R., & Zarski, J. (1989). Families, head injury, and cognitive-communicative impairments: Issues for family counseling. *Top. Lang. Disord., 9,* 78–89.

Derogatis, L., & Spencer, P. (1982). *The Brief Symptom Inventory: Administration, scoring, and procedures manual—I.* Baltimore, MD: Clinical Psychometric Research.

DiSimoni, F. G. (1978). *The Token Test for Children.* Boston, MA: Teaching Resources.

Egeland, B., Kalkoske, M., Gottesman, N., & Erickson, M. (1990). Preschool behavior problems: Stability and factors accounting for change. *J. Child Psychol. Psychiatry, 31,* 891–909.

Esser, G., Schmidt, M., & Woerner, W. (1990). Epidemiology and cause of psychiatric disorders in school-age children—Results of a longitudinal study. *J. Child Psychol. Psychiatry, 31,* 243–263.

Ewing-Cobbs, L., Levin, H., Fletcher, J., Miner, M., & Eisenberg, H. (1990). The Children's Orientation and Amnesia Test: Relationship to severity of acute head injury and to recovery of memory. *Neurosurgery, 27,* 683–691.

Finger, S., LeVere, T., Almli, C., & Stein, D. (1989). Recovery of function: Sources of controversy. In S. Finger, T. LeVere, C. Almli, & D. Stein (Eds.), *Brain injury and recovery: Theoretical and controversial issues* (pp. 351–361). New York: Plenum.

Fletcher, J., Ewing-Cobbs, L., Miner, M., Levin, H., & Eisenberg, H. (1990). Behavioral changes after closed head injury in children. *J. Consult. Clin. Psychol., 58,* 93–98.

Fletcher, J., & Levin, H. (1988). Neurobehavioral effects of brain injury in children. In D. Routh (Ed.), *Handbook of pediatric psychology* (pp. 258–295). New York: Guilford Press.

Frederick, C., Pynoos, R., & Nader, K. (1992). *Child Post-Traumatic Stress Reaction Index*. Los Angeles, CA: Department of Psychiatry, University of California.

Gaddes, W., & Crockett, D. (1975). The Spreen-Benton Aphasia Tests: Normative data as a measure of normal language development. *Brain Lang., 2,* 257–279.

Goldman, P., & Lewis, M. (1978). Developmental biology of brain damage and experience. In C. W. Cotman (Ed.), *Neural plasticity.* New York: Raven Press.

Harrington, J., & Letemendia, F. (1958). Persistent psychiatric disorders after head injuries in children. *J. Ment. Sci., 104,* 1205–1218.

Harris, B., Schwaitzberg, S., Seman, T., & Herrman, C. (1989). The hidden morbidity of pediatric trauma. *J. Pediatr. Surg., 24,* 103–106.

Hollingshead, A. (1975). *Four Factor Index of Social Status.* New Haven, CT: Yale University Press.

Hu, X., Wesson, D., Kenney, B., Chipman, H., & Spence, L. (1993). Risk factors for extended disruption of family function after severe injury to a child. *Can. Med. Assoc. J., 149,* 421–427.

Jennett, B., & Bond, M. (1975). Assessment of outcome after severe brain damage. *Lancet, 1,* 480–487.

Kaplan, E., Goodglass, H., & Weintraub, S. (1983). *Boston Naming Test* (Revised 60-item version). Philadelphia, PA: Lea & Febiger.

Kazak, A., & Marvin, R. (1984). Differences, difficulties, and adaptation: Stress and social networks in families with a handicapped child. *Fam. Relat., 33,* 67–77.

Knights, R., & Norwood, J. (1980). *Revised smoothed normative data on the Neuropsychological Test Battery for Children.* Ottawa, Ontario: Department of Psychology, Carleton University.

Kolb, B. (1989). Brain development, plasticity, and behavior. *Am. Psychol., 44,* 1203–1212.

Kovacs, M. (1981). Rating scales to assess depression in school-aged children. *Acta Paedopsychiatry, 46,* 305–315.

Kraus, J., Fife, D., Cox, P., Ramstein, K., & Conroy, C. (1986). Incidence, severity, and external causes of pediatric brain injury. *Am. J. Dis. Child., 140,* 687–693.

Levin, H., & Eisenberg, H. (1979). Neuropsychological impairment after closed head injury in children and adolescents. *J. Pediatr. Psychol., 4,* 389–402.

Levin, H., High, W. Jr., Ewing-Cobbs, L., Fletcher, J., Eisenberg, H., Miner, M., & Goldstein, F. (1988). Memory functioning during the first year after closed head injury in children and adolescents. *Neurosurgery, 22,* 1043–1052.

Lezak, M. (1987). Brain damage is a family affair. *J. Clin. Exp. Neuropsychol., 10,* 111–123.

Lindgren, S., & Lyons, D. (1984). *Pediatric Assessment of Cognitive Efficiency* (PACE). Iowa City, IA: Department of Pediatrics, University of Iowa.

Mayer, T., Matlak, M., Johnson, D., & Walker, M. (1980). The Modified Injury Severity Scale in pediatric multiple trauma patients. *J. Pediatr. Surg., 15,* 719–726.

McCormick, M., Charney, E., & Stemmler, M. (1986). Assessing the impact of a child with spina bifida on the family. *Dev. Med. Child Neurol., 28,* 53–61.

Miller, I., Bishop, D., Epstein, N., & Keitner, G. (1985). The McMaster Family Assessment Device: Reliability and validity. *J. Marital Fam. Ther., 11,* 345–356.

Moos, R., Cronkite, R., Billings, A., & Finney, J. (1987). *Health and Daily Living Form Manual.* Palo Alto, CA: Social Ecology Laboratory, Stanford University Medical Center.

Moos, R., & Moos, B. (1988). *Life Stressors and Social Resources Inventory: Preliminary manual.* Palo Alto, CA: Stanford University Medical Center.

National Center for Health Statistics. (1981). *Current estimates from the National Health Interview Survey: United States, 1980.* Hyattsville, MD: U.S. Department of Health and Human Services, National Health Survey, Series 10, no. 139.

Pendergast, K., Dickey, S., Selmar, J., & Soder, A. (1969). *Photo Articulation Test.* Danville, IL: Interstate Printers and Publishers.

Perrin, E., West, P., & Culley, B. (1989). Is my child normal yet? Correlates of vulnerability. *Pediatrics, 83,* 355–363.

Perrott, S., Taylor, H., & Montes, J. (1991). Neuropsychological sequelae, family stress, and environmental adaptation following pediatric head injury. *Dev. Neuropsychol., 7,* 69–86.

Pierce, G., Sarason, I., & Sarason, B. (1991). General and relationship-based perceptions of social support: Are two constructs better than one? *J. Pers. Soc. Psychol., 61,* 1028–1039.

Prigatano, G. (1989). Emotion and motivation in recovery and adaptation after brain damage. In S. Finger, T. LeVere, & D. Stein (Eds.), *Brain injury and recovery: Theoretical and controversial issues* (pp. 335–350). New York: Plenum.

Prior, M., Smart, D., Sanson, A., Pedlow, R., & Oberklaid, F. (1992). Transient versus stable behavior problems in a normative sample: Infancy to school age. *J. Pediatr. Psychol., 17,* 423–443.

Quittner, A., DiGirolamo, A., Michael, M., & Eigen, H. (1992). Parental response to cystic fibrosis: A contextual analysis of the diagnostic phase. *J. Pediatr. Psychol., 17,* 683–704.

Quittner, A., Glueckauf, R., & Jackson, D. (1990). Chronic parenting stress: Moderating vs. mediating effects of social support. *J. Pers. Soc. Psychol., 59,* 1266–1278.

Rivara, J., Fay, G., Jaffe, K., Polissar, N., Shurtleff, H., & Martin, K. (1992). Predictors of family functioning one year following traumatic brain injury in children. *Arch. Phys. Med. Rehabil., 73,* 899–910.

Rivara, J., Jaffe, K., Fay, G., Polisser, N., Martin, K., Shurtleff, H., & Liao, S. (1993). Family functioning and injury severity as predictors of child functioning one year following traumatic brain injury. *Arch. Phys. Med. Rehabil., 74,* 1047–1055.

Rivara, F., Thompson, R., Thompson, D., & Colonge, N. (1991). Injuries to children and adolescents: Impact on physical health. *Pediatrics, 88,* 783–788.

Rutter, M. (1981). Psychological sequelae of brain damage in children. *Am. J. Psychiatry, 138,* 1533–1534.

Rutter, M. (1983). Stress, coping, and development: Some issues and some questions. In N. Garmezy & M. Rutter (Eds.), *Stress, coping, and development* (pp. 1–42). New York: McGraw-Hill.

Rutter, M., Chadwick, O., & Shaffer, D. (1983). Head injury. In M. Rutter (Eds), *Developmental neuropsychiatry* (pp. 83–111). New York: Guilford Press.

Rutter, M., Chadwick, O., & Shaffer, D., & Brown, C. (1980). A prospective study of children with head injuries: I. Description and methods. *Psychol. Med., 10,* 633–645.

Sameroff, A., & Chandler, M. (1975). Reproductive risk and the continuum of care-taking casualty. In F. Horowitz, M. Hetherington, S. Scarr-Salapated, & G. Siegel (Eds.), *Review of child development research* (Vol. 4, pp. 187–244). Chicago: University of Chicago Press.

Semel, E., Wiig, E. H., Secord, W., & Sabers, D. (1987). *CELF-R: Clinical Evaluation of Language Fundamentals—Revised (Technical Manual)*. New York: Psychological Corporation.

Spanier, G. (1976). Measuring dyadic adjustment: New scales for assessing the quality of marriage and similar dyads. *J. Marriage Fam., 38*, 15–27.

Sparrow, S., Bolla, D., & Ciccetti, D. (1984). *Vineland Adaptive Behavior Scales*. Circle Pines, MN: American Guidance Service.

Stein, D. (1987). In pursuit of new strategies for understanding recovery from brain damage: Problems and perspectives. In T. Boll & B. Bryant (Eds.), *Clinical neuropsychology and brain function: Research, measurement, and practice* (pp. 13–55). Washington, DC: American Psychological Association.

Stein, R., & Jessop, D. (1985). *PACTS papers/AECOM: Tables documenting the psychometric properties of a measure of the impact of chronic illness on a family*. Bronx, NY: Department of Pediatrics, Albert Einstein College of Medicine.

Taylor, H., Albo, V., Phoebus, C., Sachs, B., & Bierl, P. (1987). Postirradiation treatment outcomes for children with acute lymphocytic leukemia: Clarification of risks. *J. Pediatr. Psychol., 12*, 395–411.

Taylor, H., & Schatschneider, C. (1992). Child neuropsychological assessment: A test of basic assumptions. *Clin. Neuropsychol., 6*, 259–275.

Taylor, H., Schatschneider, C., & Rich, D. (1992). Sequelae of *Haemophilus influenzae* meningitis: Implications for the study of brain disease and development. In M. Tramontana & S. Hooper (Eds.), *Advances in child neuropsychology* (Vol. 1, pp. 50–108). New York: Springer-Verlag.

Telzrow, C. (1987). Management of academic and educational problems in head injury. *J. Learn. Disabil., 20*, 536–545.

Varni, J., & Wallander, J. (1988). Pediatric chronic disabilities: Hemophilia and spina bifida as examples. In D. K. Routh (Ed.), *Handbook of pediatric psychology* (pp. 190–221). New York: Guilford Press.

Waaland, P., & Kreutzer, J. (1991). Family response to childhood traumatic brain injury. *J. Head. Trauma Rehabil., 3*, 51–63.

Waaland, P., & Raines, S. (1991). Families coping with childhood neurological disability: Clinical assessment and treatment. *Neurol. Rehabil., 1*, 19–27.

Walker, H., & McConnell, S. (1988). *The Walker-McConnell Scale of Social Competence and School Adjustment: A social skills rating scale for teachers*. Austin, TX: PRO-ED.

Wallander, J., Varni, J., Babani, L., Banis, H., & Wilcox, K. (1989). Children with chronic physical disorders: Maternal reports of their psychological adjustment. *J. Pediatr. Psychol., 13*, 197–212.

Wechsler, D. (1991). *WISC-III: Wechsler Intelligence Scale for Children—3rd edition manual*. San Antonio, TX: Psychological Corporation.

Woodcock, R., & Mather, N. (1989). *Woodcock-Johnson Tests of Achievement-Revised—Standard and supplemental batteries*. Allen, TX: DLM Teaching Resources.

Zarski, J., DePompei, R., & Zook, A. (1988). Traumatic head injury: Dimensions of family responsivity. *J. Head Trauma Rehabil., 3*, 31–41.

III

LIFE-SPAN EFFECTS, REHABILITATION, AND TREATMENT

* Journ. Nesro.
Nesrosurg. Nesropsy.
(1993)

11

Outcome of Head Injuries
from Childhood to Adulthood:
A Twenty-Three-Year Follow-Up Study

HARRY KLONOFF, CAMPBELL CLARK,
and PAMELA S. KLONOFF

(" MILD " INJury Cases)

Despite extensive research on the diverse effects of head injuries, there is a profound paucity of very-long-term outcome studies in children who have sustained traumatic brain injuries. In 1967, a prospective study of 231 children with closed head injuries was initiated. In subsequent years, a number of publications including the final results of the 5-year follow-up study were published (Klonoff & Paris, 1974; Klonoff et al., 1977). The research discussed in this chapter is a 23-year follow-up of the children included in the original project (Klonoff et al., 1993). The purpose of the investigation was to determine the relationship between trauma variables, including measures of extent of head injury, and very-long-term sequelae.

The acute neurological, cognitive, emotional, and physical sequelae of closed head injury (Levin et al., 1982, 1987), including mild head injuries (Levin et al., 1989), are well documented for children (Klonoff & Paris, 1974) and adults (Jennett & Teasdale, 1981). Recent interest has focused on the short- and long-term outcome following traumatic brain injury. Publications range from the subacute phase of 1 month after the head injury (McLean et al., 1984) to follow-up for periods up to 4 to 5 years (Brooks et al., 1986; Klonoff, P. S., et al., 1986) and late outcome studies from 6 to 15 years posttrauma (Brooks et al., 1987a,b; Costeff et al., 1988, 1990; Kraft et al., 1993; Oddy et al., 1985; Schwab et al., 1993; Tate et al., 1991; Thomsen, 1984, 1987, 1989). Aside from the research discussed in this chapter, there is only one other published study that has evaluated outcome at more than 20 years postinjury (Thomsen, 1992). Furthermore, few studies have documented the long-term consequences of head injury from childhood to adulthood in the same patient sample (Costeff et al., 1988, 1990).

In follow-up studies, enduring neuropsychological deficits have been reported (Costeff et al., 1988; Jennett & Teasdale, 1981; Thomsen, 1987). Other commonly identified problems at follow-up are in the areas of behavioral dysfunction, including anxiety, depression, and social withdrawal (Brooks et al., 1986; Klonoff, P. S., et al., 1986; Levin & Grossman, 1978; Lishman, 1986; Thomsen, 1987, 1992). It is noteworthy that families identify the behavioral changes at follow-up as more enduring and troublesome than the physical and cognitive sequelae (Thomsen, 1984, 1992).

Increasingly, studies have evaluated changes in work status and school performance following head injury. Results are variable, but most studies report a significant degree of unemployment or reduced work capacity (Brooks et al., 1987b; Kreutzer et al., 1991; McKinlay et al., 1983; Rimel et al., 1982; Thomsen, 1984). Several studies have evaluated factors affecting return to work following head injury. Decreased rates of employment have been found with increased severity of injury, as measured by length of coma (Rimel et al., 1982), initial Glasgow Coma Scale score (Klonoff, P. S., et al., 1986), and length of posttraumatic amnesia (Lewin et al., 1979). Greater cognitive and behavioral dysfunction has also been related to poorer vocational outcome (Brooks et al., 1987b; Levin et al., 1990; Rimel & Jane, 1983). A relationship between severe brain injury in childhood and reduced academic performance has been reported (Costeff et al., 1990). A growing body of literature has evaluated predictors of outcome after head injury, including severity of head injury and age at time of trauma (Levin et al., 1982; Thomsen, 1987). It has been suggested that children sustaining brain injuries show improved neurological and cognitive recovery compared to older age groups (Alberico et al., 1987; Eiben et al., 1984; Levin et al., 1982; Mahoney et al., 1983). However, one study reported no significant relationship between age and outcome (Berger et al., 1985).

Typically the recovery of patients sustaining head injury has been determined by interviewer ratings (Levati et al., 1982). The best known of these is the Glasgow Outcome Scale (Jennett & Bond, 1975). More recently, research has begun to focus on outcome based on relatives' reports (Brooks et al., 1987a), patient interviews (Klonoff, P. S., et al., 1986), and psychosocial changes in head-injured adults using questionnaire data from patients as opposed to their families (Hendryx, 1989).

Methods of Original Project

The original project in 1967 set out to investigate prospectively a head-injured group of children from the time of trauma to the fifth year after trauma within the context of antecedent factors (premorbid anomalies, age, sex), circumstances at time of head injury (extent of injury) and consequence factors (education, interpersonal transactions, sequelae). The original sample comprised 231 children—147 boys and 84 girls—with a mean age of 8.32 years at the time of the head injury. Children included in the project were consecutive admissions to two university hospitals between August 1967 and November 1968 with a diagnosis of closed

TABLE 11-1. Number of Cases Examined at Each Assessment

Examinations	Time of Trauma[a]	Follow-up Posttrauma			
		1 Year[a]	2 Years[a]	5 Years[a]	23 Years
Number	231	196	163	117	159

[a]At least equivalent numbers of matched controls were also examined.

head injury. The two clinical parameters studied were neurological and neuropsychological. For the neuropsychological data base, each head-injured child was matched on age (within 3 months) and sex with a normal control defined in terms of no neurological deficit, no physical anomalies, no profound signs of emotional disturbance, and normal school progress for those children attending school. The number of reexaminations varied from one to five, and 117 head-injured children were examined 5 years after the head injury (Table 11-1).

Methods of Long-Term Follow-up Study

During 1990–91, a variety of means were used to trace 175 (76%) of the individuals included in the original project, and 159 (91%) volunteered to participate in the current study. Of the remaining 16, contacts were made with parents or relatives, but the member of the cohort did not return telephone calls. A university-approved consent form was completed by the volunteers who were interviewed. Geographic locations of the cohort included Canada, the United States, Europe, Australia, and the Middle East. The senior author interviewed all the volunteers either in person ($n = 82$) or by telephone ($n = 77$). There was no discernible difference in response pattern related to interview format. In two instances information was provided by a parent with the volunteer, while in two additional instances only the parent provided information because of the volunteer's mental status.

A standardized interview was conducted with a predetermined format. Details of the original data base obtained during admission to hospital and on follow-up were unknown to the interviewer and the volunteer. Any difference, therefore, in subjective impressions should be randomly distributed among those with or without elicited sequelae.

Table 11-2 describes the demographic characteristics of the cohort of 159 adults at the time of trauma.

Although the Glasgow Coma Scale is now widely used to determine the severity of head injury, this project was conducted before its development in 1974. Therefore, four neurological indexes—length of unconsciousness, skull fractures, electroencephalogram (EEG) ratings, and posttraumatic seizures—and one global measure of neurological status were used as indicators of the extent of head injury. The last measure was derived from the medical opinion of one examiner. These variables and respective percentages are summarized in Table 11-3.

Each variable was rated from 1 to 3; a composite score of 5 to 15 was also

TABLE 11-2. Demographic Characteristics of
Cohort at the Time of Trauma

Characteristic		Percent
Age (years)		
Mean	7.96	
SD	3.28	
Range	2.70–15.90	
Educational placement (%)		
Preschool		29.6
Primary (lower secondary)		60.3
Secondary (upper secondary)		10.1
Occupations of fathers (%)		
Professional and semiprofessional		24.5
Clerical and skilled		44.0
Semiskilled and unskilled		27.6
Unemployed		3.8
Agent of injury (%)		
Automobile		44.0
Fall		48.0
Other		8.0
Length of hospitalization (days)		
Mean days	12.7	
Litigation (%)		21.4
Premorbid anomalies (%)		27.0
Multiple injuries (%)		26.4
Musculoskeletal		19.5
Abdomen		2.5
Ears/nose		1.9
Eyes		1.3
Skin		0.6
Respiratory		0.6

TABLE 11-3. Neurological Indicators of Extent of Head Injury

Loss of Consciousness		Neurological Status		Skull Fracture		EEG Rating		Seizure	
Indication	%	Indication	%	Indication	%	Indication	%	Indication	%
Not proven or momentary	52.2	No clinical evidence of trauma	24.5	None	59.7	Normal/ Equivocal	40.3	Absent	93.7
From 5 to <30 minutes	37.1	Unconsciousness 5 to <30 minutes, concussion, or skull fracture (simple)	60.4	Simple linear	22.0	Minimal abnormal	38.4	Petit mal	4.4
More than 30 minutes	10.7	Unconsciousness >30 minutes, concussion, or skull fracture (basal/depressed) with other symptoms (e.g., aphasia)	15.1	Basal/ depressed	18.3	Moderate/ marked abnormal	21.4	Grand mal	1.9

derived by summing the five variables. The composite score ranged from 5 to 13 with a median of 7, with the following distribution: 5 to 8 (63.5%); 9 to 10 (27.6%); 11 to 13 (8.9%).

Table 11-4 describes the current demographic and personal-social characteristics of the cohort.

TABLE 11-4.   Current Demographic and Personal-Social
Characteristics at the 23-Year Follow-up ($n = 159$)

Characteristics		Percent
Age (years)		
Mean	31.40	
SD	3.23	
Range	25–40	
Male:Female (n)	105:54	
Education (%)		
Grades 7–9 (lower secondary)		7.6
Grades 10–12 (upper secondary)		50.3
Postsecondary (tertiary vocational professional)		28.9
Bachelor's degrees		10.1
Postgraduate degrees		3.1
Grade failure (retention) (%)		25.8
Marital status (%)		
Married/common-law		59.2
Single		28.9
Divorced/separated		11.9
Occupation (%)		
Professional and semiprofessional		27.1
Clerical and skilled		38.4
Semiskilled and unskilled		27.6
Homemaker		4.4
Student		2.5
Employment status (%)		
Full-time		80.1
Part-time		7.3
Homemaker		4.4
Student		2.5
Disability unrelated to trauma		1.9
Unemployed		3.8
Interpersonal relationships (%)		
Strained relationship with spouse		11.9
Strained relationship with family members		17.9
Leisure activities restricted (%)		30.2
Alcohol problem (%)		
Past		10.1
Current		4.4
Illicit drug use (%)		
Past social		2.5
Past heavy		6.3
Current social		15.1
Current heavy		2.5
Contact with legal authorities (%)		17.0
One criminal charge		2.6
Multiple criminal charges		4.4

Results of Original Project

The data base of sequelae 1 year ($n = 196$) and then 2 years ($n = 163$) after the head injury was derived from the neurological (including EEG, a direct examination of the child, and—in most instances—an interview with a parent) and neuropsychological evaluations. Data were also obtained on educational achievement, relationships at school and at home as well as with peers, the reaction of the child to head injury, the reaction of the parents to head injury, and assignment of blame.

Sequelae were defined as involving neurological signs and/or subjective complaints. Sequelae were recorded for 40% of the group 1 year after trauma, and this figure was only slightly reduced to 39% at 2 years after trauma. The most frequent complaints reported 1 year again 2 years after trauma were personality changes, difficulties with memory and/or concentration and/or learning, headaches, irritability, dizzy spells, and visual or auditory defects. The presence of sequelae was associated with a decline in school achievement recorded 1 year after trauma and sustained 2 years after trauma.

The data base 5 years after the head injury ($n = 117$) was also derived from the neurological (including EEG, a direct examination of the child, and—in most instances—an interview with a parent) and neuropsychological evaluations. The findings indicated that 5 years after the head injury, a majority of the 117 children were well recovered. The EEG ratings had the most rapid recovery, but by the fifth reexamination there was still evidence of EEG abnormality in 12% of the children. The neuropsychological findings indicated a slower rate of recovery in that, by the fifth follow-up, 23.7% of the head-injured children still exhibited impaired neuropsychological function. Moreover, Full-Scale IQ was predictive of potential residual sequelae. The neurological parameters were least likely to show change in that 23.9% of the head-injured children still exhibited residual sequelae on both the fourth and fifth follow-up examinations. The most frequently reported complaints were personality changes, headaches, learning problems, mood changes, and problems with memory and/or concentration. Educational progress was rated as "normal" in 71.8% of the sample. Regarding the complaints, it should be noted that the rank order of complaints is distinctly similar between the first and fifth follow-up.

Results of Long-Term Follow-up Study

Health History

Subsequent (recurrent) head injuries were reported by 15.1% (8.8% with loss of consciousness) of the sample, and the number of such head injuries were as follows: 1, 10.7%; 2, 2.5%; 3, 1.3%; 4, 0.6%.

Table 11-5 summarizes the 66 intervening physical complaints (not mutually exclusive) reported as unrelated to the head injury. The physical complaints were

TABLE 11–5. Physical Complaints Unrelated to Head
Injury (*n* = 159)

System	Complaints	Frequency
Neurological	Seizures	1
	Dizzy spells	1
Musculoskeletal	Leg/back pain	20
	Arthritis	8
Head and neck	Headaches	5
	Neck pain	3
	Thyroid	2
Ears/nose	Reduced hearing	4
	Sinusitis	2
Abdomen	Colitis	1
	Crohn's disease	1
	Hepatitis	1
	Ulcers	1
	Liver	1
Skin	Psoriasis/eczema	3
Chest and lungs	Asthma	8
Lymphatic	Lymphoma	1
Heart/blood vessels	Rheumatic fever	2
Metabolism	Diabetes	1

grouped in a systems schema (Seidel, 1991). Some of these complaints, reported by 32.7% of the adults in the current study, may be related to the multiple injuries sustained at the time of the head injury or, in a number of instances, subsequent head injuries. Seizures were reported by one individual who had a severe head injury in 1989 and dizzy spells were reported by another individual who had relatively severe head injuries in 1976 and 1990.

Resolved psychological/psychiatric problems specified as unrelated to the initial head injury were reported by 31.4% of the sample. The 60 reported problems (not mutually exclusive) were categorized as emotional disorders (40.0%), problems with spouse or child (36.6%), problems with parents (15.0%), substance abuse (5.0%), and relationships in general (3.4%).

Current psychological/psychiatric problems specified as unrelated to the initial head injury were reported by 17.6% of the sample. The 33 reported problems (not mutually exclusive) were categorized as emotional disorders (42.4%), including one case of chronic schizophrenia; problems with spouse or child (21.2%); substance abuse (12.1%); problems with parents (9.1%); relationships in general (9.1%); and sleep problems (6.1%).

A comparison of the proportions in the sample listing no psychological/psychiatric problems or specifying problems both in the past and the present revealed the following: 62.3% listed no problems at any time; 11.3% listed problems both in the past and present; 20.1% listed a problem in the past but not currently; and 6.3% did not list a problem in the past but did list one currently.

Mood was determined during the interview by asking individuals to rate their mood on a scale from 1 to 10, where 1 would be very depressed and 10 very happy. The distribution was distinctly skewed toward the upper end of the scale, with a median rating of 7.

Stressors were reported by 53.5% of the sample; the number ranged from 1 to 4. The 119 identified stressors were distributed among the following: work (30.3%), spouse/child (16.8%), finances (15.1%), psychological (12.6%), relationships (8.4%), physical (7.6%), parents (5.9%), living arrangements (2.5%), and substance abuse (0.8%).

Outcome Measures

The subjective measures of outcome were derived from complaints by the respondents elicited during the interview, when they were asked whether they had noted postaccident sequelae. The reported subjective sequelae were then categorized as physical, intellectual, or emotional. The physical complaints were grouped in a systems schema (Seidel, 1991). The intellectual complaints included difficulties with learning, memory, intellectual functioning, and slowed thinking. The emotional complaints included anxiety, depressive and behavioral disorders, and problems with self-esteem and feelings of rejection.

The details of the sequelae are itemized in Table 11-6. Fifty individuals (31%) reported 96 sequelae: 36 were physical, 30 intellectual, and 30 emotional. The number of complaints among those reporting ranged from 1 (17% of the sample) to 7 (1% of the sample). Among the 50 individuals, 27 reported complaints that were exclusively intellectual and/or emotional, 12 reported complaints that were exclusively physical, and 11 reported complaints that were in all three categories.

Of the seven physical systems listed in Table 11-6, the highest number of complaints ($N = 10$) was recorded under "neurological." In this category, two individuals reported seizures; one is still on anticonvulsant medication and the seizures are currently controlled, whereas the other is not on medication and does not have a recent history of seizures. The second most frequent area of physical sequelae involved the musculoskeletal system ($N = 9$), followed by those involving the head and neck.

Among the intellectual sequelae, the most frequent complaint was difficulty in learning, followed by problems with memory or concentration. Less specific cognitive deficits were also reported. Among the emotional sequelae, depression was the most frequent complaint. Three of those reporting depression indicated a history of accompanying suicidal ideation; and of these, two were currently experiencing suicidal thoughts. Complaints of anxiety disorders followed in terms of frequency, and then problems with self-esteem, rejection by parents, and behavior disorders (pyromania and aggression) during childhood.

There was a significant relationship (Kendall's Tau 0.19, $p < 0.01$) between physical sequelae reported as directly related to the head injury and physical com-

TABLE 11-6. Types of Subjective Sequelae ($n = 50$)

Sequelae	Complaints	Frequency
Physical		
Neurological	Coordination or speed	4
	Seizures	2
	Handedness changed	2
	Dizziness	1
	Speech	1
Musculoskeletal	Arthritis/osteoarthritis	3
	Back pain	2
	Leg/hip pain	2
	Leg shorter/deformity	2
Head and neck	Headaches	3
	Plate area sensitive	3
	Neck pain	1
Eyes	Diplopia	2
	Retinal damage	1
	Fields/depth perception	2
Ears/nose	Tinnitus/sinusitis	2
Abdomen	Kidney/spleen	2
Skin	Sweating	1
Intellectual		
	Learning problems/disabilities	12
	Memory/attention/concentration	10
	Intelligence/brain affected	4
	Thinking/problem solving slowed	4
Emotional		
Anxiety disorders	Anxieties, phobias, nightmares	8
Depressive disorders	Mood disorder	6
	Depression with suicidal thoughts	3
	Depression and bereavement	3
Self-esteem problems	Insecure/self-conscious/introverted	5
Parent-child problems	Rejection by parent(s)	2
Behavior disorders	Aggression (as child)	2
	Pyromania (as child)	1

plaints identified as unrelated to the head injury. Specifically, 12.6% of the sample reported both physical sequelae related to the head injury as well as physical complaints unrelated to the trauma, and 48.4% reported neither. These findings are understandable in view of the multiple injuries sustained by 26.4% of the sample.

Relationships between Extent of Head Injury and Outcome

We first analyzed the relationships between the trauma variables and the subjective physical, intellectual, and emotional sequelae. As the reader will note in Table 11-7, the composite trauma variable (derived by rating length of unconsciousness, skull fractures, EEG, seizures, and a global measure of neurological status) was

TABLE 11-7.   Relationships between Subjective Sequelae and Trauma
Variables and Initial IQ (Kendall's Tau and t-test)

| Trauma | Subjective Sequelae | | |
Variables	Physical	Intellectual	Emotional
Unconscious	0.12	0.04	0.21[b]
Skull fracture	0.19[b]	0.20[b]	0.20[b]
EEG	−0.02	0.07	−0.06
Neurological status	0.13[a]	0.21[b]	0.35[c]
Seizure	0.20[b]	0.25[c]	0.18[a]
Composite	0.17[c]	0.23[c]	0.28[c]
Initial IQ	−0.05	−0.21[b]	−0.17[a]
Initial IQ nonsequelae group	103.5	104.7	104.2
Initial IQ sequelae group	99.9	93.3	98.6
t value	1.07	3.57[b]	2.37[a]

[a] $p < 0.05$.
[b] $p < 0.01$.
[c] $p < 0.001$.

most closely related to long-term subjective sequelae. The global measures of
neurological status, seizures, and skull fractures were also modest predictors of
reported sequelae. Unconsciousness was of limited predictive value, and the EEG
was of negligible predictive value.

The second analysis evaluated the relationship between initial IQ and subjective sequelae; these findings are also summarized in Table 11-7. Correlations of
initial IQ with reported sequelae and a comparison of those individuals who either
reported or did not report sequelae in each of the three areas revealed significantly
lower IQs for those reporting deficits in the intellectual and emotional areas.

The third analysis evaluated the relationship between selected attribute or descriptive variables and subjective sequelae, as shown in Table 11-8. While only 3
of the 21 correlations were significant, this is greater than chance expectancy. Not
surprisingly, physical sequelae were significantly related to the agent of injury and
to subsequent litigation; intellectual sequelae were related to subsequent head injuries.

The purpose of a fourth analysis was to determine whether the presence of
subjective sequelae had any measurable effects upon objective and psychosocial
measures of adaptation. The individuals reporting sequelae ($n = 50$) were compared on selected demographic, health, and psychosocial variables with individuals reporting no sequelae ($n = 109$). Significant differences were found in grade
failures/retention (40% for the sequelae group versus 19% for the nonsequelae
group, $\chi^2 = 6.65$, $p < 0.01$), work status (12% versus 2.8% of unemployed respectively, $\chi^2 = 3.89$, $p < 0.05$), current psychological/psychiatric problems (32% versus 11.9% respectively, $\chi^2 = 7.96$, $p < 0.01$) and strained relationships with family
members (24% versus 15.6% respectively, $\chi^2 = 3.95$, $p < 0.05$). No differences

were found for past but resolved psychological/psychiatric problems, physical complaints reported as unrelated to the head injury, substance abuse, or contact with legal authorities.

A fifth analysis dealt with continuity of complaints during the 23-year interval between the original project and the current study. In the 5-year follow-up study (Klonoff et al., 1977), parents of the 117 children reported an average of 0.89 complaints from the following categories: personality and mood, headaches and dizziness, memory and learning, sensory-motor, and fatigue and sleep. In the current study, the 159 adults reported an average of 0.60 sequelae, and these were categorized as physical, intellectual, and emotional. Of the 159 individuals included in the current study, 93 also had complaints in the initial project. The informants, however, were different. During the initial project, information about complaints was provided by a parent, generally the mother; whereas during the current study, information about sequelae was provided by the volunteers. Furthermore, the categories of complaints in the 5-year follow-up project were different from the sequelae in the current study. Granted these differences between the 5- and the 23- year follow-ups, the data were analyzed to determine whether a trend existed. A comparison of the presence or absence of complaints in the original project with the presence or absence of sequelae in the current study revealed a modest but significant relationship (Kendall's Tau 0.19, $p < 0.02$).

Discussion

There are few published reports that document the natural history of recovery from head injury in childhood to adulthood (Costeff et al., 1988, 1990); only the current study extends as long as 23 years after the head injury. We have demonstrated the feasibility of conducting a very long term outcome study of children who initially sustained primarily mild head injuries, with about 10% of the group having suffered a moderate or severe head injury. In some instances, the interviewer had the

TABLE 11-8.   Relationships between Subjective Sequelae and Descriptive Variables (Kendall's Tau)

Descriptive Variables	Subjective Sequelae		
	Physical	Intellectual	Emotional
Premorbid factors	0.00	0.06	−0.07
Sex	0.05	0.04	0.12
Age (trauma)	−0.08	0.06	0.04
Age (current)	0.05	−0.01	0.04
Injury agent	0.16[a]	0.03	0.05
Litigation	0.28[b]	0.08	0.11
Subsequent head injury	−0.01	0.22[b]	0.06

[a] $p < 0.05$.
[b] $p < 0.001$.

distinct impression that individuals were underreporting or minimizing effects. For example, only 2 of the 10 individuals with a history of posttraumatic seizures in the original project reported the presence of seizures in the past or at present in the follow-up study. Denial seems to be the most viable explanation. It should be emphasized that intervening life events between the initial project and the current study would have an interactive effect on long-term outcome, but the model of such interaction is complex. The health data included as an intervening variable are not intended to reflect the complexity of life events but only to sample the more obvious areas.

Given these caveats, the cardinal findings of this long-term follow-up study were as follows: (1) subjective sequelae were reported by 31% of the sample; (2) these subjective sequelae were related to the extent of head injury, initial IQ, and current measures of social adaptation. The results regarding the lack of predictiveness of the trauma variables of unconsciousness and EEG findings and the modest relationship of skull fractures to later sequelae are consistent with published predictive validity studies (Levin et al., 1989; Edna et al., 1987). In addition to the neurological variables as predictors of outcome, IQ recorded in the postacute phase was found to be a reliable predictor of long-term outcome. These relationships could not be explained by premorbid variables such as age, sex, or developmental anomalies.

This absence of a relationship between the variables of age, sex, and premorbid factors and outcome is consistent with some studies (Chadwick et al., 1981; Kraus et al., 1986; Klonoff, 1971) but not all (Annegers, 1983; Fabian & Bender, 1947). The incidence of 15.1% of recurrent head injuries reported in this study is consistent with recent research (Salcido et al., 1991) reporting recurrent brain injury rates ranging from 4.3% to 40%.

The found relationships between the presence of subjective sequelae and certain objective and psychosocial measures of adaptation—including educational lag, a higher unemployment rate, current psychological/psychiatric problems, and strained relationships with family members—further our understanding of the long-term effects of significant head injury in children. The only other identified research on outcome longer than 20 years is a study by Thomsen (1992), who reported preliminary outcome in a sample of 31 patients. These patients were age 15 to 37 at the time of injury. Thomsen reported variability in psychosocial outcome more than 20 years after the trauma. Important negative factors were severely disturbed behavior, including aggressiveness, violence, sexual disinhibition, and poor insight. Severity of injury, as measured by posttraumatic amnesia, was not a significant contributor to outcome. Differences between these data and the current study may be related to the small sample size, older age at time of injury, and greater severity of initial insult in the Thomsen study (Thomsen, 1992).

The rate of unemployment in the current study was significantly less than reported by others (Brooks et al., 1987b; Costeff et al., 1988; Thomsen, 1987). Also, the reported unemployment rate of 3.8% in the sample is substantially lower than the base rate of 7.7% of unemployment for ages 25 or older in this geographic locale. This discrepancy can be related to the other characteristics of the study sample. For example, IQ was at the 77th percentile at the last follow-up of the 5-year study. Furthermore, in the current study, educational attainment and occupational level were skewed, as 42.1% of the sample had tertiary vocational professional training or university degrees, while 27.1% reported their occupations as professional or semiprofessional. Notwithstanding the demographic characteristics of the study sample, unemployment for those with sequelae was four times higher than for those without. The rate of unemployment in studies of head injury should be interpreted in a broad context—and, in addition to the extent of the head injury and sequelae, should take into account factors such as IQ, educational attainment, occupational status, and work stability.

The natural history of recovery from a head injury in children was outlined in the 5-year follow-up study (Klonoff et al., 1977). There were immediate and very pronounced neurological, neuropsychological, and EEG effects. These effects decreased considerably, so that 5 years after the head injury, a majority of the children had improved substantially. With respect to the reconstitution process, the question posed initially was whether this was a function of the severity of head injury, individual differences in premorbid characteristics, subsequent environment, or an interaction of these variables. Based on the long-term findings of the current study, individual differences in disposition have not been identified as particularly relevant. Intervening life events, while inordinately complicated, are undoubtedly interactive; but with the available information it is not possible to go beyond this statement. However, the severity of the head injury has been identified as the primary contributory factor in the reconstitution process, and in the prediction of long-term outcome. Furthermore, the presence of long-term subjective sequelae is consistent with objective indicators of social adaptation.

Acknowledgments

We acknowledge with appreciation receiving permission from the *Journal of Neurology Neurosurgery and Psychiatry* to publish in modified form the articles which originally appeared in 1977, vol. 40, pp. 1211–1219, by Klonoff, H., Low, M. D., & Clark, C. and in 1993, vol. 56, pp. 410–415, by Klonoff, H., Clark, C., & Klonoff, P. S.

We also wish to express our gratitude to National Health Grants, Ottawa, Canada, for funding the original project and to the Insurance Corporation of British Columbia, Canada, for funding the current study. The authors wish to express their appreciation to Mrs. Vinetta Lunn, Mr. Don Gilbert, and to Mrs. Mary Klonoff for their invaluable contributions.

References

Alberico, A. M., Ward, J. D., Choi, S. C., Marmarou, A., & Young, H. F. (1987). Outcome after severe head injury: Relationship to mass lesions, diffuse injury and ICP course in pediatric and adult patients. *Neurosurg., 67*, 648–656.

Annegers, J. F. (1983). The epidemiology of head trauma in children. In K. Shapiro (Ed.), *Pediatric head trauma* (pp. 1–10). Mount Kisco, NY: Futura.

Berger, M. S., Pitts, L. H., Lovely, M., Edwards, M. S. B., & Bartkowski, H. M. (1985). Outcome from severe head injury in children and adolescents. *J. Neurosurg., 62*, 194–199.

Brooks, N., Campsie, L., Symington, C., Beattie, A., & McKinlay, W. (1986). The five-year outcome of severe blunt head injury: A relative's view. *J. Neurol. Neurosurg. Psychiatry, 49*, 764–770.

Brooks, N., Campsie, L., Symington, C., Beattie, A., & McKinlay, W. (1987a). The effects of severe head injury on patient and relative within seven years of injury. *J. Head Trauma Rehabil., 2*, 1–13.

Brooks, N., McKinlay, W., Symington, C., Beattie, A., & Campsie, L. (1987b). Return to work within the first seven years of severe head injury. *Brain Inj., 1*, 5–19.

Chadwick, O., Rutter, M., Shaffer, D., & Shrout, P. E. (1981). A prospective study of children with head injuries: IV. Specific cognitive defects. *J. Clin. Neuropsychol., 3*, 101–120.

Costeff, H., Abraham, E., Brenner, T., Horowitz, I., Apter, N., Sadan, N., & Najenson, T. (1988). Late neuropsychologic status after childhood head trauma. *Brain Dev., 10*, 371–374.

Costeff, H., Groswasser, Z., & Goldstein, R. (1990). Long-term follow-up review of 31 children with severe closed head trauma. *J. Neurosurg., 73*, 684–687.

Edna, T. H., & Cappelen, J. (1987). Late postconcussional symptoms in traumatic head injury: An analysis of frequency and risk factors. *Acta Neurochir., 86*, 12–17.

Eiben, C., Anderson, T. P., Lockman, L., Matthews, D. J., Dryja, R., Martin, J., Burrill, C., Gottesman, N., O'Brian, P., & Witte, L. (1984). Functional outcome of closed head injury in children and young adults. *Arch. Phys. Med. Rehabil., 65*, 168–170.

Fabian, A. A., & Bender, L. (1947). Head injury in children: Predisposing factors. *Am. J. Orthopsychiatry, 17*, 68–79.

Hendryx, P. M. (1989). Psychosocial changes perceived by closed-head-injured adults and their families. *Arch. Phys. Med. Rehabil., 70*, 526–530.

Jennett, B., & Bond, M. (1975). Assessment of outcome after severe brain damage. *Lancet, 1*, 480–484.

Jennett, B., & Teasdale, G. (1981). *Management of head injuries*. Philadelphia, PA: Davis.

Klonoff, H. (1971). Head injuries in children: Predisposing factors, accident conditions, accident proneness and sequelae. *Am. J. Public Health, 61*, 2405–2417.

Klonoff, H., & Paris, R. (1974). Immediate short-term and residual effects of acute head injuries in children. In R. Reitan & L. A. Davison (Eds.), *Clinical neuropsychology: Current status and applications*. Washington, DC: Winston.

Klonoff, H., Clark, C., & Klonoff, P. S. (1993). Long-term outcome of head injuries: A 23 year follow up study of children with head injuries. *J. Neurol. Neurosurg. Psychiatry, 56*, 410–415.

Klonoff, H., Low, M. D., & Clark, C. (1977). Head injuries in children: A prospective five year follow-up. *J. Neurol. Neurosurg. Psychiatry, 40*, 1211–1219.

Klonoff, P. S., Snow, W. G., & Costa, L. D. (1986). Quality of life in patients two to four years after closed head injury. *Neurosurgery, 19*, 735–743.

Kraft, J. F., Schwab, K., Salazar, A. M., & Brown, H. R. (1993). Occupational and educational achievements of head-injured Vietnam veterans at 15-year follow-up. *Arch. Phys. Med. Rehabil., 74*, 596–601.

Kraus, J. F., Fife, D., Cox, P., Ramstein, K., & Conroy, C. (1986). Incidence, severity and external causes of pediatric brain injury. *Am. J. Dis. Child., 140,* 687–693.

Kreutzer, J. S., Wehman, P. H., Harris, J. A., Burns, C. T., & Young, H. F. (1991). Substance abuse and crime patterns among persons with traumatic brain injury referred for supported employment. *Brain Inj., 5,* 177–187.

Levati, A., Farina, M. L., Vecchi, G., Rossanda, M., & Marrubini, M. B. (1982). Prognosis of severe head injuries. *J. Neurosurg., 57,* 779–783.

Levin, H. S., Benton, A. L., & Grossman, R. G. (1982). *Neurobehavioral consequences of closed head injury.* New York: Oxford University Press.

Levin, H. S., Eisenberg, H. M., & Benton, A. L. (Eds.). (1989). *Mild head injury.* New York: Oxford University Press.

Levin, H. S., Gary, H. E., Eisenberg, H. M., Ruff, R. M., Barth, J. T., Kreutzer, J., High, W. M., Portman, S., Foulkes, M. A., Jane, J. A., Marmarrou, R., & Marshall, L. F. (1990). Neuro-behavioral outcome one year after severe head injury. *J. Neurosurg., 73,* 699–709.

Levin, H. S., Grafman, J., & Eisenberg, H. M. (Eds.). (1987). *Neurobehavioral recovery from head injury.* New York: Oxford University Press.

Levin, H. S., & Grossman, R. G. (1978). Behavioral sequelae of closed head injury: A quantitative study. *Arch. Neurol., 35,* 720–726.

Levin, W., Marshall, T. F., & Roberts, A. H. (1979). Long-term outcome after severe head injury. *Br. Med. J., 2,* 1533–1538.

Lishman, W. A. (1986). Brain damage in relation to psychiatric disability after head injury. *Br. J. Psychiatry, 114,* 373–410.

McKinlay, W. W., Brooks, D. N., & Bond, M. R. (1983). Postconcussional symptoms, financial compensation and outcome of severe blunt head injury. *J. Neurol. Neurosurg. Psychiatry, 46,* 1084–1091.

McLean, A., Dikmen, S., Temkin, N., Wyler, A. R., & Gale, J. L. (1984). Psychosocial functioning at one month after head injury. *Neurosurgery, 14,* 393–399.

Mahoney, W. J., D'Souza, B. J., Haller, J. A., Rogers, M. C., Epstein, M. H., & Freeman, J. M. (1983). Long-term outcome of children with severe head trauma and prolonged coma. *Pediatrics, 71,* 756–762.

Oddy, M., Coughlan, T., Tyerman, A., & Jenkins, D. (1985). Social adjustment after closed head injury: A further follow-up seven years after injury. *J. Neurol. Neurosurg. Psychiatry, 48,* 564–568.

Rimel, R. W., Giordani, B., Barth, J. T., & Jane, J. A. (1982). Moderate head injury: Completing the clinical spectrum of brain trauma. *Neurosurgery, 11,* 344–351.

Rimel, R. W., & Jane, J. A. (1983). Characteristics of the head-injured patient. In M. Rosenthal, E. R. Griffith, M. R. Bond, & J. D. Miller (Eds.), *Rehabilitation of the head-injured adult.* Philadelphia, PA: Davis.

Salcido, R., Costich, J. F., Conder, R., & O'Shanick, G. J. (1991). Recurrent severe traumatic brain injury: Series of six cases. *Am. J. Phys. Med. Rehabil., 70,* 215–219.

Schwab, K., Grafman, J., Salazar, A., & Kraft, J. (1993). Residual impairments and work status 15 years after penetrating head injury: Report from the Vietnam head injury study. *Neurology, 43,* 95–103.

Seidel, H. M. (Ed.). (1991). *Mosby's guide to physical examination,* 2nd ed. St. Louis, MO: Mosby Year Book.

Tate, R. L., Fenelon, B., Manning, M. L., & Hunter, M. (1991). Patterns of neuropsychological impairment after severe blunt head injury. *J. Nerv. Ment. Dis., 179,* 117–126.

Thomsen, I. V. (1984). Late outcome of very severe blunt head trauma: A 10–15 year follow-up. *J. Neurol. Neurosurg. Psychiatry, 47,* 260–268.

Thomsen, I. V. (1987). Late psychosocial outcome in severe blunt head trauma. *Brain Inj., 1,* 131–143.

Thomsen, I. V. (1989). Do young patients have worse outcomes after severe blunt head trauma? *Brain Inj., 3,* 157–162.

Thomsen, I. V. (1992). Late psychosocial outcome in severe traumatic brain injury. *Scand. J. Rehabil. Med. Suppl., 26,* 142–152.

12

Recovery of Function in Adults: Lessons for the Study of Pediatric Head Injury Outcome

JORDAN GRAFMAN and ANDRES SALAZAR

How the human brain recovers from brain injury is of interest to a wide range of clinicians and researchers (Fearnside et al., 1993; Klein et al., 1992; Kunishio et al., 1993; Levin & Eisenberg, 1991; Levin et al., 1987). From a practical point of view, functional recovery has implications for employment, schooling, interpersonal relations, social responsibilities, and activities in the home. From a research perspective, an understanding of functional recovery may lead to a new awareness of the limits and potential of brain plasticity and adaptivity. Postinjury plasticity and adaptivity have been demonstrated in the adult human brain, which is in a relatively stable structural state when injury occurs. The brain of a child is still rapidly developing, so that the biological operations governing neural plasticity and recovery of function may be somewhat different than in the adult brain. Nevertheless, a brief and selective summary of what is known about recovery of function in adults may be useful for the pediatric researcher designing new studies of brain plasticity or for the clinician preparing the head-injured child and his or her family for the prospects of functional recovery (Michaud et al., 1993).

Our own interest in identifying the predictors of functional outcome following brain injury stemmed from the Vietnam Head Injury Study. This study was designed to examine the effects of preinjury, injury, and postinjury factors on functional outcome. It included 525 veterans who had suffered penetrating missile wound injuries while serving in Vietnam between 1967 and 1970 and for whom we had detailed military and Veterans Administration hospital records from the time of injury through a 5-year follow-up. Neurosurgeons in Vietnam completed registry forms denoting wound characteristics and initial neurological status of the patients. The head-injured veterans and 85 non-head-injured controls (matched for age, preinjury intelligence, and service in Vietnam) were later evaluated in a detailed 1-week, multidisciplinary, in-hospital reevaluation at Walter Reed Army

Medical Center approximately 15 years after their injuries in Vietnam. Relevant aspects of the data from this study are referred to within the chapter (and can be found elsewhere; e.g., Grafman et al., 1992).

Such studies of head-injured adults have identified a number of important potential predictor variables for recovery of function (Saneda & Corrigan, 1992; Schwab et al., 1993). These variables include age, sex, handedness, premorbid educational level, premorbid intellectual level, premorbid interpersonal functioning, severity of the head injury, topography and type of brain damage, postinjury intervention strategies, and pre- and postinjury social dynamics. Studies examining many of these variables are noted below. We also briefly discuss whether a head injury in early childhood predisposes that child for an exacerbated decline of cognitive functions in later adulthood (see Klonoff et al., this volume). The chapter concludes with a recapitulation of its major points.

Age of Patient at Time of Head Injury

It has been thought that the earlier the age of injury in the adult, the more complete and rapid recovery of function will be (Kertesz, 1988, 1992). There are at least two reasons for this view. Old age brings with it various medical illnesses. The combination of a head injury with other medical illnesses makes the recovery process more difficult. A somewhat similar explanation has been offered for the case of the otherwise healthy elderly adult who incurs a head injury. That is, noticeable cell loss begins to occur in the normal brain after the age of 40. Head injuries cause additional cell damage and loss. Therefore, the ability of the brain to recover from a head injury is slowed by the superimposed effects of the head injury upon the normal cell loss of aging. This hypothesis is known as the "threshold effect" and is discussed further below. Additionally, cell repair and other protective biological functions of the brain may be less potent in the aging brain. There is some evidence to indicate that the biological environment of the brain in the very young child (< 5 years old) may facilitate a more rapid and complete recovery than that of either the young or older adult, but few direct cross-sectional comparisons are available (Kertesz, 1992; also see Chapters 1, 5, 6, 9, and 16).

Sex of the Head-Injured Patient

There is some evidence, occasionally disputed, that the male brain is more strongly lateralized than the female brain. This sex-based topographical principle of the representation of cognitive functions suggests that female cognitive processes may be more adaptive following head injury, since their cognitive operations are more widely distributed in the brain and therefore less likely to be affected by any single focal injury.

The overwhelming majority of both closed and penetrating head injuries involve males (Levin et al., 1987). Furthermore, the smaller number of females sustaining head injuries may be a biased sample (when considering comparisons with the recovery of males). That is, females may be more likely to be the *victims* of a head injury (rather than active participants in aggressive acts). This would suggest that they are not affected by prior substance abuse and other sociodemographic variables that predict the likelihood of sustaining a head injury. This different background could predispose males to slower and more difficult recovery patterns. Females may also be likely to be more compliant with rehabilitation and to respond better to social support. These multifactorial differences between males and females who experience head injury could lead to an artifactual variability in recovery rate and patterns. The evidence for differences in recovery from head injury in children on the basis of sex is weak.

The Handedness of Head-Injured Patients

Left-handed people are thought to have a greater degree of bilateral representation of function than right-handed people, even though the majority of left-handers probably have normal laterality (i.e., left hemisphere dominance for language (Harris, 1992). True left-handers are relatively rare (< 10% of the population at large), making their participation in a head-injury study unlikely (although there are some disputed findings indicating that left-handers are more accident-prone (Halpern & Coren, 1991). In addition, left-handers are frequently eliminated from retrospective and prospective studies because of their rare numbers and potentially unusual lateralization of function. Again, the data from pediatric studies examining this variable are limited.

Premorbid Education Level of Head-Injured Patients

In the realm of premorbid experience that may protect against the ravages of head injury lies attained education level. The presumption is that greater learning results in a richer and more distributed representation of knowledge in the brain—in essence, a more complex neural network that would be more likely to absorb the effects of a head injury (Grafman et al., 1988). Since a premorbid quantitative test score is often inaccessible or lacking in adults, researchers have attempted to use education level as an index of intellectual achievement. Educational achievement is not a pure measure of intellectual functioning and may include such hard-to-quantify variables as achievement motivation and socialization needs. More studies are needed to determine whether a higher premorbid educational level is predictive of a better functional recovery following head injury (for a general discussion of predictor variables, see Aram & Eisele, 1992). Our own work with Vietnam veterans who suffered a penetrating missile injury to the brain showed that a higher premorbid educational level was particularly conducive to a better cognitive recovery when premorbid intellectual functioning (based on an intelligence test summary score) was *below* the 50th percentile, indicating that the protective effect of education may have been partially due to motivational factors (Grafman et al., 1988). Contemporary educational data are usually available for children and can be used to test hypotheses regarding the effects of premorbid educational achievement on recovery of function (Johnson, 1992).

The Effects of Premorbid Intellect in Head Injury

Particularly in young adult military populations, premorbid cognitive test data (usually in the form of a summary IQ-score equivalent) are readily available, and the same test (or a psychometric equivalent) can be administered to the subject postinjury. This particular index of premorbid intellectual reserve has proved to be a powerful predictor of postinjury recovery of function. The general findings can be conceptualized in the following way. These premorbid cognitive test scores represent intellectual capacity, which, in turn, reflects the richness of various semimodular neural networks differentially located in the brain. *Overall* lowering of *summary* achievement or IQ scores following brain damage may represent a relatively generalized impairment of cognitive functions, which is associated with *overall* brain volume loss. When *specific* subtest scores are lowered (e.g., verbal reasoning) following brain damage, there is a relatively greater association with the *specific* locus of a lesion rather than the total volume loss (Grafman et al., 1986).

The higher the premorbid intelligence test scores, the better the postinjury test results, although this finding is complicated by a general "regression to the mean," a statistical phenomenon where the subjects with the highest premorbid scores tend to show a modest decline and subjects with the lowest premorbid scores tend to show a slight increase on postinjury testing. Even a modest loss in the group of patients with the highest premorbid scores, however, may not seriously hinder their ability to have what would be classified as a "successful" outcome (Grafman et al., 1989).

Effects of Premorbid Personality Functioning on Recovery

This is an important area of investigation, given that the prefrontal cortex—which is partially responsible for modulating mood and emotion—is particularly suscepti-ble to bruising and damage in closed head injury and is a frequent target in pene-trating head injury. Unfortunately, we currently know very little about the rela-tionship of premorbid personality functioning to recovery and outcome in adults (Teuber, 1975). Information about the premorbid personality of the head-injured patient is often anecdotal, although prior school and police records can be utilized to supplement family reports. Since head injury may release previously inhibited behaviors (e.g., resulting in excessive aggressivity) or inhibit previously uncon-trolled behavior (e.g., resulting in apathy), gaining a better handle on the premor-bid personality of the patient would prove clinically useful. Questionnaires can be

administered to family members to gain their observations on the patient
ior preinjury, but they should be administered rather soon after the head
order to control for postinjury biases in responding. Teuber believed that ┌──────.
bid personality played an important role in postinjury recovery, but he had little
empirical support for his speculative thoughts (Teuber, 1975). Much more work
needs to be done in this area with both adults and children (Dikmen et al., 1993;
Schalen et al., 1994b).

Severity and Topography of the Brain Damage

It is intuitive that the more severe the head injury, the slower the recovery of
function and the poorer the outcome. Measures of severity include depth and
length of coma, severity of posttraumatic amnesia, and neuroradiological indices
of brain damage. This intuition has been validated in numerous head-injury studies
in adults (Grafman et al., 1986; Grafman & Salazar, 1987; Shigemori et al., 1992;
Stein et al., 1993; Vilkki et al., 1992). These same variables are being used
currently in studies with head-injured children (Eide & Tysnes, 1992; Levin et
al., 1992; Levin et al., 1994; Mendelsohn et al., 1992). In studies where loss of
brain tissue has been recorded, *total brain volume loss* is highly correlated with
postinjury scores on intelligence tests and is, in general, a powerful predictor of
postinjury performance on many measures of cognitive function and outcome. On
the other hand, *location of lesion* is a more powerful predictor than volume loss
when the outcome measure is relatively specific (e.g., object recognition) and
reflects the functioning of the area of brain containing the lesion. In this sense,
total volume loss is a summation of localized damage, and its effects are best
measured by a summary composite test score. Localized lesions greatly affect
local neural networks, and these effects are best measured by finely tuned cognitive tasks.

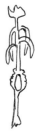

Intervention Strategies Could Affect Outcome

Both medical and psychological intervention may take place following head injury, particularly in moderate to severe head injuries (Bohnen et al., 1993; Fleming & Maas, 1994; Johnson et al., 1993; Scott-Jupp et al., 1992; Timming et
al., 1980; Wilson, 1992). These interventions are asymmetrically applied in time.
Medical interventions take place relatively close in time to the injury, whereas
most behavioral interventions are applied relatively distant in time from the injury.
The application of drugs could potentially affect a patient's rate of recovery (either
enhancing or depressing recovery) as well as helping to manage disruptive behaviors (e.g., aggressivity). The application of behavioral management techniques to
modify aberrant and unproductive behaviors or to induce appropriate behaviors
could have an effect on rate of recovery as well (Corrigan et al., 1992). Applying
cognitive techniques (such as memory retraining) may also accelerate and enhance

(and perhaps, when inappropriately applied in some cases, retard) recovery (Wilson, 1992). While the effects of medical interventions are often judged by their ability to save lives or reduce the length or severity of coma, the success of behavioral interventions is based upon the patient's ability to resume a lifestyle that resembles that which existed before the injury. The short-term results of behavioral interventions are often tangible and are reflected in changes in observed behaviors or improvement in domain-specific test scores. The long-term success of such interventions, however, is open to dispute. In any case, in measuring recovery of function, studies with children must consider the uniformity of interventions.

It was once thought that the adult brain would not show any plasticity, particularly by comparison with the functional plasticity of the young child. Recent research, however, indicates that the adult brain demonstrates plasticity under conditions of practice and learning. "Less-stimulated" brain regions may become committed to the functions subserved by active, topographically *adjacent* brain regions. This is not plasticity in the traditional sense—in which a damaged function would be incorporated by cortex previously committed to a different function—but a type of cortical imperialism (Di Piero et al., 1992; Weiller et al., 1993).

Since tasks can be accomplished by a variety of means, it is likely that brain-damaged individuals shift their reliance from one neural configuration (with one or more damaged neural networks) to another (with relatively intact neural networks) in order to accomplish a task-related goal. This shift in strategic operations may take place in an environmental context that includes rehabilitation interventions, which can bias the subject toward using a particular adaptive neural configuration (i.e., set of cognitive processes). Therefore, on both biological and cognitive grounds, it would be important to standardize treatment exposures as much as possible in children being studied for their outcome from head injury.

Socioeconomic Factors May Influence Outcome

Optimal rehabilitation requires familial and health care resources to work in tandem. Unfortunately, resources may vary greatly among hospitals, clinics, and, not surprisingly, families. The typical health insurance policy in the hands of a family with few financial resources and exposed to less than optimal health care systems may result in less than optimal rehabilitation care. The more closely the study subjects can be matched for socioeconomic status and hospitalization (e.g., duration of stay) variables, the more successful the outcome study should be (Schalen et al., 1994a).

Neuroplasticity

Reorganization of the adult brain following brain damage has been inferred from neuroimaging studies, experimental cognitive probes (such as dichotic listening and split-field tachistoscopic studies), rapid-rate transcranial magnetic stimulation (rTMS), and similar techniques (Di Piero et al., 1992; Grafman et al., in press; Kertesz, 1992; Lewine et al., 1994; Pascual-Leone et al., 1994; Pascual-Leone et al., 1993; Ramachandran, 1993). The evidence certainly indicates that a modified pattern of neural activity is often found during and following recovery of function. While no strict conclusions can be drawn about structural reorganization in the brain from these data, it is clear from the postinjury patterns of functionally related neural activity that other areas of the brain may become unusually active relative to the typical brain areas (now damaged) committed to subserving performance on a particular task. Furthermore, functional magnetic resonance and other neuro-imaging studies may be able to denote the rate of recovery in a particular damaged brain area by indicating the functional activity levels of that network longitudinally.

Some limited studies using rTMS have noted that when one regional neural network is partially damaged, the functions that activate adjacent neural networks may also activate a subset of those cells in the damaged area that lie closest to the neighboring intact neural network. This suggests that something akin to an "imperialism" of the cortex occurs after one region has been damaged. That is, adjacent cortical regions assume primary control over some of the remaining neurons in the damaged network(s). These plastic changes may depend on relatively increased use of adjacent cortical functions, a passive neurobiological imperative when a brain region is partially damaged, or some combination of the two. Using rTMS, it is possible to demonstrate that in normal adults, cortical plasticity may be rapid, learning a skill affects the topography of cortical maps, and primary neural network responsibility for performance of a task may fluctuate depending on the nature of the information that is to be processed. Of course, the demands of any task may be fluid, with different aspects of a stimulus being focused upon at different times during the task.

The implication of all these findings for adult brain-damaged patients is that:

1. Some recovery may occur in the area of damage.
2. Brain regions topographically adjacent to the area of damage may co-opt some of the cells from the damaged neural network for their own purposes.
3. Compensatory strategies may lead to a different neural network configuration becoming principally responsible for performance on a task. This configuration may not always be the optimal one but at least may allow for an improvement in functional capabilities.
4. There is little evidence of a literally substitutive plasticity, where another brain region assumes exactly the same computational and informational properties of the damaged area.

Very little of this kind of work has been done with children, however, thus limiting the generalizability of the findings. In particular, we do not know whether these same principles of plasticity of structure and function apply to children or whether children have some neurobiological advantages for neural plasticity—so that, under a certain age, spared cortical areas can, in fact, assume the exact computational properties of the damaged area. This hypothesis has had some support on the basis of research with very young children who have been longitudinally followed after a brain injury (Maratsos & Matheny, 1994; Thal et al., 1991).

Exacerbated Decline

In recent years, many adult survivors of childhood acute paralytic poliomyelitis (polio) have reported new muscle weakness in previously affected (and sometimes even unaffected) muscles. One possible explanation for this exacerbated decline in motor function is that, while the original polio episode in childhood permanently affected selected motor neurons, compensatory processes in surviving motor neurons hid any functional sequelae. During the normal process of aging, motor neuron function declines. This decline in polio survivors may reach a functional threshold before that in unaffected adults due to the partial loss of effective motor neurons in childhood. The postpolio patient, therefore, reports declining motor function much earlier than a normally aging adult (Grafman et al., in press).

Corkin developed this idea in the context of head injury outcome (Corkin et al., 1989). She studied older adults who had suffered a head injury during combat in World War II or the Korean War and found that the head injury incurred in young adulthood led to an exacerbated decline in cognitive functions in the older adult. This decline did not resemble a dementia but an accelerated loss of certain cognitive abilities.

The lesson for the study of recovery from childhood head injury is that some of the late effects of such an injury may be *very* late, not appearing until the child reaches age 60 or later. On the other hand, if plasticity is more operational in children that in adults, perhaps we would not see such an exacerbated decline in adults whose injury occurred before the age 5.

Discussion

Longitudinal outcomes research is notoriously difficult to do when outcome is defined by functional status. The few studies that have merged longitudinal study with outcome in adult head-injury patients have shown that a variety of variables may contribute to predicting outcome (Levin, 1992). These variables include the severity and locus of the lesion, preinjury education and intelligence, age, and intervention therapies. Less is known about the predictive effects of gender, handedness, personality, and socioeconomic factors. It is probable that some of these same variables would be relevant for the prediction of outcome following pediatric head injury. While it is not always possible to control strictly for such variables, addressing their presence or absence in an outcome study of pediatric head injury would enhance its interpretability.

Of course, the brain of a child has some special qualities. Foremost among these is the purported relative plasticity (compared to adults) of their brains in conjunction with their emotional immaturity and limited knowledge base (compared to adults). While these qualities can be viewed as compromising for a study, the more optimistic view is that we can learn even more about brain plasticity in the young brain as long as we carefully control for such confounding influences upon outcome. The use of sophisticated neuroimaging techniques in conjunction with behavioral and performance measures will help investigators to make inferences about brain plasticity. While the use of some of these technologies, like positron emission tomography, may not be advisable with children (because of radiation exposure), other techniques like functional magnetic resonance imaging may be more suitable for use with the young brain (Cohen & Bookheimer, 1994; Rueckert et al., 1994).

It is safe to say that the combination of new functional imaging and mapping technologies and neuropsychological testing will enable clinicians and researchers to make advances in our understanding of the factors that contribute to recovery of function. A more intensive effort to study recovery of function in children using the same methods applied in adult studies will undoubtedly lead to a more complete understanding of the limitations and possibilities of brain plasticity.

References

Aram, D. M., & Eisele, J. A. (1992). Plasticity and recovery of higher cognitive functions following early brain injury. In F. Boller & J. Grafman (Eds.), *Handbook of neuropsychology* (Vol. 6, pp. 73–92). Amsterdam: Elsevier Science Publishers.

Bohnen, N. I., Twijnstra, A., & Jolles, J. (1993). A controlled trial with vasopressin analogue (DGAVP) on cognitive recovery immediately after head trauma. *Neurology, 43,* 103–106.

Cohen, M. S., & Bookheimer, S. Y. (1994). Localization of brain function using magnetic resonance imaging. *Trends Neurosci., 17,* 268–276.

Corkin, S., Rosen, T. J., Sullivan, E. V., & Clegg, R. A. (1989). Penetrating head injury in young adulthood exacerbates cognitive decline in later years. *J. Neurosci., 9,* 3876–3883.

Corrigan, J. D., Mysiw, W. J., Gribble, M. W., & Chock, S. K. (1992). Agitation, cognition and attention during post-traumatic amnesia. *Brain Inj., 6,* 155–160.

Di Piero, V., Chollet, F. M., MacCarthy, P., Lenzi, G. L., & Frackowiak, R. S. (1992). Motor recovery after acute ischaemic stroke: A metabolic study. *J. Neurol. Neurosurg. Psychiatry, 55,* 990–996.

Dikmen, S., Machamer, J., & Temkin, N. (1993). Psychosocial outcome in patients with moderate to severe head injury: 2-year follow-up [see comments]. *Brain Inj., 7,* 113–124.

Eide, P. K., & Tysnes, O. B. (1992). Early and late outcome in head injury patients with radiological evidence of brain damage. *Acta. Neurol. Scand., 86,* 194–198.

Fearnside, M. R., Cook, R. J., McDougall, P., & Lewis, W. A. (1993). The Westmead Head Injury Project: Physical and social outcomes following severe head injury. *Br. J. Neurosurg., 7,* 643–650.

Fleming, J. M., & Maas, F. (1994). Prognosis of rehabilitation outcome in head injury using the Disability Rating Scale. *Arch. Phys. Med. Rehabil., 75,* 156–163.

Grafman, J., Clark, K., Richardson, D., Dinsmore, S., Stein, D., & and Dalakas, M. C.

(In press). Neuropsychology of post-polio syndrome. In M. C. Dalakas, H. Bart-field, & L. T. Kurland (Eds.), *The post-polio syndrome: Advances in the pathogenesis and treatment.* New York: New York Academy of Science.

Grafman, J., Jonas, B. S., Martin, A., Salazar, A. M. Weingartner, H., Ludlow, C., Smutok, M. A., & Vance, S. C. (1988). Intellectual function folowing penetrating head injury in Vietnam veterans. *Brain, 111,* 169–184.

Grafman, J., Jonas, B., & Salazar, A. (1992). Epilepsy following penetrating head injury to the frontal lobes: Effects on Cognition. In P. Chauvel & A. V. Delgado-Escueta etal. (Eds.) *Frontal lobe seizures and epilepsies: Advances in neurology* (Vol. 57, pp. 369–378). New York: Raven Press.

Grafman, J., Lalonde, F., Litvan, I., & Fedio, P. (1989). Premorbid effects on recovery from brain injury in humans: Cognitive and interpersonal indexes. In J. Schulkin (Ed.), *Preoperative events: Their effects on behavior following brain damage.* (pp. 277–304). Hillsdale, NJ: Erlbaum.

Grafman, J., Pascual-Leone, A., Wasserman, E., & Hallett, M. (In press). Identification and plasticity of human cortical maps revealed by transcranial magnetic stimulation. *Behav. Brain Res.*

Grafman, J., & Salazar, A. M. (1987). Methodological considerations relevant to the comparison of recovery from penetrating and Closed head injuries. In H. S. Levin, J. Grafmn, & H. Eisenberg (Eds.), *Neurobehavioral recovery from head injury* New York: Oxford University Press.

Grafman, J., Salazar, A., Weingartner, H., Vance, S., & Amin, D. (1986). The relationship of brain-tissue loss volume and lesion location to cognitive deficit." *J. Neurosci., 6,* 301–307.

Halpern, D. F., & Coren, S. (1991). Handedness and life span. *N. Engl. J. Med., 324,* 998.

Harris, L. J. (1992). Left-handedness. In F. Boller & J. Grafman. (Eds.), *Handbook of Neuropsychology* (Vol. 6, pp. 145–208). Amsterdam: Elsevier Science Publishers.

Johnson, D., Roethig-Johnston, K., & Richards, D. (1993). Biochemical parameters of recovery in acute severe head injury. *Br. J. Neurosurg., 7,* 53–59.

Johnson, D. A. (1992). Head injured children and education: A need for greater delineation and understanding. *Br. J. Educ. Psychol., 62,* 404–409.

Kertesz, A. (1988). Recovery of language disorders: Homologous contralateral or connected ipsilateral compensation. In S. Finger, T. E. Levere, C. R. Almli, and D. G. Stein (Eds.), *Brain injury and recovery: Theoretical and controversial issues.* (pp. 307–322). New York: Plenum.

Kertesz, A. (1992). Behavioral and cognitive disorders. In R. W. Evans, D. S. Baskin, & F. M. Yatsu (Eds.), *Prognosis of Neurological Disorders* (pp. 681–692). New York: Oxford University Press.

Klein, S. K., Masur, D., Farber, K., Shinnar, S., & Rapin, I. (1992). Fluent aphasia in children: Definition and natural history. *J. Child Neurol., 7,* 50–59.

Kunishio, K., Matsumoto, Y., Kawada, S., Miyoshi, Y., Matsuhisa, T., Moriyama, E., Norikane, H., & Tanaka, R. (1993). Neuropsychological outcome and social recovery of head-injured patients. *Neurol. Med. Chir., 33,* 824–829.

Levin, H. S. (1992). Neurobehavioral recovery. *J. Neurotrauma, 9,* 5359–5373.

Levin, H. S., Aldrich, E. F., Saydjari, C., Eisenberg, H. M., Foulkes, M. A., Bellefleur, M., Luerssen, T. G., Jane, J. A., Marmarou, A., & Marshall, L. F. (1992). Severe head injury in children: Experience of the Traumatic Coma Data Bank. *Neurosurgery, 31,* 435–443.

Levin, H. S. & Eisenberg, H. M., (1991). Management of head injury: Neurobehavioral outcome. *Neurosurg. Clin. North Am., 2,* 457–472.

Levin, H. S., Grafman, J., & Eisenberg, H. (1987). *Neurobehavioral recovery from head injury.* New York: Oxford University Press.

Levin, H. S., Mendelsohn, D., Lilly, M. A., Fletcher, J. M., Culhane, K. A., Chapman, S. B., Harward, H., Kusnerik, L., Bruce, D., & Eisenberg, H. M. (1994). Tower of London Performance in relation to magnetic resonance imaging following closed head injury in children. *Neuropsychology, 8,* 171–179.

Lewine, J. D., Astur, R. S., Davis, L. E., Knight, J. E., Maclin, E. L., & Orrison, W. W. Jr. (1994). Cortical organization in adulthood is modified by neonatal infarct: A case study. *Radiology, 190,* 93–96.

Maratsos, M., & Matheny, L. (1994). Language specificity and elasticity: Brain and clinical syndrome studies. *Annu. Rev. Psychol., 45,* 487–516.

Mendelsohn, D. B., Levin, H. S., Harward, H., & Bruce, D. (1992). Corpus callosum lesions after closed head injury in children: MRI, clinical features and outcome. *Neuroradiology, 34,* 384–388.

Michaud, L. J., Duhaime, A. C., & Batshaw, M. L. (1993). Traumatic brain injury in children. *Pediatr. Clin. North Am., 40,* 553–565.

Pascual-Leone, A., Grafman, J., & Hallett, M. (1994). Modulation of cortical motor output maps during development of implicit and explicit knowledge. *Science 263,* 1287–1289.

Pascual-Leone, A., Houser, C. M., Reese, K., Shotland, L. I., Grafman, J., Sato, S., Valls-Sole, J., Brasil-Neto, J. P., Wassermann, E. M., Cohen, L. G., & Hallett, M. (1993). Safety of rapid-rate transcranial magnetic stimulation in normal volunteers. *Electroencephalogr. Clin. Neurophysiol., 89,* 120–130.

Ramachandran, V. S. (1993). Behavioral and magnetoencephalographic correlates of plasticity in the adult human brain. *Proc. Natl. Acad. Sci: U.S.A., 90,* 10413–10420.

Rueckert, L., Appollonio, I., Grafman, J., Jezzard, P., Johnson, R., Jr., Le Bihan, D., & Turner, R. (1994). Magnetic resonance imaging functional activation of left frontal cortex during covert word production. *J. Neuroim., 4,* 67–70.

Saneda, D. L., & Corrigan, J. D. (1992). Predicting clearing of post-traumatic amnesia following closed-head injury. *Brain Inj., 6,* 167–174.

Schalen, W., Hansson, L., Nordstrom, G., & Nordstrom, C. H. (1994b). Psychosocial outcome 5–8 years after severe traumatic brain lesions and the impact of rehabilitation services. *Brain Inj., 8,* 49–64.

Schalen, W., Nordstrom, G., Nordstrom, C. H. (1994a). Economic aspects of capacity for work after severe traumatic brain lesions. *Brain Inj., 8,* 37–47.

Schwab, K., Grafman, J., Salazar, A. M., & Kraft, J. (1993). Residual impairments and work status 15 years after penetrating head injury: Report from the Vietnam Head Injury Study. *Neurology, 43,* 95–103.

Scott-Jupp, R., Marlow, N., Seddon, N., & Rosenbloom, L. (1992). Rehabilitation and outcome after severe head injury [see comments]. *Arch., Dis. Child, 67,* 222–226.

Shigemori, M., Kikuchi, N., Tokutomi, T., Ochiai, S., & Kuramoto, S. (1992). Coexisting diffuse axonal injury (DAI) and outcome of severe head injury. *Acta. Neurochir. Suppl., 55,* 37–39.

Stein, S. C., Spettell, C., Young, G., & Ross, S. E. (1993). Delayed and progressive brain injury in closed-head trauma: radiological demonstration. *Neurosurgery 32,* 25–30.

Teuber, H. -L. (1975). Recovery of function after brain injury in man. In R. Porter (Ed.),

Outcome of severe damage to the central nervous system (pp. 151–191). Ciba Foundation Symposium 34. Amsterdam: Elsevier.

Thal, D. J., Marchman, V., Stiles, J., Aram, D., Trauner, D., Nass, R., & Bates, E. (1991). Early lexical development in children with focal brain injury. *Brain Lang., 40*, 491–527.

Timming, R. C., Cayner, J. J., Grady, S., Grafman, J., Haskin, R., Malec, J., & Thornsen, C. (1980). Multidisciplinary rehabilitation in severe head trauma. *Wisc. Med. J., 79*, 49–52.

Vilkki, J., Holst, P., Ohman, J., Servo, A., & Heiskanen, O. (1992). Cognitive test performances related to early and late computed tomography findings after closed-head injury. *J. Clin. Exp. Neuropsychol., 14*, 518–532.

Weiller, C., Ramsay, S. C., Wise, R. J., Friston, K. J., & Frackowiak, R. S. (1993). Individual patterns of functional reorganization in the human cerebral cortex after capsular infarction. *Ann. Neurol., 33*, 181–189.

Wilson, B. (1992) Recovery and compensatory strategies in head injured memory impaired people several years after insult. *J. Neurol. Neurosurg. Psychiatry, 55*, 177–180.

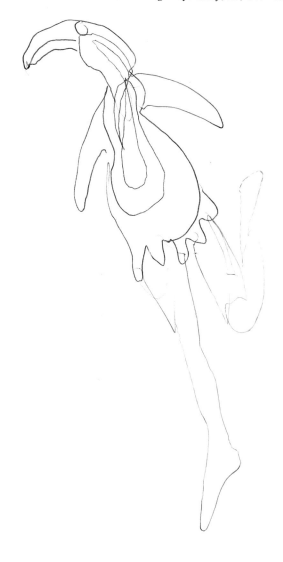

13

Evaluating Efficacy of Rehabilitation after Pediatric Traumatic Brain Injury

LINDA J. MICHAUD

Traumatic brain injury (TBI) is the most common cause of acquired disability in childhood and thus the focus of major effort in pediatric rehabilitation. Rehabilitation for pediatric TBI is associated with high human and economic costs. Jaffe and colleagues reported that rehabilitation costs accounted for 37% of the total costs of medical care in a cohort of children with mild, moderate, and severe TBI, in which 21% required inpatient rehabilitation (Jaffe et al., 1993). While rehabilitation costs account for a significant proportion of the total economic costs of pediatric TBI, the efficacy of rehabilitative efforts for children with TBI remains poorly documented. With the current emphasis on cost containment, it becomes increasingly necessary to demonstrate the effectiveness of rehabilitation strategies.

To claim that an intervention is efficacious, one should be able to demonstrate that it produced the desired outcome. This is a challenge that remains largely unanswered for most of the commonly accepted interventions in pediatric rehabilitation, including those for children with TBI. The purpose of this chapter is to discuss some of the major reasons that interventions in pediatric rehabilitation for children with TBI remain "unproven" and to suggest possible future strategies for development of a research foundation on which to base clinical practice.

Several factors that have been demonstrated to be associated with the occurrence of pediatric TBI and/or its outcome are independent of rehabilitative interventions. Such factors, which are discussed individually, include those that exist prior to injury, injury-related factors, acute management factors, factors in the postrehabilitation environment, and developmental factors. Some of these factors can confound the results of studies attempting to evaluate the effects of rehabilitation on outcome and therefore should be recognized in order to adequately design and carry out such studies.

Preinjury Factors

Many investigators have linked behavioral problems—including aggressiveness, high activity levels, or discipline problems—with a predisposition to injury (Bijur et al., 1986; Davidson et al., 1988; Langley et al., 1983; Matheny et al., 1971). Differences in temperament, activity levels, and attentiveness by 1 year of age were observed by Matheny and associates in twins with higher rates of injury (Matheny et al., 1971). Factors within the child appeared to contribute more to injury incidence than environmental factors. Psychosocial or environmental conditions may also predispose some children to head injury (Craft et al., 1972; Klonoff et al., 1971) and confound the association between head injury and behavioral disorders. Increased risk of head injury in children has been associated with lower socioeconomic status and parental marital instability (Klonoff, 1971).

Preinjury function can have a significant impact on outcome after pediatric TBI (Rivara et al., 1993). It is important to recognize preexisting factors in the child or environment because these factors may be erroneously attributed to the injury and also because they may independently affect long-term outcome after pediatric TBI.

Injury-Related Factors

Severity of TBI is the major factor associated with outcome. There is a strong association of severity of injury as estimated by the Glasgow Coma Scale (GCS), used as described by Teasdale and Jennett (1974), with outcome (Braakman et al., 1980; Humphreys, 1983; Jennett et al., 1979; Langfitt & Gennarelli, 1982; Lokkeberg & Grimes, 1984; Mayer & Walker, 1982; Miller et al., 1981). In particular, the motor response score of the GCS has been observed to be a better predictor of outcome than the total GCS score after severe brain injury (Braakman et al., 1980; Jagger et al., 1983). Glasgow Coma Scale scores obtained during the first few days after severe brain injury are better predictors of severity of disability in survivors than admission GCS scores (Michaud et al., 1992; Teasdale et al., 1979). The duration of coma is an important indicator of TBI severity; longer duration of coma is associated with less favorable outcome (Filley et al., 1987). In one study of children and young adults with severe TBI (Eiben et al., 1984), if coma duration was less than 21 days, 73% of patients regained independent function, whereas after coma persisting over 21 days, 78% remained dependent. The duration of posttraumatic amnesia, during which the patient is unable to store and recall ongoing events, was observed by Ewing-Cobbs and coworkers to be a better predictor of verbal and nonverbal memory in children with TBI than the GCS score (Ewing-Cobbs et al., 1990).

The type of brain injury is also an important predictor of neurological outcome. Depth of lesion is one indicator of severity, with greater force required to produce progressively deeper lesions extending from the cortical surface to the brainstem (Ommaya & Gennarelli, 1974). Several investigators have identified intracranial hematomas as contributory to poor outcome (Berger et al., 1985; Mayer & Walker, 1982; Miller et al., 1981). When epidural hematomas in children are rapidly evacuated, however, the outcomes are usually good, in contrast to those of children with subdural hematomas, who have worse outcomes even following prompt surgical evacuation (Raimondi & Hirschauer, 1984). Outcomes are worse in children with diffuse injury in addition to focal lesions compared with outcomes in children with diffuse injury alone (Filley et al., 1987). Diffuse axonal injury with multiple scattered axonal tears throughout the brain is associated with prolonged coma and poor outcome.

In addition to the primary lesions resulting from acute mechanical forces, secondary brain injuries may result from hypoxia or hypotension, brain swelling or edema, infarction, delayed hemorrhage, or pressure necrosis from displacement and herniation of the brain (Gentry et al., 1988). The presence of secondary brain injury is associated with worse outcome. Specifically, diffuse brain swelling with increased intracranial pressure has been demonstrated to increase the likelihood of poor outcome by many investigators (Berger et al., 1985; Walker et al., 1985). Extracranial injuries frequently complicate acute TBI and can influence outcome. In one study, 60% of children with severe TBI had at least one associated injury of intermediate or greater degree of severity to another organ system (Michaud et al., 1992). Severity of total injuries, including both brain and associated injuries, was the best predictor of survival in that study. In survivors, the presence of a chest injury was associated with worse outcomes. Hypoxia, hypercarbia, and hypotension have been associated with multiple trauma by a number of investigators (Langfitt et al., 1982; Mayer and Walker, 1982; Miller et al., 1981); these factors can contribute to secondary brain injury and worse outcomes.

Studies designed to evaluate efficacy of rehabilitation must include and control for factors such as severity, type and extent of primary and secondary brain injuries, and nature and severity of associated extracranial injuries. The outcome in a child with TBI will be significantly influenced by these factors as well as by rehabilitative procedures.

Factors in Acute Management

Acute medical and surgical interventions for the primary and secondary brain injuries and associated extracranial injuries can also have an impact on outcome in the child with TBI. For example, timely surgical evacuation of a subdural hematoma or good control of intracranial pressure can have positive effects on functional outcome independently of subsequent rehabilitation. Discussion of acute management in pediatric TBI is beyond the scope of this chapter; the reader is referred to Ghajar and Hariri's recent review (1992) and to Bruce, this volume.

There is evidence from animal studies that calcium-mediated toxicity, excitotoxicity, acidosis, and enhanced free-radical production contribute to secondary brain injury that can be ameliorated with pharmacological intervention (Siesjö, 1992). Should these experimental therapies be demonstrated in clinical trials to be efficacious following TBI in children, any such early intervention will also need to be considered in the evaluation of the effectiveness of subsequent rehabilitation.

Postrehabilitation Factors

The factors in the child or environment that predispose a child to injury, as reviewed above, are likely to remain operative following injury. Quality of parental supervision or intrafamilial stress factors in the preinjury period, for example, are likely to continue to be factors in the postacute rehabilitation environment of the child. These are also factors that need to be considered in the evaluation of variability in children's responses to subsequent rehabilitation and education programs.

After the period of acute rehabilitation, family and social support, availability and quality of outpatient rehabilitative services (provided either through the medical or educational systems), and access to optimal educational programming may all have significant influences on the long-term outcome of a child with TBI. Parents vary in ability and desire to function as advocates for children with TBI. This becomes an important factor for the child in making the transition from rehabilitation to an appropriate school program and in obtaining further rehabilitation services. Family functioning has been demonstrated by Rivara and colleagues to correlate significantly with the child's global and adaptive functioning 1 year following TBI (Rivara et al., 1993).

Public Law 101-476, the Individuals with Disabilities Education Act (IDEA) of 1990, recognized TBI as a specific category of disability within special education. As yet, neither the necessary training of educators nor material resources have been made available to implement this legislation to a major extent. In addition to special education, other rehabilitative services may be included in the child's individualized educational program, including physical, occupational and/or speech-language therapies, behavior management, counseling, and other special services as needed. Variations in effectiveness of special educational and rehabilitive interventions provided through the school systems may also contribute to variability in outcome in children with TBI.

The importance of the above sources of variability that follow acute rehabilitation can be expected to increase with longer intervals from rehabilitation to the time of follow-up. As the interval from rehabilitation to follow-up increases, the number of potential intervening variables increases, and it therefore becomes more difficult to evaluate the effect of rehabilitation on outcome in the child with TBI.

Developmental Factors

Developmental changes may confound assessment of the effects of rehabilitative interventions in children with TBI. Unlike adults, in whom independent function is usually the baseline that precedes onset of acquired disability due to TBI, the level of preinjury independence in children may be less than complete, but nonetheless appropriate for age, in the various domains of function. The normal baseline level of independent function in children changes with developmental age. During rehabilitation, it may be difficult to determine the proportion of increased independence due to rehabilitation alone.

Cerebral water content, extent of myelination, degree of brain development, stage of development of localization of cortical function, and neurochemical content vary in children of different ages. Each of these factors may have an impact on brain "plasticity" and potential recovery of function in children. Mechanisms of neurological and functional recovery following TBI are not well understood for any age group.

The effect of age on outcome following TBI in children may also depend on which domains of function are assessed. Brink and coworkers (1970) did not observe a significant difference in motor recovery as a function of age at injury but did find increased impairment in intellectual function with younger age at injury. Much remains to be learned about potential independent effects of age and developmental level at the time of injury on functional outcome following pediatric TBI.

Acute Rehabilitation

Rehabilitation may be defined as "development of a person to the fullest physical, psychological, social, vocational, avocational, and educational potential consistent with his or her physiological or anatomical impairment and environmental limitations" (DeLisa et al., 1988). As such, it is not a standardized, readily quantifiable process that can be prescribed in discrete, consistent units. Rehabilitation programs are individualized for each patient and consist of many components, most of which have subjective as well as objective elements.

Rehabilitation following severe TBI in children is an interdisciplinary process, involving physicians, nurses, physical and occupational therapists, speech and language pathologists, psychologists, social workers, and special educators. Family members are also important participants in the rehabilitation process for their child. Rehabilitative interventions for children with TBI are directed toward maximizing physical, communicative, cognitive, behavioral, social, and emotional function as appropriate for the age of the child. In general, this is accomplished by preventing secondary complications, retraining lost skills, and training in developing compensatory strategies. While lacking scientific "proof," professionals involved in pediatric rehabilitation believe that their efforts for children with TBI are effective based on their own training and their clinical experience. The evidence, however, has not been systematically evaluated.

Each child has individualized, specific goals targeted to his or her pattern of deficits. Sequelae vary in children with TBI depending on the location, type, and severity of injury to the brain. Deficits may be present in motor, sensory, communicative, cognitive, behavioral, and/or emotional domains of function. Motor problems following severe TBI in children most commonly include spasticity, incoordination, and ataxia (Brink et al., 1970; Costeff et al., 1990), depending upon the location of injury to the motor pathway. Visual and/or hearing impairment as well as other sensory and perceptual deficits, may result from TBI in children, depending on site of injury. Disorders of speech and language are very common, especially following severe injury. Language disorders may be expressive, receptive, or mixed, and may involve oral and/or written language. Neuropsychological deficits may include impairments in attention, memory, information processing, motor speed, problem-solving skills, ability to process abstract information, organizational abilities, and judgment. These deficits may be interrelated and may vary in severity. Traumatic brain injury may also cause neurobehavioral changes, most commonly aggression, hyperactivity, disinhibition, poor anger control, and social withdrawal.

Deficits in multiple domains of function typically follow severe TBI, with variability in the combinations of the types and severities of each area of dysfunction. There may be interactions among deficits in the effects on the child's overall function. Children with cognitive and motor deficits, for example, may, due to such problems as inattention to task or inability to understand and follow directions, have limitations in their abilities to participate optimally in physical therapy programs directed toward ameliorating motor deficits.

Recovery of function following TBI in children may vary in different functional domains. Brink and colleagues, for example, have observed that motor function may be recovered to a greater degree than language and other cognitive functions (Brink et al., 1970).

Significant variability exists among and within rehabilitation programs on inpatient units that care for children with TBI. Within each discipline contributing to the rehabilitation program, there are variations in clinical practice in the nature, timing, duration, and frequency of specific interventions. Inter- and intratherapist variability exists, and personal interactions of individual therapists with individual patients may vary and affect the child's responses to the interventions.

Even were it possible to standardize the specific components of rehabilitative interventions, the effects of different patients would introduce variability. As discussed above, preinjury backgrounds and injury-related factors are likely to differ between patients. The effects of similar therapeutic strategies can also vary in the same patient at different stages of recovery.

Acute rehabilitation provided in an inpatient setting may be followed by outpatient rehabilitation in a day hospital program or by a variable range of further outpatient services. Comprehensive, coordinated, interdisciplinary pediatric rehabilitation programs for children with TBI are not available in all communities. Regional variations exist in access to inpatient versus outpatient programs. Outpatient rehabilitative services vary in comprehensiveness along a spectrum from day rehabilitation hospital programs through outpatient services provided to supplement a school-based program to no outpatient rehabilitation services at all. For those children who do receive intensive inpatient rehabilitation following TBI, there is wide variation among communities in the availability and quality of subsequent rehabilitative services. Many of the services provided in the rehabilitation setting are subsequently continued in the educational setting, especially when, as is typically the situation, the child's deficits have implications for his or her ability to benefit maximally from the educational program, as discussed above.

Research Designs

Many threats to validity must be addressed in the designs of studies that attempt to evaluate whether or not rehabilitative interventions are efficacious in children with TBI. In order to claim that the intervention produced the effect on outcome, the investigators must ensure that other factors extraneous to the treatment did not produce the effect. In view of the above discussion, this is a significant challenge. The natural history of neurological recovery following TBI, especially in the acute period following injury, may be such that return of function would have occurred even in the absence of the intervention.

In the typical acute rehabilitation setting, multiple interventions are provided concurrently. Stimulation is provided by the family and nursing staff in addition to the activities in which the child participates in formal sessions in physical, occupational, and speech-language therapies. It may be difficult to demonstrate with certainty that a specific therapeutic intervention resulted in a specific effect. For example, increased length of utterances in speech may not be due only to the amount of time spent in therapeutic activities during formal speech-language therapy sessions but may reflect other experiences in the therapeutic environment, all superimposed on the process of neurological recovery. This may especially be true in coordinated interdisciplinary settings in which the speech-language pathologist may enlist the efforts of other members of the rehabilitation team, including the family, to integrate speech-language therapy goals into the daily routine. Similarly, improvements in strength, coordination, or balance are not likely to be entirely attributable to number of minutes of participation in appropriate exercises in physical therapy, especially if the therapists provide recommendations for incorporation of their goals into the activities of other members of the rehabilitation team.

Studies to evaluate efficacy of specific components of the total rehabilitation program for children with TBI might be expected to be more feasible than those aiming to evaluate efficacy of the total interdisciplinary effort. But the more challenging problem of evaluating overall effectiveness should not be dismissed because of challenging measurement issues. The most relevant research questions in pediatric rehabilitation for TBI are not likely to be those that can be easily answered. Development of standardized measures of pediatric functional outcome would contribute a critical link to the process of evaluating efficacy of rehabilitative interventions (Haley et al., 1991).

Most studies of outcome that include rehabilitation for TBI in children are descriptive and are not designed to demonstrate the efficacy of rehabilitation. They generally lack control groups and certainly do not include groups of children with TBI matched for severity of injury and randomized not to receive intervention.

True experimental designs are unlikely to be used in evaluating efficacy of pediatric rehabilitation for children with TBI. Ethical issues would be raised, as pediatric rehabilitation team members believe that their current standards of care for children with TBI result in preventing secondary complications and in facilitating maximal recovery of function.

Because it is neither likely nor desirable that experimental, randomized studies of rehabilitative intervention be designed and carried out, consideration should be given to the use of "natural experiments" to study the effectiveness of rehabilitation following TBI in children. The research design would not control which patients receive intervention, but patients would be "randomized" or grouped through some other mechanism such as access to the intervention or regional variations in standards of practice. It may then be feasible to locate and compare patients with similar characteristics who have received a particular intervention with others who have not. Even if it were possible to "match" children with TBI on salient characteristics, however, it is not likely that true randomization occurs with regard to rehabilitation for children with TBI. Although barriers to access exist, some level of rehabilitative intervention is likely to be available in most regions of the United States, at least for the most severely brain-injured children. Referrals of children with TBI to inpatient pediatric rehabilitation units occur, involving long distances between the child's residence and the rehabilitation center. It is probable that referrals of children with TBI for rehabilitation vary by nonrandom factors, such as socioeconomic status or the family's ability to advocate for the child.

Such quasi-experimental designs, in which assignments for rehabilitation are not random, can, however, be useful. But caution should be exercised in the design and interpretation of these studies. Nonrandom assignment for intervention may introduce confounding variables into the study, with factors that increase the likelihood for selection for rehabilitation having important independent effects on outcome. Although variations in access to pediatric rehabilitation services, coverage for rehabilitative services by third-party payers, and geographic variations in practices provide potential for studies to evaluate differences in outcomes for children with TBI who have received differing levels of rehabilitation intervention, this author is not aware of any such studies.

Longitudinal studies of cohorts of children with TBI, done either prospectively or retrospectively, may be helpful. Natural history may become better known with changes in health care systems. Variations in rehabilitative interventions that are determined by payers rather than physicians may result in groups of children with similar injuries receiving inpatient versus outpatient services. Varying levels of services received may allow some assessment of "dose-response" effects. Cross-sectional studies of children with TBI who have received variable levels of rehabilitative services may also be useful.

As an alternative to between-group research designs, single-case designs provide a methodological approach that is appropriate for investigations of individual patients or groups of patients (Kazdin, 1982). Single-subject methodology would appear to have great potential in the evaluation of efficacy of rehabilitation. A number of single-subject strategies have been described that would be appropriate for use in a rehabilitation setting. These include A-B-A-B [alternating a baseline phase with no intervention (A phase) with an intervention (B phase)], multiple baselines, changing criterion, and alternating treatment designs. These strategies are well described by Kazdin (1982), Ottenbacher (1986), and Payton (1988).

Single-subject experimental designs can be successfully implemented with children with TBI during acute rehabilitation in the inpatient pediatric rehabilitation unit setting, as demonstrated by Slifer and associates (Slifer et al., 1993). These investigators used single-case methodology to demonstrate effects of treatment on behavior problems including agitated, disruptive, aggressive, and noncompliant behaviors. Payton (1988) and Ottenbacher (1986) provide examples of single-case experimental designs applied to a variety of patient populations other than TBI in a variety of settings other than inpatient rehabilitation units. Among these examples are several that address the types of target behaviors that may be seen in children with TBI in rehabilitation settings, such as motor deficits or self-care problems. It would appear that a wide range of motor, communicative, cognitive, and social behaviors that are the targets of rehabilitative interventions in children with TBI could be studied using this methodology. Characteristics of the interventions such as nature, timing, frequency, duration, or setting could be varied and the effect on the target behavior assessed.

Limitations in the generalizability of the results of studies using single-case designs are acknowledged (Ottenbacher, 1986). These designs are, nonetheless, appropriate for evaluation of treatment effectiveness through either replicating several single-subject designs or substituting small groups of subjects for the individual subject (Ottenbacher, 1986).

Conclusion

Outcomes in survivors of pediatric TBI range from complete recovery to severe disability associated with physical and cognitive deficits. Multiple preinjury, injury-related, acute management, and postinjury factors, many of which are interrelated, can influence outcome following pediatric TBI and thus potentially confound assessment of efficacy of rehabilitative interventions. Evidence that rehabilitative interventions are efficacious in improving functional outcome in children with TBI has not been systematically evaluated. While the role of traditional experimental designs in clinical investigations may be limited, a variety of research methods involving group and single-case designs may be appropriate for assessing the effectiveness of pediatric rehabilitative interventions following TBI.

The nature, intensity, and quality of rehabilitative interventions contribute to the variability in short- and long-term outcomes in children with TBI. We who are concerned with pediatric rehabilitation must strive to meet the challenge of assessing and improving efficacy.

References

Berger, M. S., Pitts, L. H., Lovely, M., Edwards, M. S. B., & Bartkowski, H. M. (1985). Outcome from severe head injury in children and adolescents. *J. Neurosurg., 62,* 194–199.

Bijur, P. E., Stewart-Brown, S., & Butler, N. (1986). Child behavior and accidental injury in 11,966 preschool children. *Am. J. Dis. Child., 140,* 487–492.

Braakman, R., Gelpke, G. J., Habbema, J. D. F., Maas, A. I. R., & Minderhoud, J. M. (1980). Systematic selection of prognostic features in patients with severe head injury. *Neurosurgery, 6,* 362–370.

Brink, J. D., Garrett, A. L., Hale, W. R., Woo-Sam, J., & Nickel, V. L. (1970). Recovery of motor and intellectual function in children sustaining severe head injuries. *Dev. Med. Child Neurol., 12,* 565–571.

Costeff, H., Groswasser, Z., & Goldstein, R. (1990). Long-term follow-up review of 31 children with severe closed head trauma. *J. Neurosurg., 73,* 684–687.

Craft, A. W., Shaw, D. A., & Cartlidge, N. E. F. (1972). Head injuries in children. *Br. Med. J., 4,* 200–203.

Davidson, L. L., Hughes, S. J., & O'Connor, P. A. (1988). Preschool behavior problems and subsequent risk of injury. *Pediatrics, 82,* 644–651.

DeLisa, J. A., Martin, G. M., & Currie, D. M. Rehabilitation medicine: Past, present, and future. In J. A. DeLisa (Ed.), *Rehabilitation medicine: Principles and practice* (p. 3). Philadelphia, PA: Lippincott, 1988.

Eiben, C. F., Anderson, T. P., Lockman, L., Matthews, D. J., Dryja, R., Martin, J., Burrill, C., Gottesman, N., O'Brian, P., & Witte, L. (1984). Functional outcome of closed head injury in children and young adults. *Arch. Phys. Med. Rehabil., 65,* 168–170.

Ewing-Cobbs, L., Levin, H. S., Fletcher, J. M., Miner, M. E., & Eisenberg, H. M. (1990). The Children's Orientation and Amnesia Test: Relationship to severity of acute head injury and to recovery of memory. *Neurosurgery, 27,* 683–691.

Filley, C. M., Cranberg, L. D., Alexander, M. P., & Hart, E. J. (1987). Neurobehavioral outcome after closed head injury in childhood and adolescence. *Arch. Neurol., 44,* 194–198.

Gentry, L. R., Godersky, J. C., & Thompson, B. (1988). MR imaging of head trauma: Review of the distribution and radiopathologic features of traumatic lesions. *Am. J. Neuroradiol., 9,* 101–110.

Ghajar, J., & Hariri, R. J. (1992). Management of pediatric head injury. *Pediatr. Clin. North Am., 39,* 1093–1125.

Haley, S. M., Coster, W. J., & Ludlow, L. H. (1991). Pediatric functional outcome measures. *Phys. Med. Rehabil. Clin. North Am. 2,* 689–723.

Humphreys, R. P. (1983). Outcome of severe head injury in children. In A. J. Raimondi (Ed.), *Concepts in pediatric neurosurgery* (Vol. 3, pp. 191–201). Basel: Karger.

Jaffe, K. M., Massagli, T. L., Martin, K. M., Rivara, J. B., Fay, G. C., & Polissar, N. L. (1993). Pediatric traumatic brain injury: Acute and rehabilitation costs. *Arch. Phys. Med Rehabil., 74,* 681–686.

Jagger, J., Jane, J. A., & Rimel, R. (1983). The Glasgow Coma Scale: To sum or not to sum? *Lancet, 2,* 97 (letter).

Jennett, B., Teasdale, G., Braakman, R., Minderhoud, J., Heiden, J., & Kurze, T. (1979). Prognosis of patients with severe head injury. *Neurosurgery 4,* 283–289.

Kazdin, A. E. (1982). *Single-case research designs: Methods for clinical and applied settings.* New York: Oxford University Press.

Klonoff, H. (1971). Head injuries in children: Predisposing factors, accident conditions, accident proneness and sequelae. *Am. J. Public Health, 61,* 2405–2417.

Langfitt, T. W., & Gennarelli, T. A. (1982). Can the outcome from head injury be improved? *J. Neurosurg., 56,* 19–25.

Langley, J., McGee, R., Silva, P., & Williams, S. (1983). Child behavior and accidents. *J. Pediatr. Psychol., 8,* 181–189.

Lokkeberg, A. R., & Grimes, R. M. (1984). Assessing the influence of non-treatment variables in a study of outcome from severe head injuries. *J. Neurosurg. 61,* 254–262.

Matheny, A. P., Brown, A. M., & Wilson, R. S. (1971). Behavioral antecedents of accidental injuries in early childhood: A study of twins. *J. Pediatr. 79,* 122–124.

Mayer, T., & Walker, M. L. (1982). Emergency intracranial pressure monitoring in pediatrics: Management of the acute coma of brain insult. *Clin. Pediatr., 21,* 391–396.

Michaud, L. J., Rivara, F. P., Grady, M. S., & Reay, D. T. (1992). Predictors of survival and severity of disability after severe brain injury in children. *Neurosurgery, 31,* 254–264.

Miller, J. D., Butterworth, J. F., Gudeman, S. K., Faulkner, J. E., Choi, S. C., Selhorst, J. B., Harbison, J. W., Lutz, H. A., Young, H. F., & Becker, D. P. (1981). Further experience in the management of severe head injury. *J. Neurosurg., 54,* 289–299.

Ommaya, A. K., & Gennarelli, T. A. (1974). Cerebral concussion and traumatic unconsciousness: Correlation of experimental and clinical observations on blunt head injuries. *Brain, 97,* 633–654.

Ottenbacher, K. J. (1986). *Evaluating clinical change: Strategies for occupational and physical therapists.* Baltimore, MD: Williams & Wilkins.

Payton, O. D. (1988). *Research: The validation of clinical practice,* 2nd ed. Philadelphia, PA: Davis.

Raimondi, A. J., & Hirschauer, J. (1984). Head injury in the infant and toddler: Coma scoring and outcome scale. *Childs Brain, 11,* 12–35.

Rivara, J. B., Jaffe, K. M., Fay, G. C., Polissar, N. L., Martin, K. M., Shurtleff, H. A., & Liao, S. (1993). Family functioning and injury severity as predictors of child functioning one year following traumatic brain injury. *Arch. Phys. Med. Rehabil., 74,* 1047–1055.

Siesjö, B. K. (1992). Pathophysiology and treatment of focal cerebral ischemia: Part II. Mechanisms of damage and treatment. *J. Neurosurg., 77,* 337–354.

Slifer, K. J., Cataldo, M. D., Babbitt, R. L., Kane, A. C., Harrison, K. A., & Cataldo, M. F. (1993). Behavior analysis and intervention during hospitalization for brain trauma rehabilitation. *Arch. Phys. Med. Rehabil. 74,* 810–817.

Teasdale, G., & Jennett, B. (1974). Assessment of coma and impaired consciousness: A practical scale. *Lancet, 2,* 81–84.

Teasdale, G., Parker, L., Murray, G., Knill-Jones, R., & Jennett, B. (1979). Predicting the outcome of individual patients in the first week after severe head injury. *Acta Neurochir. Suppl. (Wien), 28,* 161–164.

Walker, M. L., Mayer, T. A., Storrs, B. B., & Hylton, P. D. (1985). Pediatric head injury—factors which influence outcome. In P. H. Chapman (Ed.), *Concepts in pediatric neurosurgery* (Vol. 6, pp. 84–97). Basel: Karger.

14

The Prospect of Pediatric Clinical Trials: Experience with Adult Trials

JOHN DAVID WARD

It is well known that trauma is the leading killer of children by a factor of 2 to 3 depending on the age group (Guyer & Ellers, 1990). It is further known that head injury is the major cause of death following trauma in children (Tepas et al., 1990). Brain injury is clearly a serious health problem in children. What is not so well known is that there have been few therapeutic trials aimed primarily at children with severe head injury. To date, most of the published data on pediatric head-injured patients have been descriptive in nature. While this is useful, the treatment of pediatric head injury can be improved only through prospective randomized, controlled therapeutic trials. Unfortunately, there are no large-scale clinical trials currently ongoing that are designed to improve the care of *children* with moderate and severe head injury. The reasons for this are multifaceted. In this chapter, we will look at some of the problems that must be considered when carrying out clinical head injury treatment trials in children. We will examine past and current trials in head-injured adults to see how they may apply to children, see what lessons and principles can be extracted, and sketch the prospects for future clinical trials in head-injured children. Finally, recommendations for pediatric head injury trials are offered.

Problems in Children

It is not due to lack of interest that there are few clinical head injury trials in children. Many problems face anyone preparing to do such a study. Some of the more common difficulties that must be considered are changes in the developing nervous system, unknown effects of drugs, definition of end points, and legal and ethical issues as well.

The pediatric brain, especially in the very young, may not only be physiologically different (Muizelaar et al., 1991) but may also react differently to injury

258

(Lou et al., 1979). These differences must be considered when any clinical trial in children is designed. The pediatric brain is in varying stages of development depending upon the age of the child. The injury may impose profound developmental delay in a very young child, while its effect may be quite different in the more mature brain. The newborn and infant are different from the toddler and preschooler who, in turn, are probably different from school-age children and adolescents (Luerssen et al., 1988). These groups differ in response to injury, type of injury, and the outcome they can achieve. One obvious answer is to group children by age when studying a particular therapy. This grouping, however, dilutes patient numbers and complicates trial implementation and analysis. Significant age differences cannot be ignored and necessitate sample stratification when doing a study.

Another problem encountered early in the design of clinical studies is that some classes of drugs commonly used in adults may have an unacceptable or unknown effect on development in the young child. It might be expected that those compounds that most mimic what already occurs in the body, such as superoxide dismutase or vitamin E, might be less inclined to have an adverse effect. We must realize however, that many of these drugs have not undergone the required animal and human testing to allow us to make accurate statements concerning their effect and use in children.

The presence or absence of appropriate and reasonable end points can make or break a clinical trial in any age group. The primary end point in most adult head injury trials is the Glasgow Outcome Score (GOS) (Jennett & Bond, 1975). In addition, some trials include other end points, such as the Disability Rating Scale (DRS) (Rappaport et al., 1983). These end points may or may not be appropriate for children. It may be that measuring rate of recovery or a drug's effect on development will be a more appropriate indication of outcome. As complex as this is, appropriate end points are pivotal to the successful completion of a clinical trial in terms of its ability to evaluate the efficacy of a compound. There have been suggestions recently about establishing earlier end-point determinations in order to complete trials more quickly. This will be quite difficult to do in the pediatric age group.

There are also complex legal and ethical issues that arise whenever a child participates in a clinical trial. Although it may differ from place to place, most states have statutes that make persons and companies involved with the care of a child legally liable until the child reaches the ages of 18 to 21 years. In addition, the ethical issues of informed consent and the responsibility of the physician investigators to protect the child pose unique and serious considerations. While these conditions are accepted by providers of health care for children, industry remains free to choose how much legal and ethical exposure it will assume. For example, in certain areas—such as the treatment of specific childhood diseases that require anticonvulsants or vaccinations—there is a large market, and industry has been willing to assume some degree of risk. In the case of severe head injury, however, where the patient population is small and includes both pediatric and adult patients, any success in the development of therapies may not be worth the expense and the potential risks as industry sees it. Therefore, the impetus to study children is lessened. When all issues are considered, the result is that today, children with a head injury receive "trickle-down" therapy. That is, drugs and therapeutic endeavors shown to be effective in adults are, without adequate testing and evaluation, being used in pediatric patients who have head injuries. That is not to say that the pediatric patients have not benefited from adult trials. However, separate evaluation of most therapies has not been done in the pediatric population. There are many complex issues facing investigators who wish to do a clinical trial dedicated to head-injured children. These challenges, though formidable, are not insurmountable.

Review of Adult Closed Head Injury Trials

The study of head injury has progressed from initially gathering a large amount of data about head-injured patients to current attempts to alter basic pathological processes with specific compounds. This transformation, from the collection of epidemiological data to the focus on altered physiology, has been the direct result of increased understanding through the study of experimental head injury. It is of value to examine some of the resultant clinical trials in adult patients to see what lessons can be applied to the planning of trials for the treatment of pediatric head injury.

Basically, most clinical trials can be grouped by how the treatment is expected to affect the pathology or process of the head injury. These groupings are (1) therapies that treat a specific aspect of the head injury, such as elevated intracranial pressure; (2) therapies that change the brain's immediate environment, as with hyperventilation or hypothermia; or (3) treatment regimens that include a compound or drug in the study protocol (i.e., steroids, barbiturates, tromethamine (THAM), superoxide dismutase (PEG-SOD), 21-aminosteroids (tirilazad), calcium channel blockers (nimodipine), or NMDA-receptor antagonists. Each of these groups of therapies is briefly examined to see if they included children and what the results of these clinical trials yielded in terms of new and improved therapies.

Early on, a system of head injury treatment was proposed that gradually became the standard of care (Becker et al., 1977). It consisted of rapid transport of the head-injured patient to a level I trauma center, aggressive resuscitation, prompt diagnosis and removal of mass lesions, and high-quality intensive care. Currently, almost all children with head injury undergo this type of systematic care. This approach is often coupled with monitoring of intracranial pressure (ICP) and control of elevated ICP. More recently emphasis has been on controlling cerebral perfusion pressure (CPP) rather than ICP alone (Rosner & Coley, 1986). There has been no report of a prospective, randomized trial of this mode of ICP control in adults or children, though children seem to benefit from this type of monitoring and treatment.

Two trials have attempted to improve outcome by altering the brain milieu. The first was an attempt to treat acidosis by decreasing $PaCO_2$ with hyperventilation and the second was by decreasing the brain's temperature to alter certain pathological processes. A trial of chronic prophylactic hyperventilation down to a $Paco_2$ of 24 was reported in 1991 by Muizelaar and associates (Muizelaar et al., 1991). When initially carried out, this form of therapy was part of a three-armed trial, with a group treated with tromethamine (THAM) (Wolf et al., 1993), a hyperventilation group, and a control group. This was one of the few trials that enrolled children; however, no subject was below the age of 3 years, and the total number of children was small. The results in the hyperventilation trial showed that chronic hyperventilation did not improve outcome but in fact, in some cases, retarded recovery.

Hypothermia has been used for many years as a means of protection for organs such as the heart, but only recently have investigators organized trials in head injury (Marion et al., 1993). Such trials have not yet been reported in children.

The use of specific drugs to treat head injury is predicated on the theory that once a head injury occurs certain pathological processes are set into motion. If these processes are interrupted before extensive tissue damage occurs, outcome can be improved. Initially, the more common drugs already on the market were studied; more recently, new investigational compounds are being tested.

One of the first drug trials carried out in head-injured patients tested the use of high-dose steroids. Steroids had long been used in patients with tumors, and although the precise reason for improvement was unknown, it was felt that patients with severe head injury would also benefit. As shown in Table 14-1, two prospective studies were performed. In the study by Braakman, children were included and received a smaller dose than adults. There was no improvement in outcome (Braakman et al., 1983). In a similar fashion. Dearden's study included

TABLE 14-1. Drug Treatment Clinical Trials

Drug	Reference	Lowest Age	Results
Steroids	Braakman et al., 1983	3 years	No effect
	Deardon et al., 1986	3 years	No effect
Barbiturates	Ward et al., 1985	12 years	No effect
	Eisenberg et al., 1988	15 years	Better ICP control, better survival 1 month
Triomethamine (THAM)	Wolf et al., 1993	3 years	Counteracts bad effect of chronic hyperventilation
Nimodipine	Teasdale et al., 1992	18 years	No effect
Tirilazad	N/A	18 years	Unknown
Superoxide dismutase (Peg-SOD)	Muizelaar et al., 1993	15 years	Phase II trial—may be helpful
NMDA receptor antagonist	N/A	16 years	Unknown

children down to the age of 3 years, with dose calculation done as a function of weight. They too found no improvement in outcome (Dearden et al., 1986).

The next drug to be tested was pentobarbitol. This drug was administered in two different ways in two different trials. First, a trial of prophylactic administration of barbiturates was performed by Ward and associates (Ward et al., 1985). The second trial was performed by a group of investigators in comprehensive trauma centers where barbiturates were given only if needed to control intracranial pressure (Eisenberg et al., 1988). The trial of prophylactic barbiturate administration included children down to the age of 12 years but none younger. The trial failed to demonstrate any effectiveness in improving outcome and cautioned about the possible occurrence of occasional hypotension with the use of this treatment. The second trial showed that ICP could be controlled with acute barbiturate therapy, with a significant improvement in mortality at 1 month. It was unclear whether outcome improved at 1 year. The youngest patient in this trial was 15 years of age.

The THAM trial, aimed at treating acidosis, was one arm of the hyperventilation trial, as mentioned earlier. This trial also failed to yield significant improvement in outcome, although THAM did counteract the harmful effects of chronic hyperventilation (Wolf et al., 1993). This was one of the few trials that included children down to the age of 3 years.

All of the head injury trials mentioned so far utilized conventional therapies or common drugs already on the market. The following trials have used new compounds under development by pharmaceutical companies and have had to go through the classic phase I, phase II, and phase III trial process. None of these trials have included children under the age of 15 years.

The use of the calcium channel blocker nimodipine was studied in Europe in two trials: HIT 1 and HIT 2 (Teasdale et al., 1992). These multicenter trials had a large number of patients but none below the age of 18 years. Results indicated that nimodipine did not improve outcome in patients with a severe head injury.

Superoxide dismutase (SOD) is a naturally occurring enzyme that, for this therapy, has been joined with a polyethylene glycol (PEG) shell to decrease antigenicity and lengthen shelf life. Hence the name PEG-SOD. It has been shown in experimental animals that free radicals are generated after head injury and that SOD quenched the free radicals and improved survival (Kontos & Wei, 1986). The phase II trial reported by Muizelaar in head injury patients was quite encouraging (Muizelaar et al., 1993). There seemed to be improved survival if the population was split into only two outcome categories: dead and vegetative versus severe, moderate, and good (rather than the five categories of GOS). Intracranial pressure was also favorably affected. There were not enough patients to draw any definite conclusions, but the results were encouraging enough to allow the investigators to go forward with a full phase III trial. The trial is in progress and will probably be completed in the near future. The phase II trial and the current phase III trial do not include any children under the age of 15 years. The 21-aminosteroid tirilazad has been shown to improve outcome in animals subjected to a head injury (Dimlich et al., 1990) and has been in phase III trials in the

United States and Europe. The European trial is completed and the American trial is reaching its conclusion, but there are no reported results as yet. No children were included in the tirilazad trials. Whether, if successful, this compound will be used in children remains to be seen. As far as we know, no safety or toxicity studies have been performed with tirilazad in children.

The final class of drugs are the NMDA-receptor antagonists, the prototype being MK-801. This drug has not been brought to clinical trials for head injury because of its side effects. Another drug of this class, the Ciba Geigy compound CG 19755, has shown a beneficial effect and relative safety in preliminary studies (Stewart et al., 1993). It is currently in a phase II trial and will soon go into phase III testing with both European and North American participation. The compound is aimed at blocking the harmful excitatory effects of the amino acid glutamate. This excitatory amino acid has been shown to be present in the brain in significant excess after trauma. In experimental head injury, this excess in glutamate causes abnormal fluxes of ions, especially calcium, resulting in cellular injury. We will have to wait until the trials are completed before any conclusions can be drawn. In the current NMDA-receptor antagonist phase II trial, only patients 16 years of age or older are included.

Lessons Learned from Adult Trials

Although there are many difficulties and obstacles to the performance of pediatric head injury trials, valuable lessons have been learned from previous clinical head injury trials. It is essential that information gleaned from these previous trials be incorporated into any future pediatric study.

The selection of any therapeutic modality should be based on sound scientific data. Available experimental evidence should indicate at least a reasonable chance of clinical effectiveness. Unfortunately, for a variety of reasons as mentioned above, some potentially effective newer compounds may not be available for use in children. This means that only the more common compounds that are readily available and are considered safe for children will be used. This limits the selection of compounds and impedes progress in treating children with severe head injury.

There must be measurable and meaningful endpoints. These end points must be clean, unambiguous, obtainable, and truly reflective of the outcome of the patient. The end points selected should represent different categories of outcome and should be sensitive enough to discern any real differences between groups. In children as opposed to adults, the end point may actually be the effect of the injury on rate of development rather than, or in addition to, the more traditional measures of outcome.

The quality or reliability of the data must be good and the quantity or scope of the study must be appropriate. The data collected must be sufficient to achieve the purpose of the trial and to answer associated scientific and regulatory questions. At the same time, data should not become so voluminous that collection is impractical. Trials focused in their scope are much more likely to be completed than those that try to collect large amounts of data.

There must be a sufficient number of patients to answer defined questions of efficacy of any proposed therapy. Since large patient numbers are usually required, a multicenter trial model is necessary. The issue of patient numbers needs to be addressed up front. Most centers tend to overestimate the number of eligible patients who will actually be included in a trial. Ideally, an appropriate number of centers needs to be included to accrue a sufficient number of patients for conducting a trial over a 1- to 3-year period.

In order for a clinical trial to succeed, there must be adequate personnel and resources to handle data entry forms, ensure the quality of the data, enter the data in the correct manner, analyze the data, and also ensure that the trial is run efficiently and safely. Appropriately run head injury trials are expensive, and there is stiff competition for funding. In today's climate of limited resources, sufficient funding poses a significant hurdle. It is most wasteful, however, to try to perform a trial that, due to inadequate funding or an insufficient number of patients, does not yield conclusive results.

Possible Future Trials

Because of the difficulties, mentioned above, in using unproven drugs and compounds in children, it is most likely that any trial in the near future will involve some therapy or compound that is already in common use. This current situation actually limits what would be available for a future trial in pediatric patients with head injuries. Hypothermia has been used in the care of patients for many years. More specifically, pediatric patients with significant cardiac disease have been cooled during the repair of their cardiac anomalies. There have been some preliminary data in adults, and there is currently an adult hypothermia trial (Marion et al., 1993). It would probably be appropriate to apply this technique to the pediatric population with moderate and severe head injury.

A drug that might be useful is dextromethorphan (Duhaime, 1994), a commonly used antitussive drug in both children and adults. Although the dosage would be significantly higher for patients with brain injury, dextromethorphan has been around a long time, its effects are known, and it has a reasonable chance of success. Vitamin E, desferrioxamine, indomethacin, and magnesium all represent other common compounds that are currently in widespread use for other diseases. Each of these, at one time or another, has been shown to successfully block harmful pathological processes in experimental head injury. Potentially harmful side effects would have to be carefully studied, especially in the very young, before beginning clinical trials.

What the future will hold for clinical trials in pediatric head injury is unknown. There are several possible scenarios. The first would be that the study of drugs for head injury will continue as it is now being practiced. That is, drugs will be developed and tested in adult head injury, and—without further testing—it will be automatically assumed that they are useful in pediatric head injury as well. Therefore their use will gradually trickle down to the pediatric population. The second scenario would be that, although drugs may be useful in adult head injury, they will be withheld from injured children pending appropriate drug safety and efficacy studies. Since these studies are quite difficult and expensive, it may be that meaningful therapies would be denied to children with severe head injury. A third scenario would be that investigators and pharmaceutical companies, while recognizing the risk involved, would try to develop and test new compounds in the pediatric patient. This third scenario is the most desirable and would ultimately lead to the best and safest approach to the care of the head-injured child.

Recommendations

Recommendations made concerning pediatric head injury trials must take into account the significance of the problem to be studied, the feasibility of the trial, and the potential resources available. With these points in mind, the following recommendations seem reasonable:

Head injury is a major medical and public health problem in the pediatric age group and therefore deserves study.

While the newer protective compounds would probably be more efficacious, the reality is that most pharmaceutical companies are unwilling to subject them to a clinical trial in the pediatric age group. Because of this, drugs that are in common use and established techniques will most likely be tested first.

All pediatric clinical head injury trials must involve multiple centers to obtain a sufficient number of patients. These multicenter trials will require sophisticated data collection, data analysis, and trial coordination.

Decisions will have to be made about the focus of the trial and what questions should be answered before beginning patient accrual.

Suitable end points that measure efficacy in a pediatric trial will have to be selected. This means not only a static determination of level of functioning but also the effect of the treatment on development.

Likely treatments that could be studied now are hypothermia, dextromethorphan, or a free radical scavenger. Sufficient safety data in defined age groups would have to be obtained prior to a full phase trial.

Funding should be sufficient to perform the trial adequately. Using small amounts of resources to conduct trials that have no hope of answering crucial questions is a waste of valuable time and scarce resources.

Treatment specifically aimed at the pediatric population must be developed. There are significant hurdles to be overcome, but with the information and experience from past trials, we should be in a position to successfully complete trials that yield improved outcomes for children with serious head injury.

References

Becker, D. P., Miller J. D., Ward, J. D., Greenberg, R. P., Young, H. F., & Salakas, R. (1977). The outcome from severe head injury with early diagnosis and intensive management. *J. Neurosurg., 47,* 491–502.

Braakman, R., Schouten, J. H. D., van Dishoeck, B. M., & Minderhould, J. M. (1983). Megadose steroids in severe head injury: Results of a prospective double blind clinical trial. *J. Neurosurg., 58,* 326–330.

Dearden, N. M., Gibson, J. S., McDonwall, D. G., Gibson, R. M., M., & Cameron, M. M. (1986). Effect of high dose dexamethasone on outcome from severe head injury. *J. Neurosurg., 64,* 81–88.

Dimlich, R. V., Tornheim, P. A., Kindel, R. M., Hall, E. D., Braughler, J. M., & McCall, J. M. (1990). Effects of a 21-aminosteroid (U-74006F) on cerebral metabolites and edema after severe experimental head trauma. *Adv. Neurol. (U.S.), 52,* 365–375.

Duhaime, H. C. (1994). Exciting your neurons to death: Can we prevent cell loss after brain injury? *Pediatr Neurosurg., 21,* 117–122.

Eisenberg, H. M., Frankowski, R. F., Contant, C. F., Marshall, L. F., Walker, M. D. & the Comprehensive Central Nervous System Trauma Centers. (1988). High-dose barbiturate control of elevated intracranial pressure in patients with severe head injury. *J. Neurosurg., 69,* 15–23.

Guyer, B., & Ellers, B. (1990). Childhood injuries in the United States: Mortality, morbidity, and cost. *Am. J. Dis. Child., 144,* 649–652.

Jennett, B., & Bond, M. R. (1975). Assessment of outcome after severe brain damage: A practical scale. *Lancet, 1,* 480–484.

Kontos, H. A., & Wei, E. P. (1986). Superoxide production in experimental head injury. *J. Neurosurg., 64,* 803–807.

Lou, H. C., Lassen, N. A., & Fris-Hansen, B. (1979). Impaired autoregulation of cerebral blood flow in the distressed newborn infant. *J. Pediatr., 94,* 118–121.

Luerssen, T. G., Klauber, M. R., & Marshall, L. F. (1988). Outcome from head injury related to patient's age: A longitudinal prospective study of adult and pediatric head injury. *J. Neurosurg., 68,* 409–416.

Marion, D. W., Obrist, W. D., Carlier, P. M., Penrod, L. E., & Darby, J. M. (1993). The use of moderate therapeutic hypothermia for patients with severe head injuries: A preliminary report. *J. Neurosurg. (U.S.), 79,* 354–362.

Muizelaar, J. P., Marmarou, A., DeSalles, A. A., Ward, J. D., Zimmerman, R. S., Li, Z., Choi, S. C., & Young, H. F. (1989). Cerebral blood flow in severely head-injured children: Part I. relationship with GCS score, outcome, ICP, and PVI. *J. Neurosurg., 71,* 63–71.

Muizelaar, J. P., Marmarou, A., Ward, J. D., Kontos, H. A., Choi, S. C., Becker, D. P., Greumber, H., & Young, H. F. (1991). Adverse effects of prolonged hyperventilation in patients with severe head injury: A randomized clinical trial. *J. Neurosurg., 75,* 731–739.

Muizelaar, J. P., Marmarou, A., Young, H. F., Choi, S. C., Wolf, A., Schneider, R. L., & Kontos, H. A. (1993). Improving the outcome of severe head injury with the oxygen radical scavenger polyethylene glycol-conjugated superoxide dismutase: A Phase II trial. *J. Neurosurg., 78,* 375–382.

Rappaport, M., Hall, K. M., Hopkins, K., Belleza, T., & Cope, D. N. (1983). Disability rating scale for severe head trauma: Coma to community. *Arch. Phys. Med. Rehabil., 63,* 118–123.

Rosner, M. J., & Coley, I. B. (1986). Cerebral perfusion pressure intracranial pressure and head elevation. *J. Neurosurg., 65,* 636–641.

Stewart, L., Bullock, R., Jones, M., Kotake, A., & Teasdale, G. M. (1993). The cerebral haemodynamic and metabolic effects of the competitive NMDA antagonist CGS 19755 in humans with severe head injury. *J. Neurotrauma 10*(S1), S104.

Teasdale, G., Bailey, I., Bell, A., Gray, J., Gullan, R., Heiskanan, O., Marks, P. V., Marsh, H., Mendelow, D. A., Murray, G., et al. (1992). A randomized trial of nimodipine in severe head injury: HIT I. British/Finnish Co-operative Head Injury Trial Group. *J. Neurotrauma (U.S.), 9*(suppl 2), S545–S550.

Tepas, J. J., DiScala, C., Ramenofsky, M. L., & Barlow, B. (1990). Mortality and head injury. *J. Pediatr. Surg., 25,* 92–95.

Ward, J. D., Becker, D. P., Miller, J. D., Choi, S. C., Marmarou, A., Wood, C., Newlon, P. G., & Keenan, R. (1985). Failure of prophylactic barbiturate coma in the treatment of severe head injury. *J. Neurosurg., 62,* 383–388.

Wolf, A. L., Marmarou, A., Ward, J. D., Muizelaar, J. P., Choi, S. C., Young, H. F., Rigamonti, D., & Robinson, W. L. (1993). Effect of THAM upon outcome in severe head injury: A randomized prospective clinical trial. *J. Neurosurg., 78,* 54–59.

IV

COMMENTARY

15

Implications for Clinical
Care and Cognitive Neuroscience

BENNETT A. SHAYWITZ

This book addresses two distinct but closely linked audiences, each with a different focus of interest. The first is clinical—that is, those professionals caring for children with traumatic brain injury (TBI): pediatricians, child neurologists, neurosurgeons, neuropsychologists, developmental psychologists. To clinicians, the causes and, most important, the outcome of TBI represent a serious problem; from this perspective, the volume offers a rich series of essays that provide the reader with a state-of-the-art view of TBI in children.

The second audience is potentially much broader, comprising scientists who represent the disciplines of cognitive psychology, developmental neurology, and basic neurosciences—scientists who see studies of TBI as a unique opportunity to discern brain function by observing the pattern of behavior in individuals with lesions to particular brain regions. From this perspective, studies of children with TBI can serve as a model for developmental cognitive neuroscience. Distinct from the clinical issues, studies of children with TBI represent an opportunity "to better understand how development proceeds in a child with brain injury . . . how behavior is mediated by the normal and injured brain" (Fletcher, Ewing-Cobbs, Francis, & Levin, this volume). Thus, TBI provides an opportunity to study cognitive function in humans by examining the effects of brain injury on neural function, the classic "lesion" strategy developed in the nineteenth century but which now can exploit the tremendous power of modern neuroscience. Each of these perspectives is examined in this chapter.

Clinical Issues in Traumatic Brain Injury

For the clinician, this book will quickly bring the reader into the mainstream of the often confusing literature of TBI, particularly the studies examining outcome. In no small measure this confusion has been fostered by the failure to critically consider sources of variability in reports of outcome, and it is to this issue that Fletcher and his associates devote the first and perhaps defining chapter of this volume. Because the interpretation of nearly every other one of these chapters depends upon an understanding of the factors discussed in the first, it is considered in some detail.

Fletcher and coworkers begin by identifying three potential sources of variability in studies of outcome: (1) how outcome is measured; (2) the varying nature and severity of both the injury itself and its measurement and the effects of varying conditions existing both prior to the injury—such as the premorbid personality of the child—and the environment to which the child returns; (3) the variability inherent in development, which is unique in studying children.

It should come as no surprise that the assessment of outcome reflects how outcome is measured. In general, Fletcher and colleagues consider assessment measures within three broad domains: (1) clinical judgments of the child by an examiner, which may range from dichotomous categories such as survival versus death to more quantitative assessments such as the Glasgow Outcome Scale; (2) psychometric assessments of the child (representing a range of cognitive and neuromotor abilities); and (3) rating scales and interviews of parents or caregivers about the child's behavior. Fletcher and coworkers highlight two particular measures, the Vineland Adaptive Behavior Scales and the Personality Inventory for Children—Revised, but the reader should recognize that a wide variety of such scales are used to assess a range of behaviors, and that these are administered to both parents (e.g., Shaywitz et al., 1992) and teachers (e.g., Atkins & Pelham, 1992).

Also embedded within this discussion is the decades-old debate over the type of model used to define a clinical disorder such as TBI (i.e., a categorical or a dimensional model). Categorical disorders are characterized as highly discrete entities, that are discontinuous with and sharply demarcated from the normal distribution. Such disorders typically occur as all-or-none phenomena and have distinct cut points that separate affected individuals from the rest of the population; examples include Duchenne muscular dystrophy, cystic fibrosis, and Down's syndrome. Dimensional disorders occur along a continuum that blends into the normal distribution and requires the imposition of often arbitrary cutoff points for identification. Hypertension and obesity represent two of the most common dimensional disorders.

Fletcher and associates make a real contribution in bringing the issue of conceptual model to the attention of clinicians and investigators interested in TBI. Consideration of the most appropriate model to represent TBI, which is not often brought to the fore, in truth plays a critical role in shaping our conceptualization of and approach to this disorder. That is, the model within which a disorder (such as TBI) is viewed provides a conceptual framework for defining and then considering the most critical questions (i.e., diagnosis, epidemiology, treatment, and outcome) necessary to characterize and understand that particular disorder. Thus, the conceptual model (categorical versus dimensional) within which TBI is considered will set the parameters for definition and be inextricably linked both to the clinical care of patients and the strategies chosen to investigate the disorder itself. The interested reader will find this issue discussed in even further detail elsewhere (Blashfield, 1984; Fletcher et al., 1992).

Not surprisingly, variations in both the nature and severity of the injury and how these are measured contribute significantly to variability in outcome. However, while the particular characteristics of the injury are typically factored into considerations of outcome, what is often overlooked is the key role that factors related to measurement may play in influencing data on outcome. Such potential sources of variation may range from differences in the particular point in time that the injury is assessed to the specific measures, clinical and anatomic, used to quantify severity. Thus, variation may result from factors as simple as differences in when the child is assessed (e.g., in the emergency room versus 24 hours later) or from the measures used to assess clinical severity (e.g., Glasgow Coma Scale or duration of posttraumatic amnesia). Even a measurement that appears to be as discrete and objective as determination of the extent of brain injury, even as assessed by modern neuroimaging techniques, is confounded by an often unappreciated group of factors relating both to subject characteristics and selection of anatomic landmarks; this issue is discussed in more detail later. Other sources of variability are external to the injury itself; they are what Fletcher and colleagues broadly consider "environmental sources," encompassing such diverse components as the premordid characteristics of the child and the child's postinjury environment. Awareness of this wide range of potential sources of variation, reflected in the planning of future studies as well as in the interpretation of reported outcomes, should contribute significantly to increasing comparability across studies and to bringing a sense of order and discipline to an often confusing literature.

Finally, Fletcher and coworkers note that the variability inherent in development represents an often unsuspected source of variation, and they devote the final portion of their chapter to a description of a new methodology for determining the measurement of change over time. The notion of change incorporated within previous measurement approaches relied on difference scores in which change was represented as the difference between what was known at two points of measurement. In this view, the acquisition of knowledge, as in children recovering from TBI, was considered from the perspective of change as discrete and incremental, "as the quantized acquisition of skills, attitudes, and beliefs. It is as though the individual is delivered of a quantum of learnings in the time period that intervenes between the premeasure and the postmeasure, and that our only concern should be with the size of the 'chunk' " (Willett, 1988, p. 347).

In contrast, the conceptualization of change embodied by Fletcher and coworkers represents a radically different perspective—one that views change in learning as an ongoing and *continuous process*. Furthermore, the focus is on change over time as a characteristic of *individuals* in contrast to change as a characteristic of groups. It is this reconceptualization of change from an incremental to a continuous process as well as the reshifting of focus from change within a group to change within an individual that allows investigators to examine the trajectories describing this process in individual subjects. Rather than emphasizing the scores, the specific amount of learning that such scores represent at a particular point in time, or the change or increment in scores from one point in time to another, models of individual growth curves seek to define the underlying developmental function—that is, the mathematical function that best describes the ongoing learning process for a particular characteristic or skill. In such a view, any single score represents a point in time reflective of a more basic, ongoing process of change. Such an approach is liberating in many ways: it is very flexible, enabling growth-curve models to accommodate linear/nonlinear as well continuous/discontinuous processes. It is also generalizable; such models are not limited in interpretation to current scores and to the time period being assessed. By describing the underlying developmental function, statements can be made that extend beyond the time frame of the particular measurements. Use of individual growth-curve models allows the investigator to go beyond the specific details of scores and to begin to comprehend the nature of the ongoing learning process underlying performance at each of the time points measured and at points beyond.

The method is summarized briefly here, but Fletcher and his associates provide more detailed descriptions elsewhere (Francis et al., 1994; Shaywitz & Shaywitz, 1994). Individual growth-curve models allow a dynamic view of learning that emphasizes individual change and correlates of change. With the focus on individual growth curves for each particular child, intraindividual differences can be isolated and studied. As illustrated by Fletcher and colleagues, the methodology seems ideally suited to studying the outcome of TBI in children.

With this framework in place, the range of contributions can be better appreciated. Part I serves as a clinical overview of the epidemiology and pathogenesis of TBI. As Kraus's review indicates, TBI represents a serious public health problem. Depending on the vagaries of subject selection, the prevalence of TBI is established at 100–300 per 100,000, with fatality rates varying between 2 and 14 per 100. Injuries associated with transport or resulting from falls account for the great bulk of TBI; significant sex differences are also seen, so that by school age, boys are significantly more likely than girls to suffer TBI.

The mechanisms of brain injury and measures taken to reverse these effects are reviewed by Bruce. He notes that the current state of the art assumes that the primary injury to the brain cannot be modified and that therefore interventions are directed at secondary effects of the injury: systemic hypotension and shock, hypoxia, hypercarbia, and increased intracranial pressure. In addition, Bruce notes that newer studies implicate free radicals as well as excitotoxins in the secondary effects of ischemia. Studies in progress in adults are evaluating the effects of interventions such as hypothermia and a variety of pharmacological agents (e.g., superoxide dismutase designed to quench free radicals, NMDA receptor antagonists, and newer steroids, such as tirilazad).

Clinicians who treat children with head injuries will no doubt find discouraging the paucity of data relating to "safe" limits of cerebral perfusion pressure in children. The cerebral perfusion pressure (CPP) represents the difference between the mean arterial blood pressure and the intracranial pressure. Studies in adults indicate that cerebral blood flow remains constant as long as cerebral perfusion pressure remains above 70 mm Hg. Early data suggested that in children, the critical value may be considerably lower, with cerebral blood flow remaining constant as long as cerebral perfusion pressure remained above 50 mm Hg. Bruce, an experienced clinician and investigator, seems to suggest that the latter belief may be ill founded. The therapeutic implications are significant, and it may be that clinicians should try to maintain CPP above 70 mm Hg even in pediatric populations.

Part II comprises recent empirical studies designed to address outcome after head injury. Shaffer reviews the classic British studies performed in the 1970s on the relationship between head injury and psychiatric illness. Using posttraumatic amnesia as the criterion of severity, these studies found that TBI in children was associated with a variety of psychiatric disorders. While these studies were limited because they did not screen for previous psychiatric disorders, their importance lay with the suggestion that outcome may be potentiated by preexisting psychiatric symptoms as well as a poor psychosocial environment postinjury. As such, these studies provide the only previous evidence to support the interaction of environment and outcome after head injury. Such issues are addressed as well in Chapter 10. Taylor and his associates begin to examine questions of the relationship between environment and head injury in a prospective study, using an interactive model. Though preliminary and a study in progress, its findings provide "the strongest support to date for family influences on the behavioral sequelae of traumatic injury in children."

Mild head injury represents one of the most common clinical problems in pediatrics, and it is reassuring that two chapters examining the outcome of mild head injury find, in general, no permanent effects from such an injury. Taken together, these two reports demonstrate the value of a stringent definition of mild head injury. Asarnow and his associates (Chapter 7) report findings on prospectively studied children (at 12 months) with mild closed head injuries (defined as a Glasgow Coma Scale score of 12 or higher); the great majority of these had periods of unconsciousness of less than 30 minutes. A major innovation in this study was the incorporation of preinjury factors assessed 1 month postinjury; in fact, the inclusion of preinjury functioning proved critical in the conclusion. Bijur and Haslum (Chapter 8) report findings from the British Birth Cohort Study. Although these reports of head injury were retrospective, the authors had available cognitive and behavioral data that preceded the injury as well as comparison groups of children with other types of injuries. Although their results suggest that reading achievement test scores were 2 to 3 points lower in head-injured children than in controls (consistently but not statistically different from controls), these findings were comparable to scores in children with other injuries (burns, fractures, lacerations), suggesting that the differences were not specific to TBI. Children with TBI differed from controls on just one measure—the teacher's report of the child's hyperactivity, which was rated as significantly greater in children with head injury even after controlling for preexisting hyperactivity. However, children with other types of injuries were also rated by their teachers as more hyperactive than children with no injuries. Bijur and Haslum suggest that "the observed differences between the head injured and controls may be largely due to factors that increase the risk of any injury, rather than due to adverse sequelae of damage associated with head trauma." In general, these results are consonant with those of Asarnow and associates. However, a somewhat contrary view is presented by Klonoff and coworkers (Chapter 11), who followed for 23 years a cohort of over 100 children who sustained head injuries at age 8. The majority of these children exhibited mild head injury. About one-third of the sample reported subjective sequelae related to head injury. However, Klonoff and associates did not have the advantage of contemporary approaches to injury characterization; thus, the subjects were not screened for preexisting disorders nor was a control group included. Such methodological problems make it difficult to interpret these findings.

Therapeutic Implications

The experienced clinician and clinical investigator cannot come away from this book without the feeling that tremendous progress has already been made in the study of TBI in children. Thus, empirically based operational definitions have been elaborated and strategies for assessment have been developed that take into consideration a wide range of cognitive and behavioral domains. The elaboration of methods for assessing individual growth curves offers the possibility of quantifying the effects of TBI on development as well as quantifying the inevitable variation in outcome for any single child.

Yet despite the obvious progress that has been made in the field, a number of the authors comment that children have not been included in any of the pharmacological treatment trials of TBI. One suspects that many others share Ward's belief that in "today's current economic, medical, legal, and ethical environment," many investigators are reluctant to include children in clinical trials until the effects of the agents under investigation are established in adults. I suggest that such a view, regarded by West as nonoptimal, may be misguided. There is certainly no scientifically valid reason to continue to exclude children from therapeutic trials. As the papers in this volume attest, the investigators represented here have been able to develop methodologies that can reliably measure outcome, and they have recognized the need to include methods to control for preexisting conditions. Furthermore, the development of models that measure growth curves of specific cognitive functions offer for the first time the possibility of accounting for the variability inherent in development. Given these methodological advances in the investigation of TBI in children, there can be no scientific justification for continuing to exclude children from therapeutic trials. One might turn Ward's question around and ask whether, in today's legal and ethical environment, it is justifiable to continue to exclude subjects from therapeutic trials solely because of their age. The well-intentioned belief that we are "protecting" children by excluding them from studies until all potential risks are established means that we may be excluding children from the potential positive and significant benefits of therapy. We should remember the lessons learned from studies that arbitrarily and capriciously excluded females and minority subjects. Children must be permitted to participate in significant numbers in and benefit from any rational, well-designed therapeutic trials for TBI.

Traumatic Brain Injury as a Model System for Developmental Cognitive Neuroscience

Studies of the localization of cognitive function in brain-damaged individuals represent the basis of the modern doctrine of cerebral localization, and while connectionist models are increasingly being used to explain neural function, cerebral localization continues to represent one of the core tenets of cognitive neuroscience. Historically, the doctrine of cerebral localization generally credited to Broca (though, in fact, the roots of this concept originated a generation before with the work of Franz Joseph Gall) was based on the study of individuals with injuries to specific brain regions (Young, 1990). Our current views represent a continuation and extension of these theories and, until very recently, were all still based upon studies of individuals with brain lesions. From this perspective, studies of children with TBI (assuming one could determine which brain regions were injured) could serve as a model for developmental cognitive neuroscience—an opportunity to illuminate neural mechanisms involved in higher cortical functions in the developing human.

The development of modern neuroimaging techniques allows investigators to begin to try to relate neural function with brain structure in children with TBI, and Chapter 5 serves as a model for such studies. Levin and associates examine the hypothesis that abnormalities on neuropsychological measures generally assumed to reflect frontal lobe function are related to the degree of injury of frontal lobes as determined by neuroimaging. The degree and localization of brain injury is determined independently by a neuroradiologist based upon coronal magnetic resonance imaging (MRI) sections in children recovering from TBI, and these anatomic changes are then related to cognitive measures. Findings suggest that damage to left frontal regions relates to verbal fluency and inhibitory control; right frontal damage is related to semantic performance, verbal fluency, and inhibitory control. In contrast, extrafrontal lesions are not related to performance on any of these cognitive measures. Using a similar strategy, Chapman suggests that damage to frontal regions may be related to performance on measures of discourse processing, though these findings are somewhat tenuous, since they are based on very small numbers of subjects. These findings are reassuring in that they support current dogma relating disinhibition to frontal lobe damage. But they are also quite novel in relating specific deficits in linguistic function to particular brain regions—for example, in demonstrating that abnormalities in semantic processing and verbal fluency are related to anatomic abnormalities in frontal regions.

Not surprisingly, there is no free lunch, and despite these advances in imaging technology, investigators are just beginning to recognize the complexities involved in attempting to relate anatomic changes in the brain to neural function. Thus, recent evidence suggests that differences in subject characteristics (e.g., sex, age, handedness, and variability in the severity of TBI) as well as methodological variations in the landmarks used to define anatomic regions of interest, such as the frontal lobes, may all significantly influence morphometric measures of brain (Schultz et al., 1994). It seems reasonable to suggest that subsequent investigations of TBI in children should, at the very least, incorporate important subject-related characteristics (e.g., sex, age) into the study design.

Traumatic brain injury may also be a useful model to better define and understand the neural basis of particularly difficult psychological constructs, such as attention and attention-deficit hyperactivity disorder (ADHD). Psychologists have been intrigued by the construct of attention for almost a century (James, 1898) and have elaborated a number of conceptual models of the construct, models that vary in their relatedness to one another and to the cognitive and behavioral syndrome of inattention following TBI (Cooley & Morris, 1990; Kinchla, 1992; Mirsky et al., 1991; Posner, 1988; Posner & Petersen, 1990; for a recent review, see Barkley, 1994). Many investigations over the past decade have focused on the ecological validity of laboratory measures commonly used to assess "attention." In these studies, researchers have examined the relationship between performance on laboratory tests of the psychological construct "attention" [e.g., the Continuous Performance Test (CPT) or Cancellation Tasks] and the symptoms referred to as inattention (generally assessed in naturalistic settings by rating scales or observational measurements) reflecting the core symptoms in ADHD. Overall, investigators have not been able to demonstrate consistently strong relationships between measures relating to the psychological construct and those used to diagnose the clinical syndrome; they continue to be frustrated by the apparent lack of ecological validity for the laboratory measures of attention (Achenbach et al., 1987; Barkley, 1991, 1994; Kazdin et al., 1983).

While this background serves to frame the interrelationships between ADHD and measures of attention, what do we know of the associations between ADHD and TBI? At one level, ADHD may be considered as a *predisposing factor* for TBI, as suggested by data from studies such as Bijur's. At another level, abnormalities in attentional processes may represent a significant *cognitive outcome* of TBI, and it is within this context that Chapter 9 should be considered. Dennis and her associates employ two measures of attention in children with brain injury: focused attention (vigilance), as measured by a continuous performance test, and selective attention, a similar measure but one that incorporates distractors. Their results indicate differences in performance between normal children and subjects with TBI. Clearly, the next step will be to determine how performance on these measures relates to cerebral localization and to the behaviors generally considered as inattention or distractibility.

Future Directions

Investigations designed to explore the reorganization of the brain following TBI in children offer an opportunity to elucidate some of the most fundamental questions of modern neuroscience. Studies incorporating modern connectionist views of brain organization have begun, and in Chapter 12 Grafman and Salazar review such studies in adults, using a technique (in this case, transcranial magnetic stimulation) that allows, in contrast to static views of brain anatomy using MRI, the dynamic assessment of neural function. To date, functional studies have not been performed in children, but clearly they are now possible. The development of functional imaging methods using positron emission tomography (Demonet, Wise & Frackowiak, 1993; Petersen & Fiez, 1993) and of perhaps more relevance in children, functional MRI (Shaywitz et al., 1995a; Shaywitz et al., 1995b) opens new vistas to the study of brain function in the developing nervous system—studies which could combine lesion studies (TBI) with functional imaging measures to better understand the cognitive organization of the child's brain and its reorganization following injury. These technologies offer, for the first time, an opportunity to examine the relationship between performance on specific cognitive and behavioral measures and the functional (as opposed to the static anatomic) localization of activity in particular brain regions. The challenge for the field is how best to combine these remarkable new technologies with careful studies of individual children who have suffered traumatic brain injury, studies which may ultimately lead to more specific and effective therapies for one of the most significant clinical problems of childhood.

References

Achenbach, T. M., McConaughy, S. H., & Howell, C. T. (1987). Child/adolescent behavioral and emotional problems: Implications of cross informant correlations for situational specificity. *Psychol. Bull., 101,* 213–232.

Atkins, M. S., & Pelham, W. E. (1992). School-based assessment of attention deficit-hyperactivity disorder. In S. E. Shaywitz & B. S. Shaywitz (Eds.), *Attention deficit disorder comes of age: Toward the twenty-first century* (pp. 69–88). Austin, TX: Pro-Ed.

Barkley, R. A. (1991). The ecological validity of laboratory and analogue assessment methods of ADHD symptoms. *J. Abnorm. Child Psychol., 19,* 149–178.

Barkley, R. A. (1994). The assessment of attention in children. In G. Reid Lyon (Ed.), *Frames of reference for the assessment of learning disabilities* (pp. 69–102). Baltimore, MD: Paul H. Brookes.

Blashfield, R. K. (1984). *The classification of psychopathology: NeoKraepelinian and quantitative approaches.* New York: Plenum.

Cooley, E. L., & Morris, R. D. (1990). Attention in children: A neuropsychologically based model for assessment. *Dev. Neuropsychol., 6,* 239–274.

Demonet, J. F., Wise, R., & Frackowiak, R. S. J. (1993). Language functions explored in normal subjects by positron emission tomography: A critical review. *Human Brain Mapping, 1,* 39–47.

Fletcher, J. M., Morris, R. D., & Francis, D. J. (1992). Methodological issues in the classification of attention-related disorders. In S. E. Shaywitz & B. S. Shaywitz (Eds.), *Attention deficit disorder comes of age: Toward the twenty-first century* (pp. 13–28). Austin, TX: Pro-Ed.

Francis, D. J., Shaywitz, S. E., Stuebing, K. K., Shaywitz, B. A., & Fletcher, J. M. (1994). The measurement of change: Assessing behavior over time and within a developmental context. In G. R. Lyon (Ed.), *Frames of reference for the assessment of learning disabilities: New views on measurement issues* (pp. 29–68). Baltimore, MD: Paul H. Brookes.

James, W. (1898). *Principles in psychology*. Chicago: University of Chicago Press.

Kazdin, A. E., Esveldt-Dawson, K., & Loar, L. L. (1983). Correspondence of teacher ratings and direct observations of classroom behavior of psychiatric inpatient children. *J. Abnorm. Child Psychol., 11,* 549–564.

Kinchla, R. A. (1992). Attention. *Annu. Rev. Psychol., 43,* 711–742.

Mirsky, A. F., Anthony, B. J., Duncan, C. C., Ahearn, M. B., & Kellam, S. G. (1991). Analysis of the elements of attention: A neuropsychological approach. *Neuropsychol. Rev., 2,* 109–145.

Petersen, S. E., & Fiez, J. A. (1993). The processing of single words studied with positron emission tomography. *Annu. Rev. Neurosci., 16,* 509–530.

Posner, M. (1988). Structures and functions of selective attention. In T. Boll & B. K. Bryant (Eds.), *Clinical neuropsychology and brain function: Research, measurement, and practice* (pp. 169–202). Washington, DC: American Psychological Association.

Posner, M., & Peterson, S. (1990). The attention system of the human brain. *Annu. Rev. Neurosci., 13,* 25–42.

Schultz, R. T., Cho, N. K., Staib, L. H., Kier, L. E., Fletcher, J. M., Shaywitz, S. E., Shankweiler, D. P., Katz, L., Gore, J. in normal and dyslexic children: The influence of sex and age. *Ann. Neurol., 35,* 732–742.

Shaywitz, B. A., Pugh, K. R., Constable, R., Shaywitz, S. E., Bronen, R. T., Fulbright, R. K., Shankweiler, D. P., Katz, L., Fletcher, J. M., Skudlarski, P., & Gore, J. C. (1995a). Localization of semantic processing using functional magnetic resonance imaging. *Hum. Brain Map., 2,* 1–10.

Shaywitz, B. A., and Shaywitz, S. E. (1994). Measuring and analyzing change. In G. Reid Lyon (Ed.), *Frames of reference for the assessment of learning disabilities: New views on measurement issues* (pp. 59–68). Baltimore, MD: Paul H. Brookes.

Shaywitz, B. A., Shaywitz, S. E., Pugh, K. R., Constable, R. T., Skudlarski, P., Fulbright, R. K., Bronen, R. A., Fletcher, J. M., Shankweiler, D. P., Katz, L., Gore, J. C. (1995b). Sex differences in the functional organization of the brain for language. *Nature, 373,* 607–609.

Shaywitz, S. E., Holahan, J. M., Marchione, K. E., Sadler, A. E., & Shaywitz, B. A. (1992). The Yale Children's Inventory: Normative data and their implications for the diagnosis of attention deficit disorder in children. In S. E. Shaywitz, & B. B. Shaywitz (Eds.), *Attention deficit disorder comes of age: Toward the twenty-first century* (pp. 29–68). Austin, TX: PRO-ED.

Willett, J. B. (1988). Questions and answers in the measurement of change. *Rev. Res. Ed., 15,* 345–422.

Young, R. M. (1990). *Mind, brain and adaptation in the nineteenth century*. New York: Oxford University Press.

16

A Summing Up

ARTHUR BENTON

This volume documents the substantial progress that has been achieved in recent years in our understanding of the etiology, mechanisms, and consequences of traumatic brain injury in children. These advances are due in no small part to the efforts of the investigators and clinicians whose contributions were presented in the workshop that gave rise to this book. With perhaps one exception (namely, the formidable issue of prevention), all the facets of this major health problem have been covered thoroughly and with uncommon insight.

No one needs to be told that the prevalence of traumatic brain injury in children has reached an alarming height, even though the majority of cases are classified as "mild." The epidemiological analyses of Kraus (chapter 2) give us some indication of the impressive breadth and depth of the problem. Bruce reports that head injury is the single most frequent condition he is called upon to treat in his pediatric neurosurgical practice. A particularly poignant note is sounded by his observations that head injury is now the leading cause of death in children and that child abuse is now the leading cause of fatal injury in infants. Remarkable advances in the neurosurgical management of head injury in children have resulted in a very significant decrease in mortality. However, for the most part, this has meant a corresponding increase in morbidity, as it has in the comparable field of extreme prematurity (Hack et al., 1989, 1991).

Etiology and Pathology

Bruce (Chapter 3) has described the modes of action of physical forces that lead to traumatic brain injury (e.g., acceleration and deceleration, impact). These forces produce diffuse or focal injury that can take a number of forms, including hematomas, contusions, injury to blood vessels, brain swelling, and axonal injury. The application of magnetic resonance imaging now permits the timely identification of these changes, which can be followed by interventions that may prevent adverse complications such as intracranial hypertension. Bruce has presented a frank picture of the complexities of the situation facing the neurosurgeon and of the many issues that still require clarification. Both he and Ward (Chapter 14) raise incisive questions about some of the assumptions that guide current neurosurgical practice.

A noteworthy development in recent years is the enhanced appreciation of the significance of axonal injury. It was on the basis of her autopsy studies of patients who did not survive their injuries that Sabina Strich introduced this concept in 1956, and her observations on "diffuse degeneration of the white matter" in non-surviving patients were confirmed in the 1960s. The advent of MRI, which allowed visualization of white matter in the living patient, made it clear that "shearing," as it came to be called, was a common result of closed head injury and that it was by no means confined to patients who did not survive or in whom the outcome was a severe dementia or vegetative state. Instead, it is frequently found in patients with mild and moderate injuries (Povlishock et al., 1983, 1992; Dixon et al., 1993). Moreover, associations between focal axonal injury and cognitive deficits during the chronic epoch have been demonstrated (Levin et al., 1985). However, axonal injury does occur within the context of other brain changes, and it is not altogether clear that it is axonal injury per se that is responsible for the observed behavioral changes. More often than not, one finds focal axonal injury in the surviving children, who are our primary interest, whatever significance diffuse axonal injury may have for survival or the persistent vegetative state.

Experimental study in animals of the neurochemical alterations that take place in the traumatically injured brain has become a research area of increasing importance (Becker et al., 1987; Stein & Sabel, 1988; Hayes et al., 1989). Attention has focused largely on the action of neurotransmitters on receptor neurons. There is substantial evidence that one effect of brain trauma is to liberate excessive amounts of acetylcholine. A major guiding hypothesis is that the release of acetylcholine modifies agonist-receptor interactions and that these changes lead to behavioral impairment, usually temporary but sometimes long-standing. This research effort is still in a preliminary stage and its possible implications for therapeutic application to human patients have still to be worked out.

Ward (Chapter 14) and Fletcher and colleagues (Chapter 1) have pointed out some of the distinctive problems posed by head injury in children as contrasted to that in adults. The organism with a developing nervous system may react differently to trauma, and specific interventions may have to be modified in view of their implications for a child's future development. Ward has outlined the requirements that clinical trials have to meet if valid findings are to be secured, and he has specified the directions such trials might take.

The chapters by Bruce, Levin and colleagues, and Ward reflect the noteworthy advances of recent years in the treatment of acute head injury in children. In addition, they have presented valuable recommendations for investigative work that will resolve unanswered questions and enhance the effectiveness of treatment. There is now clear recognition of the diverse factors that must be taken into account in alleviating the effects of the injury and preventing the occurrence of secondary complications.

The Behavioral Consequences

From a behavioral standpoint, we often divide the consequences of childhood head injury into the cognitive domain, the affective-emotional domain, the influence of the family and social support systems on the course of recovery, and finally the injured child's effect on the fortunes of the family itself. Divisions like these are necessary to achieve progress. However, as Fletcher and his coauthors emphasize, these domains are interrelated and interactive. Cognitive impairment disrupts emotional responsiveness, and emotional disturbance has cognitive consequences. Sometimes it is difficult to decide whether a behavioral manifestation (for example, disinhibition) should be viewed as an "emotional" or a "cognitive" defect. It is reasonable to anticipate that a supportive family setting will foster recovery to the extent that this is possible, but in some instances the heavy burden of caring for a brain-injured child may disrupt that nurturant function. Thus, in interpreting the diverse behavioral consequences of head injury, it is well for both the clinician and the investigator to keep the total picture in mind. It will surely affect their remediation efforts and their interpretations of symptoms.

A broad spectrum of cognitive deficits in moderately and severely head-injured children is clearly demonstrated in the studies of Chapman, Ewing-Cobbs, Fletcher, and Levin (Chapters 1, 5, and 6). Overall intellectual impairment (with, however, marked interindividual variation) is indicated by Verbal and Performance Scale IQs that are much below those of controls in the severely injured and less strikingly (but significantly) so in children who have sustained moderate injury. More focused measures—such as, for example, those assessing attention, verbal learning, nonverbal visual memory, and problem solving—show even larger intergroup differences.

In themselves the findings are not surprising; in the main, they confirm the indications of widespread and varied intellectual defects found in earlier reports. What is new about these studies is that they are guided by hypotheses based on current conceptions of brain-behavior relationships and that they generate specific predictions.

Attention

Attention is an old concept in psychology and its importance has always been recognized. Attention underpins learning and retention. Its disruption is responsible at least in part for the academic difficulties that head-injured children experience, particularly those whose overall intelligence level as measured by conventional IQ tests would predict better school progress.

But it has been an unwieldy concept that was defined differently by different authors, was difficult to formulate in a useful way, was not readily separated from other cognitive processes, and posed formidable problems of measurement. Although clinical examiners have often treated it as such, attention is not a unitary process. In recent years great progress has been made in fractionating "attention" into its components, in the development of neuropsychologically meaningful classifications of types of attention, and in relating these types to underlying neural systems and physiological events. The work of Posner (1989; Posner & Rafal, 1987; Posner & Petersen, 1990) and Van Zomeren (1981; Van Zomeren & Brouwer, 1994) exemplifies the advances that have been made in theoretical analysis and clinical application in the field.

Dennis has adopted one such classification in her studies of attention in children with closed head injury. Three types are investigated: *focused attention* (sometimes called sustained attention, concentration, or vigilance), reflecting the capacity to maintain a preparatory set over time; *selective* attention, reflecting the capacity to maintain the preparatory set in the face of competing stimuli or distractors; and *response inhibition,* reflecting the capacity to respond appropriately only at a given point in time. Some salient findings were that measures of selective attention generated greater differences between the head-injured and normal children than did measures of focused attention and that children with documented bifrontal damage showed particularly severe impairment on the response inhibition task, an observation which is consistent with well-known findings in the literature on the behavioral correlates of frontal lobe disease in adults. It was also found that head injury sustained before the age of 7 years produced more severe impairment of attentional processes than did injury incurred at a later age. As a number of authors have pointed out, this may be because the prefrontal region is still incompletely developed at this early age.

In Chapter 9 Dennis and colleagues make it clear that the assessment of attentional processes is a promising field for both investigation and clinical evaluation. Their report provides fairly sensitive measures of brain dysfunction that are minimally affected by cultural factors. It can be used in the initial workup as well as to monitor the course of recovery and to assess outcome. One would hope that it could be used to guide the selection of rehabilitation procedures.

Reaction time (RT) was the primary measure (along with incorrect and omitted responses) used in the Dennis studies, as it is in most studies of attention. Most RT tasks measure either focused attention or selective attention. It may prove to be useful, however, to distinguish between the concepts of attention and speed of information processing. Some RT tasks (e.g., simple visual RT under optimal conditions of presentation with a warning signal as well as the most favorable time interval between the warning signal and the presentation of the stimulus) make only modest demands on focused attention. Yet simple visual RT effectively discriminates adult patients with brain disease from control patients; indeed, in some studies it has been found to be as effective a discriminator as more demanding and complex RT tasks (Blackburn & Benton, 1955; Klentsch, 1973; Van Zomeren & Deelman, 1976). Comparison of the performances of a head-injured child on different RT tasks may help to identify the locus of any impairment, permit inferences about the status of the underlying neural networks, and guide the selection of reeducation procedures. It is worth repeating that these tasks are largely "culture free," which is an advantage in a society where "cultural diversity" is currently such a popular theme.

Learning and Retention

There is general agreement that impairment in new learning is the type of deficit that is most frequently encountered in head-injured children as well as in adults. The studies reported by Levin, Ewing-Cobbs, and Eisenberg (Chapter 5) provide abundant support for this belief. The learning and retention of both verbal and nonverbal material appear to be equally affected. As with other behavioral functions, the degree of impairment is significantly related to the severity of the injury. The vulnerability of learning and retention abilities is reflected in the finding that almost all children with injuries rated as moderate or severe show defective performances. The degree to which attentional disturbance, as compared to difficulty in consolidation and storage of information, contributes to failure on learning tasks must be analyzed in the individual case.

Language Abilities and Judgment

Impairment in language functions—as assessed by tests of vocabulary, confrontation naming, repetition, and verbal understanding—was found by Levin, Ewing-Cobbs, and Eisenberg (Chapter 5) to be relatively infrequent in children with a history of mild or moderate head injury. Such defects as were found were in the realm of expressive rather than receptive language. Nor does it appear that reading ability is particularly vulnerable to traumatic head injury. In contrast, writing to dictation and arithmetic calculation are typically more severely affected (Levin & Benton, 1986; Chapter 5).

The findings of these carefully designed studies may be accepted at face value. However, as the investigations on discourse and the pragmatics of language described by Chapman (Chapter 6) indicate, the relationship of these test findings to the language behavior of the head-injured child in situations more closely approximating those of real life needs to be clarified. "Discourse" may be defined as the employment of language abilities to express ideas and to achieve effective communication—"the use of words in the service of thought," as Hughlings Jackson once phrased it. The work of Chapman and the earlier studies cited by her suggest that defective narrative discourse may persist for an extraordinarily long time after apparent recovery from a head injury. That this should be the case is not surprising, since narrative discourse (e.g., telling a complicated story) involves the participation of a number of cognitive capacities such as short-term memory, integration of elements of information, and discriminating between the important and the unimportant, any one of which may still be residually impaired. In these preliminary studies, Chapman has found that in children with severe head injuries, both the number of words and sentences employed and the amount of information in their narratives are markedly lower than in control children. In contrast, no differences between children with mild/moderate injuries and controls on any of these measures were obtained. Thus there is as yet no evidence that analysis of narrative discourse will add specific incremental information to an initial diagnostic evaluation. However, since discourse is such a vital ingredient of effective communication, its assessment does have a direct bearing on plans for the management and rehabilitation of head-injured children.

Brain-Behavior Relationships

The advent of modern neurodiagnostic techniques created new possibilities for understanding the neurological basis for the diverse behavioral deficits shown by head-injured children. Foremost among the investigators who have employed these techniques are Harvey Levin and his coworkers, some of whose findings are reported in this volume. Abnormalities on magnetic resonance imaging (MRI) are invariably observed in children who have sustained injuries that on clinical grounds were classified as severe. The well-known predilection for head trauma to affect the anterior region of the brain has been strikingly confirmed; in fact, trauma that involves nonfrontal areas exclusively is rather uncommon. Further analysis indicated that correlations between focal injury and specific cognitive deficits could be demonstrated (e.g., between size of lesion in the left frontal region and controlled word association performance). Levin and colleagues consider their findings to be only of a preliminary nature; there is little doubt that future study will disclose other significant brain-behavior associations.

Familial and Social Factors

Fletcher and coworkers note the reciprocal relationship between the head-injured child and his or her environment, particularly the family and school. Although data on the issue are scarce, there can be little doubt that the quality of the environment significantly affects behavioral outcome in mild and moderate head injury. In a related area, that of "minimal brain dysfunction" (MBD), there is substantial evidence that social and familial factors have a determining influence on such symptoms as aggressive behavior, hyperactivity, and attention disorder (Paternite et al., 1976; Paternite & Loney, 1980; Werner, 1980). General factors such as socioeconomic status and more specific factors such as marital harmony and level of parental concern appear to be decisive in the symptom picture, not only in childhood but also later, in the adolescent years. Paternite and coworkers found that aggressive behavior in MBD children was correlated with ratings of one or both of their parents as being "too short-tempered," "too strict," and "too busy." Confirmatory findings on the influence of social, familial, and educational factors on outcome in at-risk children have been reported in more recent studies (Wilson, 1985; Sameroff et al., 1987; Leonard et al., 1990; Korhonen et al., 1993). Thus it is reasonable to conclude that at least some of the behavioral sequelae of brain dysfunction, traumatic and nontraumatic, are not an invariant effect of a child's neurological status but rather the product of an interaction between neurological and environmental factors.

However, the relationship between head injury and the social and familial environment must be viewed as bidirectional. The presence of a head-injured child in the household—with its special demands of increased attention and care, its effect on expectations about the future of the child, its bias toward differential treatment of siblings, and its strain on financial resources—may create a stressful situation to which both parents and siblings may react adversely.

The carefully designed prospective study of Taylor and his coworkers addresses this issue of the impact of childhood head injury on family functioning. Only preliminary data are available, since the investigation is still in progress; however, coupled with the findings of an earlier study by Perrott and associates (1991), the results are highly suggestive. Parents experience significantly higher stress in dealing with their head-injured children than in their interactions with their normal children. A primary source of this undue stress is the head-injured child's social behavior—in addition to poor academic achievement, which is often below the level that his or her psychometrically assessed cognitive capacities would predict. While we must await the more definitive outcome of this comprehensive study, it seems likely that it will provide evidence for a circular interactive process in which the child's behavior induces parental stress, which, in turn, reinforces the child's poor psychosocial adjustment.

Mild Head Injury

"Mild head injury" is a topic of paramount importance, since some 80% to 90% of reported cases are placed in this category. The term generally refers to the condition of a child with an initially high Glasgow Coma Scale score of 13 to 15 who is usually sent home after examination or may be hospitalized for injuries not involving the central nervous system. However, the defining criteria have differed somewhat from one study to another, particularly with respect to the variable of duration of coma (Dikmen & Levin, 1993). Moreover, it is not at all clear that the Glasgow Coma Scale score is an adequate measure of the severity of brain injury (see Beers, 1992; and Taylor et al., this volume).

The findings of the studies reported by Asarnow (Chapter 7) and Bijur and Harlum (Chapter 8) as well as by Shaffer (Chapter 4) of the earlier studies of the Rutter group are almost entirely negative on the question of the occurrence of behavioral disabilities reasonably ascribable to mild head injury. The study of Fay and coworkers (1993) confirms these negative results. From a methodological standpoint, these recent large-scale investigations represent a distinct advance over earlier studies that did not include matched control groups but instead depended upon published normative standards for interpreting the performances of head-injured children. Taking account of the diverse factors that affect the empirical findings, these studies control (about as well as one can) the variables that are likely to add noise to the system as well as those that would bias the results in one direction or another. Their samples are community-based and account is taken of *preinjury status,* which is clearly related to postinjury status.

As we know, there have historically been two warring camps on this issue of the sequelae of mild head injury in children—which was so often beclouded by claims for compensation for disabilities allegedly resulting from the injury. A hard-boiled negatavistic school viewed the complaints at best as arising from parental anxiety and at worst as being simply fraudulent. But a more liberal school of neurologists and psychiatrists was at least willing to entertain the possibility that apparently trivial head trauma could produce brain injury leading to behavioral impairment. Generally they had no hard evidence to support their position. Rather, clinical intuition told them that the patient's behavior and disabilities had an unmistakably "organic" flavor. Now it is clear that the findings of recent studies have come down in favor of the negativistic school.

Since mild head injury in children is far more frequent than moderate or severe injury, the generally negative results of these excellent studies are gratifying. Yet it would be unfortunate if this led to a casual dismissal of the testimony of parents or teachers of a child who has sustained an apparently trivial injury. The overall findings do not exclude the possibility that as a consequence of a "mild" head injury, some children in fact have suffered behavioral disability that only becomes evident as they are confronted by increasing intellectual, academic, and social demands with advancing age.

The only truly long-term study relevant to the question is the 23-year follow-up reported in the chapter by Klonoff and associates. As they point out, this study dealing with children, the great majority of whom were considered to have sustained a "mild" injury, is fairly limited in scope. Moreover, the less than adequate control of a number of determining variables makes interpretation of the findings difficult. Yet this pioneer study demonstrates that long-term follow-up studies can be undertaken, and the findings are of interest in suggesting that apparently mild injury can sometimes have long-term sequelae. In any case, delayed deterioration after a symptom-free period, although hardly qualifying as a remote effect, is a well-known phenomenon (Snoek, 1989).

The literature on adults indicates that a latent or asymptomatic period after head injury can be followed by very serious disability. Perhaps the most striking example is the "dementia pugilistica" of professional boxers. The classic study of Corsellis and associates (1973) documented obvious brain pathology at autopsy in boxers who for years had shown no obvious signs of mental deterioration. A typical picture is that of a veteran boxer who retires from the ring, usually after a few defeats attributable to reduced physical stamina and slowing of complex reaction time, but without obvious decline from his level of intellectual function. Then, after some years of stability, a progressive deterioration (often accompanied by parkinsonian features) sets in, reaching an end state of at least moderate and more often severe dementia.

Another study of adults suggesting that early brain injury may have at least moderately adverse remote effects is that of Corkin and coworkers (1989), in which World War II veterans with penetrating head injuries were reexamined 30 years after their initial examination at a mean age of 32 years. The essential finding was that these brain-injured veterans (mean age 62 years at reexamination) showed a somewhat steeper decline in mental ability than did a control group of veterans with peripheral nerve injuries. There was also an indication that the decline first began to manifest itself when the veterans were in their forties (i.e., some 10 years after the initial assessment).

There are too many distinctive characteristics of the adult cases to warrant an analogy with mild childhood head injury. Nevertheless, these findings in adult cases suggest that comparable long-term studies of asymptomatic mildly head-injured children and their controls should be carried out to determine whether or not there are adverse remote effects of the early injury. It is quite possible that a significant "silent" effect of traumatic head injury is to reduce "brain reserve capacity," with the consequence that overt behavioral impairment appears only in later life under the stress created by increased environmental demands (see Satz, 1993, for a discussion of this concept).

Rehabilitation

Michaud has provided a realistic evaluation of the efficacy of current intervention and rehabilitation techniques in dealing with the sequelae of head injury in children. The considerable variability of the posttraumatic course noted by Fletcher and colleagues in children (Chapter 1) and by Grafman and Salazar in adults (Chapter 12) makes it extremely difficult to disentangle the effects of treatment from those of other determinants of course and outcome. This uncertainty is, of course, not restricted to the field of head injury. For example, the effectiveness of psychotherapy is still a contentious issue and the value of aphasia rehabilitation in stroke patients is still debated.

The Road Ahead

The contributions to this volume not only present detailed analyses of our present status of knowledge of the diverse determinants of outcome in children with head injury but also emphasize the gaps and limitations in our knowledge. In many instances the specific investigative approaches and strategies that need to be adopted to advance our understanding are identified.

"Outcome," the theme of this volume and the workshop on which it is based, itself requires adequate definition in terms of measurement and duration of observation. As Fletcher and coworkers point out, the variation in judgments about what constitutes a "good" or a "bad" outcome is quite striking. Generally speaking, neurosurgeons and neurologists, who have been concerned primarily with the survival and prevention of gross disability in an acutely head-injured child, are more liberal in their assessments than are psychologists, psychiatrists, and educators, whose primary concern is with the life adjustment and academic progress of the child during the chronic epoch. The evaluation of the modification of the Glasgow Outcome Scale (GOS) applied to head-injured children by Miner and colleagues (1986) shows that it was not useful for assessing the posttraumatic status of the school-age head-injured child. Too many children whose condition was rated as "good" were in fact experiencing serious academic difficulties. This is not to say that the GOS is without merit; it has its place as a first approximation. But obviously the "good" category must be fractionated into a number of levels.

There are a number of psychometric tests and rating scales that have been used occasionally to assess posttraumatic abilities and the quality of life and adjustment, but none has been widely employed. There is a definite need to evaluate the usefulness of these instruments as well as for the development of new instruments that would provide cogent assessments of the behavioral capacities of head-injured children. Standardized measures that enjoy wide use would foster effective communication among workers in the field and provide realistic guides for management and rehabilitation. One would hope that these instruments would be of reasonable length and free of the time-consuming redundancy that characterizes so many assessment protocols.

Recent advances in the neurosurgical management of acute head injuries have resulted not only in a remarkable increase in survival rate but also in a reduction of the secondary complications that are so often the primary determinants of posttraumatic status. It is, of course, not possible to predict the extent to which progress in surgical intervention and pharmacological treatment will further mitigate the effects of acute head injury. But the advances that have been made bode well. Substantial support should be provided to resolve the questions that have been posed and to undertake the clinical trials that have been discussed. This is almost certainly the most fruitful area in which research efforts should be concentrated. Irreversible traumatic brain damage is a process that takes place over time. Surely early intervention is the next best thing to prevention.

Study of the behavioral consequences of head injury has now moved from the descriptive level, in which diverse deficits were identified, to a truly neuropsychological level in which correlations between specific disabilities and lesional variables (e.g., frontal lobe dysfunction) are being established. This multidisciplinary investigative approach has already led to a deeper understanding of the neurological basis of the behavioral deviations seen in traumatically injured children. Research of this type deserves strong encouragement. Its findings cannot help but lead to more useful interpretations of the behavior of the head-injured child, and these, in turn, may be expected to improve management and rehabilitation.

It was stated at the beginning of this chapter that with perhaps one exception all the major aspects of childhood head injury were dealt with in this book and in the preceding workshop. That exception is the problem of preventing the occurrence of head injury in the first instance. The ultimate goal of medicine and public health is the prevention of disease and disability. Contemporary medicine reflects this conviction in its strong emphasis on such measures as the control of diet, cessation of smoking, and prophylactic medication and fluoridation to thwart or at least retard the development of cardiovascular, neoplastic, and dental disease.

Preventive intervention takes a number of forms. There are legally mandated measures such as fluoridation, specifications for the design of automobiles, and the prohibition of smoking in public and private establishments. There are educational programs designed to give individuals the motivation and knowledge to change their behavior in a desirable direction. There is direct intervention to alleviate familial dysfunction and help individuals cope with their problems through home visits and individual counseling, the assumption being that successful intervention will reduce the probability of the development of physical and mental disorders.

The major risk factors for head injury in children are fairly well known. They are physical abuse in infants and young children, sports and roughhousing in schoolchildren, and vehicular accidents and gunshot wounds in children of all ages. Should not those specialists who are most intimately concerned with alleviating the consequences of childhood head injury take the lead in promoting the legal, social, and educational measures that, if implemented, would significantly reduce these risk factors?

References

Becker, D. P., Jenkins, L. W., & Rabow, L. (1987). The pathophysiology of head trauma. In T. A. Miller & B. J. Rowlands (Eds.), *The physiological basis of modern surgical care.* St. Louis, MO: Mosby.

Beers, S. R. (1992). Cognitive effects of mild brain injury in children and adolescents. *Neuropsychol. Rev., 3,* 281–320.

Blackburn, H. L., & Benton, A. L. (1955). Simple and choice reaction time in cerebral disease. *Confinia Neurologica, 15,* 327–338.

Corkin, S., Rosen, T. J., Sullivan, E. V., & Clegg, R. A. (1989). Penetrating head injury in young adulthood exacerbates cognitive decline in later years. *J. Neurosci., 9,* 3876–3883.

Corsellis, J. A. N., Bruton, C. J., & Freeman-Browne, D. (1973). The aftermath of boxing. *Psycholog. Med., 3,* 270–301.

Dikmen, S. S., & Levin, H. S. (1993). Methodological issues in the study of mild head injury. *J. Head Trauma Rehabil., 3,* 30–37.

Dixon, C. E., Taft, W. C., & Hayes, R. L. (1993). Mechanisms of mild traumatic brain injury. *J. Head Trauma Rehabil., 8,* 1–12.

Fay, G. C., Jaffe, K. M., Polissar, N. L., Liao, S., Maftin, K. M., Shurtleff, H. A., Rivara, J. B., & Winn, H. R. (1993). Mild pediatric traumatic brain injury: A cohort study. *Arch. Phys. Med. Rehabil., 74,* 895–901.

Hack, M., & Fanaroff, A. A. (1989). Outcomes of extremely low birth-weight infants between 1982 and 1988. *N. Engl. J. Med., 320,* 1642–1647.

Hack, M., Horbar, J. D., Malloy, M. H., Tyson, J. E., Wright E., & Wright, L. (1991). Very low birth weight outcomes of the National Institute of Child Health and Human Development Neonatal Network. *Pediatrics 87,* 587–597.

Hayes, R. L., Lyeth, B. G., & Jenkins, L. W. (1989). Neurochemical mechanisms of mild and moderate head injury: Implications for treatment. In H. S. Levin, H. M. Eisenberg, & A. L. Benton (Eds.), *Mild head injury.* New York: Oxford University Press.

Klentsch, H. (1973). Die diagnostische Valenz der Reaktionszeitmessung bei verschiedenen zerebralen Erkrankungen. *Fortschr. Neurol. Psychiatr., 41,* 575–581.

Korhonen, T. T., Vähä-Eskell, E., Sillanpää, M., & Kero, P. (1993). Neuropsychological sequelae of perinatal complications: A 6-year follow-up. *J. Clin. Child Psychol., 22,* 226–235.

Leonard, C. H., Clyman, R. I., Piecuch, R. E., Juster, R. P., Ballard, R. A., & Behle, M. B. (1990). Effects of medical and social risk factors on outcome of prematurity and very low birth weight. *J. Pediatr., 116,* 620–626.

Levin, H. S., & Benton, A. L. (1986). Developmental and acquired dyscalculia in children. In I. Flehmig & L. Stern (Eds.), *Child development and learning behavior.* Stuttgart: Gustav Fischer Verlag.

Levin, H. S., Handel, S. F., Goldman, A. M., Eisenberg, H. M., & Guinto, F. C. Jr. (1985). Magnetic resonance imaging after "diffuse" nonmissile injury. *Arch. Neurol., 42,* 963–968.

Miner, M. E., Fletcher, J. M., & Ewings-Cobb, L. (1986). Recovery versus outcome after head injury in children. In M. E. Miner & K. A. Wagner (Eds.), *Neural trauma: Treatment, monitoring and rehabilitation issues.* Stoneham, MA: Butterworth.

Paternite, C. E., & Loney, J. (1980). Child hyperkinesis: Relationships between symptomatology and home environment. In C. B. Whalen & B. Henker (Eds.), *Hyperactive children.* New York: Academic Press.

Paternite, C. E., Loney, J., & Langhorne, J. E. (1976). Relationship between symptomatology and SES-related factors in hyperactive/MBD boys. *Am. J. Orthopsychiatry, 46,* 291–301.

Perrott, S. B., Taylor, H. G., & Montest, J. L. (1991). Neuropsychological sequelae, familial stress, and environmental adaptation following pediatric head injury. *Dev. Neuropsych., 7,* 69–86.

Posner, M. I. (1989). *Foundations of cognitive science.* Cambridge, MA: MIT Press.

Posner, M. I., & Petersen, S. E. (1990). The attention system of the human brain. *Annu. Rev. Psychol., 13,* 182–196.

Posner, M. I., & Rafal, R. D. (1987). Cognitive theories of attention and the rehabilitation of attentional deficits. In M. J. Meier, A. Benton, & L. Diller (Eds.), *Neuropsychological rehabilitation.* Edinburgh: Churchill Livingstone.

Povlishock, J. T., Becker, D. P., Cheng, C. L. Y., & Vaughan, G. W. (1983). Axonal change in minor head injury. *J. Neuropathol. Exp. Neurol., 42,* 225–242.

Povlishock, J. T., Erb, D. E., & Astruc, J. (1992). Axonal response to traumatic brain injury: Reactive axonal change, deafferentation, and neuroplasticity. *J. Neurotrauma, 9* (suppl.), S189–S200.

Sameroff, A. J., Seifer, R., Barocas, R., Zax, M., & Greenspan, S. (1987). Intelligence quotient scores of 4-year-old children: Social-environmental risk factors. *Pediatrics 79,* 343–350.

Satz, P. (1993). Brain reserve capacity on symptom onset after brain injury: A formulation and review of evidence for threshold theory. *Neuropsychology, 7,* 273–295.

Snoek, J. W. (1989). Mild head injury in children. In H. S. Levin, H. M. Eisenberg, & A. L. Benton (Eds.), *Mild Head Injury.* New York: Oxford University Press.

Stein, D. G., & Sabel, B. A. (1988). *Pharmacological approaches to the treatment of brain and spinal cord injury.* New York: Plenum.

Strich, S. J. (1956). Diffuse degeneration of the cerebral white matter in severe dementia following head injury. *J. Neurol. Neurosurg. Psychiatry, 19,* 163–185.

Van Zomeren, A. H. (1981). *Reaction time and attention after cerebral injury.* Lisse, The Netherlands: Swets Publishing.

Van Zomeren, A. H., & Brouwer, W. H. (1994). *Clinical neuropsychology of attention.* New York: Oxford University Press.

Van Zomeren, A. H., & Deelman, B. G. (1976). Differential effects of simple choice reaction after closed head injury. *Clin. Neurol. Neurosurg., 79,* 81–90.

Werner, E. E. (1980). Environmental interactions in minimal brain dysfunctions. In H. E. Rie & E. D. Rie (Eds.), *Handbook of minimal brain dysfunctions*. New York: Wiley.

Wilson, R. S. (1985). Risk and resilience in early mental development. *Dev. Neuropsychol., 21*, 795–805.

Index